Handbook of
PEDIATRIC
DENTISTRY

For Elsevier:

Commissioning Editor: Michael Parkinson/Alison Taylor
Development Editor: Ailsa Laing
Project Manager: Emma Riley
Designer: George Ajayi
Illustration Manager: Merlyn Harvey
Illustrator: Joanna Cameron

Handbook of
PEDIATRIC
DENTISTRY

Editors

Angus C Cameron BDS (*Hons*) MDSc (*Syd*) FDSRCS (*Eng*) FRACDS FICD

Head, Department of Paediatric Dentistry and Orthodontics, Westmead Hospital
Clinical Associate Professor and Head, Paediatric Dentistry, University of Sydney
Visiting Senior Specialist, Children's Hospital at Westmead, Sydney, Australia

Richard P Widmer BDSc (*Hons*) MDSc (*Melb*) FRACDS FICD

Head, Department of Dentistry, Children's Hospital at Westmead
Clinical Associate Professor, Paediatric Dentistry, University of Sydney
Senior Consultant, Paediatric Dentistry, Westmead Hospital, Sydney, Australia

THIRD EDITION

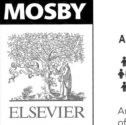

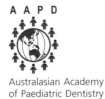

Australasian Academy
of Paediatric Dentistry

EDINBURGH LONDON NEW YORK OXFORD PHILADELPHIA ST LOUIS SYDNEY TORONTO 2008

MOSBY
ELSEVIER

First edition 1997
Second edition 2003
Third edition 2008

ISBN 978 0 7234 3452 8

British Library Cataloguing in Publication Data
A catalogue record for this book is available from the British Library

Library of Congress Cataloging in Publication Data
A catalog record for this book is available from the Library of Congress

Note
Knowledge and best practice in this field are constantly changing. As new research and experience broaden our knowledge, changes in practice, treatment and drug therapy may become necessary or appropriate. Readers are advised to check the most current information provided (i) on procedures featured or (ii) by the manufacturer of each product to be administered, to verify the recommended dose or formula, the method and duration of administration, and contraindications. It is the responsibility of the practitioner, relying on their own experience and knowledge of the patient, to make diagnoses, to determine dosages and the best treatment for each individual patient, and to take all appropriate safety precautions. To the fullest extent of the law, neither the Publisher nor the Editors assume any liability for any injury and/or damage to persons or property arising out or related to any use of the material contained in this book.

The Publisher

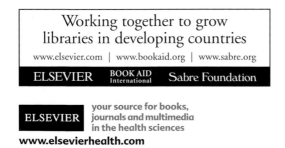

Working together to grow
libraries in developing countries

www.elsevier.com | www.bookaid.org | www.sabre.org

ELSEVIER   BOOK AID International   Sabre Foundation

ELSEVIER   your source for books, journals and multimedia in the health sciences

www.elsevierhealth.com

The publisher's policy is to use **paper manufactured from sustainable forests**

Printed in China

Contributors

Paul Abbott
BDSc (*WA*) MDS (*Adel*) FRACDS (Endo) FPFA FADI FICD FACD
Professor of Clinical Dentistry, Head, School of Dentistry, Director, Oral Health Centre of WA, and Deputy Dean, Faculty of Medicine and Dentistry, University of Western Australia, Perth, Australia

Eduardo A Alcaino
BDS (*Hons*), MDSc, FRACDS GradDipClinDent (Sedation and Pain Control)
Specialist Paediatric Dentist, Private Practice, Specialist Clinical Associate, Sydney University and Visiting Specialist, Westmead Centre for Oral Health and Sydney Dental Hospital, Sydney, Australia

Michael J Aldred
BDS PhD GradCertEd (QUT) FDSRCS FRCPath FFOP (*RCPA*)
Oral Pathologist, Dorevitch Pathology, Melbourne, Australia

Wendy J Bellis
MSc BDS
Specialist Paediatric Senior Dental Officer and Assistant Clinical Director for the Community Dental Service of Camden and Islington Primary Care Trusts, London, UK

Louise Brearley Messer
BDSc LDS MDSc PhD FRACDS FICD
Emeritus Professor, School of Dental Science, University of Melbourne, Melbourne, Australia

Michael G Cooper
MB BS FANZCA FFPMANZCA
Senior Anaesthetist, Department of Anaesthesia and the Pain and Palliative Care Service, The Children's Hospital at Westmead, Westmead, Sydney, Australia

Peter J Cooper
MB ChB BSc MRCP FRACP DHL
Staff Specialist, Respiratory Medicine, The Children's Hospital at Westmead, Westmead, Sydney, Australia

Peter J M Crawford
BDS MScD FDS RCS (*Edin and Eng*) FRCPCH FHEA
Consultant Senior Lecturer in Paediatric Dentistry, Head of Division in Child Dental Health, University of Bristol Dental School, UK

Julia Dando
BDS (*Wales*) FDSRCS (*Edin*) MMSci (*Sheff*) MOrthRCS (*Eng*)
Staff Specialist, Department of Orthodontics, Westmead Centre for Oral Health, Westmead Hospital, Westmead, Sydney, and Sydney Private Practitioner, Evolution Orthodontics, Blacktown, New South Wales, Australia

Bernadette K Drummond
BDS (*Otago*) MS (*Roch*) PhD (*Leeds*) FRACDS
Associate Professor of Paediatric Dentistry, University of Otago, Dunedin, New Zealand

John Fricker
BDS MDSc GradDipEd(Adult) MRACDS(Orth) FRACDS FADI FPFA
Specialist Orthodontist, Canberra, ACT, Australia

Roger K Hall OAM
MDSc (*Melb*) FRACDS FICD FADI
Emeritus Dental Surgeon, Royal Children's Hospital, Visitor, Department of Pharmacology, University of Melbourne, Melbourne and Honorary Fellow Genetic Health Services, Victoria, Australia

Kerrod B Hallett
MDSc MPH FRACDS FICD
Senior Paediatric Dentist, Royal Children's Hospital, Brisbane, Australia

Andrew A C Heggie
MB BS MDSc FRACDS (OMS) FACOMS FFDRCS
Associate Professor and Head, Section of Oral and Maxillofacial Surgery, Department of Plastic and Maxillofacial Surgery, Royal Children's Hospital of Melbourne, Melbourne, Australia

Timothy Johnston
BDSc (*WA*) MDSc (*Melb*) FRACDS FADI
Specialist Paediatric Dentist, Consultant Paediatric Dentist, Princess Margaret Hospital, and Clinical Lecturer, University of Western Australia, Perth, Australia

Om P Kharbanda
BDS (*Lucknow*) MDS (*Lucknow*) MOthRCS (*Edin*) MMEd (*Dundee*) Fellow Indian Board of Orthodontics Honoris Causa FAMS MAMS FICD
Professor and Head, Division of Orthodontics, and Medical Superintendent Centre for Dental Education and Research (CDER), All India Institute of Medical Sciences, and Adjunct Faculty and Coordinator, KL Wig Centre for Medical Education and Research, New Delhi, India

v

Nicky Kilpatrick
BDS PhD FDS RCPS FRACDS (Paed)
Associate Professor and Director, Department of
Dentistry, Royal Children's Hospital, Melbourne,
Australia

Nigel M King
BDS Hons (*Lond*), MSc Hons (*Lond*), PhD (*HK*),
FHKAM (Dental Surgery), FCDSHK (Paediatr Dent),
FDS RCS (*Edin*), LDS RCS (*Eng*)
Professor in Paediatric Dentistry, Faculty of
Dentistry, University of Hong Kong, Pokfulam,
Hong Kong SAR

Jane McDonald
MB BS (*Hons*) UNSW FANZCA
VMO Anaesthetist, Westmead Hospital and The
Children's Hospital at Westmead, Westmead,
Sydney, Australia

Cheryl B McNeil
PhD
Professor of Psychology, West Virginia University,
Morgantown, West Virginia, USA

Daniel W McNeil
PhD
Professor of Psychology, Clinical Professor of Dental
Practice and Rural Health, Eberly Professor of Public
Service, West Virginia University, Morgantown,
West Virginia, USA

Erin Mahoney
BDS (*Otago*) MDSc PhD FRACDS
Specialist Paediatric Dentist, Hutt Valley District
Health Board, and Clinical Senior Lecturer,
University of Otago, Wellington, New Zealand

David Manton
BDSc MDSc FRACDS
Senior Lecturer and Convenor, Paediatric Dentistry,
Growth and Development, School of Dental Science,
University of Melbourne, Melbourne, Australia

Kareen Mekertichian
BDS (*Hons*) MDSc FRACDS FPFA FICD
Specialist Paediatric Dentist, Private Practice,
Chatswood and Honorary Specialist, Westmead
Centre for Oral Health, Westmead, Sydney, Australia

Christopher Olsen
MDSc (*Melb*) FRACDS
Senior Lecturer, Child Dental Health, University of
Melbourne, Paediatric Dentist, Royal Dental
Hospital, Melbourne, Australia

Sarah Raphael
BDS MDSc GradCert(Higher Ed) FRACDS FICD
Specialist Paediatric Dentist and Consultant,
Colgate Oral Care, Sydney, Australia

Julie Reid
BAppSc (*LaTrobe*) Grad Dip (*Syd*) PhD (*LaTrobe*)
Senior Clinician (Cleft Palate/Craniofacial Team),
Speech Pathology Department, Royal Children's
Hospital, Melbourne, Australia

Mark Schifter
BDS MDSc MSND RCS (*Edin*) MOM RCS (*Edin*) FFD
RCSI (*Oral Med*) FRACDS (*Oral Med*), FICD
Head, Department of Oral Medicine, Oral
Pathology and Special Care Dentistry, Westmead
Centre for Oral Health, Westmead Hospital,
Sydney, Australia

Sarah Starr
BAppSc (Speech Path) MHealthSc (Educ)
Speech Pathologist, Speech Pathology Services,
Burwood, NSW

Neil Street
MB BS (*NSW*) MAppSci (*UTS*) FANZCA
Specialist Anaesthetist, The Children's Hospital at
Westmead, Westmead, Sydney, Australia

Meredith Wilson
MB BS FRACP MBioeth
Senior Staff Specialist and Head, Department of
Clinical Genetics, The Children's Hospital at
Westmead, Westmead, Sydney, Australia

John Winters
BDSc MDSc
Chairman and Consultant Paediatric Dentist,
Princess Margaret Hospital, Private Specialist
Practitioner in Paediatric Dentistry, Perth, Australia

Contributors to previous editions

The Editors would like to acknowledge the great support and contributions made to the earlier editions by the following people who have made this book possible.

Roland Bryant
MDS (*Syd*) PhD FRACDS
Professor of Conservative Dentistry, University of
Sydney, Sydney, Australia

Santo Cardaci
BDSc (*Hons*) (*WA*) MDSc (*Adel*) FRACDS
Specialist Endodontist, Perth, Australia

Peter Gregory
BDSc MDSc (*WA*) FRACDS
Specialist Paediatric Dentist and Visiting
Paedodontist, Princess Margaret Hospital for
Children and Clinical Lecturer, University of
Western Australia, Perth, Australia

Fiona Heard
BDSc (*Melb*) LDS MDSc (*Syd*) FRACDS
Specialist Endodontist and Visiting Dental Officer,
Westmead Hospital, Westmead, Sydney, Australia

Justine Hemmings
BAppSc (Speech Path)
Senior Speech Pathologist, Royal Alexandra Hospital
for Children, Westmead, Sydney, Australia

David Isaacs
MBBChir MD MRCP FRACP
Associate Professor and Head, Department of
Immunology, Royal Alexandra Hospital for Children,
Westmead, Sydney, Australia

Tissa Jayasekera
MDSc (*Melb*) MDS (*Syd*) FRACDS
Specialist Orthodontist, Bendigo, Victoria and
Visiting Dental Officer (Paediatric Dentistry),
Westmead Hospital, Westmead, Sydney, Australia

Allison Kakakios
MB BS (*Hons*) FRACP
Staff Specialist, Paediatric Immunology, Royal
Alexandra Hospital for Children, Westmead,
Sydney, Australia

Peter King
MDS (*Syd*)
Specialist in Special Needs Dentistry and former
Head, Special Care Dentistry, Westmead Hospital,
Westmead, Sydney, Australia

Linda Kingston
BAppSci (Speech Path)
Formerly Senior Speech Pathologist, Royal Alexandra
Hospital for Children, Westmead, Sydney, Australia

Judy Kirk
MB BS (*Syd*) FRACP
Staff Specialist Cancer Genetics, Medical Oncology,
Westmead Hospital, Westmead, Sydney, Australia

Sandy Lopacki
MA (Speech Path) (*Northwestern*) CCC-ASHA
Formerly Senior Speech Pathologist, Westmead
Hospital, Westmead, Sydney, Australia

James Lucas
MDSc (*Melb*) MS (*LaTrobe*) FRACDS LDS
Deputy Director, Department of Dentistry, Royal
Children's Hospital, Melbourne, Melbourne,
Australia

Stephen O'Flaherty
MBChB FRACP FAFRM
Head, Department Paediatric Rehabilitation, Royal
Alexandra Hospital for Children, Westmead,
Sydney, Australia

Tony Sandler
BDS (*Witw*) HDDent (*Witw*)
Specialist Endodontist, Perth, Australia

W Kim Seow
BDS (*Adel*) MDSc (*Qld*) DDSc PhD FRACDS
Associate Professor, Paediatric Dentistry, University
of Queensland, Queensland, Australia

Margarita Silva
CD (*Mexico*) MS (*Minn*)
Specialist Paediatric Dentist, Melbourne, Victoria

Joe Verco
BDS (*Adel*) LDS (*Vic*) BScDent (*Hons*) MDS FAAPD
Specialist Paediatric Dentist, Adelaide, Australia

Peter Wong
BDS (*Hons*) MDSc (*Syd*) FRACDS
Specialist Paediatric Dentist, Canberra ACT and
Visiting Dental Officer (Paediatric Dentistry),
Westmead Hospital, Westmead, Sydney, Australia

Foreword

This excellent and user-friendly text, already translated into several other languages, has firmly established itself as the foremost available comprehensive handbook on paediatric dentistry. The third edition has been updated in all areas, with new illustrations, and has, in addition, some new sections, such as that on recent changes in the care of the child with a complex medical disorder. Each chapter shows evidence of thorough careful revision. The editors, two of Australia's most eminent clinicians and academics, who have established international reputations, together with specialist contributors from the Australasian Academy of Paediatric Dentistry, again most well known internationally, are to be congratulated on their continuing contribution to knowledge in all aspects of the expanding world of paediatric dentistry.

Although the oral health of children continues to improve, there may be something of a plateau at the present time, whereby the influence of multimedia food and drink advertising targeted at children is leading to the increased consumption of cariogenic, high-calorie foods, which are to some extent countering the protective effect of fluorides from various sources. In addition, a new type of enamel maturation defect (molar–incisor hypomineralization) has recently emerged, challenging both diagnosis and management. The day-to-day management of dental caries and developmental tooth defects therefore continues, now hand-in-hand with the management of anomalies of facial growth and development and the diagnosis of less common oral pathology.

Most orofacial disorders in children have a developmental component to their origin. We now recognize a genetic basis for many disorders which were previously not understood or thought to have a different cause. Common 'congenital' disorders such as cleft lip and palate are now routinely diagnosed in utero during the first trimester prenatal screening. Paediatric dentists working with medical, surgical and specialist dental colleagues now form an integral part of the interdisciplinary teams that are necessary for the management of complex craniofacial disorders in infants and young children. Paediatric dentists are best placed of all the team members to follow these children frequently and long term. This handbook provides the necessary background and sets out the essentials of management for conditions such as clefting disorders, haematological and endocrine disorders, congenital cardiac disease, disorders of metabolism, organ transplantation and cancer in children, in addition to the more familiar problems of dental trauma, oral infections and dental caries.

This text is now well recognized as an essential chairside and bedside companion for all those practitioners caring for children, from undergraduate students of dentistry to general dental practitioners, specialist paediatric dentists, orthodontists and paediatricians. Family medical practitioners will also find this book useful as an occasional, authoritative reference source. The information provided in this book is needed and used on a daily basis by all the practitioners mentioned.

The book is a pleasure to read and use and I commend it to all those involved in the clinical oral care of children.

Roger K Hall OAM

Emeritus Paediatric Dental Surgeon, Royal Children's Hospital, Melbourne, Australia
Visitor, Department of Pharmacology, University of Melbourne, Australia
Honorary Fellow, Genetic Health Victoria, Australia
Foundation President, Australasian Academy of Paediatric Dentistry
Foundation President Australian and New Zealand Society of Paediatric Dentistry

Foreword

Oral health for infants, children and adolescents plays a very important part in the overall health of children. Even though there has been remarkable progress in the promotion of oral health, it will be some time before oral diseases are wholly eradicated and most likely this will never occur. Those diseases known as caries and periodontal disease remain in varying degrees throughout the world. It is therefore extremely important that all dentists be prepared to deal with the most common oral problems encountered in the paediatric population. As in all clinical specialties, new advances are made almost daily and it is difficult for the student or practitioner to keep abreast of these changes.

Both the busy practitioner and dental student frequently require a quick reference to a topic, a clinical procedure, or to an oral finding. However, although there are many excellent text books in paediatric dentistry, it may not always be easy to find the information required.

The Handbook is very comprehensive and in this 3rd edition the authors have expanded the behaviour management and fluoride implementation chapters. They have included the new international guidelines to manage trauma and enhanced the section on oral pathology and dental anomalies. Finally they have included new chapters on cariology, restorative dentistry and primary pulp therapy.

The handbook is written in an outline fashion, which allows for quick reference and easy reading; it is also profusely supplemented with colour photographs which aid greatly in the understanding of conditions. The appendices are lengthy and provide the reader with information that is often difficult to find and which can, therefore, be overlooked.

I congratulate the authors, Drs Cameron and Widmer, for their vision in taking departmental notes out of the classroom and organizing them into a handbook version, now available in a 3rd edition to the entire profession. This achievement will further promote the importance of oral healthcare for all paediatric patients and increase the availability of professional care.

Arthur J Nowak DMD MA
Diplomate, American Academy of Pediatric Dentistry
Professor Emeritus, Departments of Pediatric Dentistry and Pediatrics
Colleges of Dentistry and Medicine, University of Iowa
Iowa City, USA

Preface

On retiring after completing his final round at the British Open at St Andrews in 2005, the golfer Jack Nicklaus commented:

> a lot of players say you can't play that course. That's a bunch of junk. A good player can play any course. You adapt your game to the golf course. You don't adapt the course to your game.

This quotation from the great man struck the authors as the perfect metaphor for paediatric dentistry. When we hear our colleagues comment that they cannot treat children, particularly the more challenging ones, we urge them to use their basic knowledge of paediatric dentistry and adapt themselves to cope with the child or clinical issue at hand. That is 'to change their game'! In preparing ourselves for this, the third edition, we have had time to reflect on possible changes in content and layout as we change our game to embrace and reflect the development of our specialty.

For many years, those treating children were seen only to be fixing little holes, in little teeth, of little people, a rather narrow and mechanistic view. We regard these important restorative aspects of treating children as 'paedodontics' and the term 'paediatric dentistry' more properly expressing the broad scope of child dental health, which is the basis of most specialist work.

We have perceived the need for a paediatric dentistry handbook, specializing in the important but often hard to find information about current paediatric dental practice. Children are not little adults; and as more children with chronic disease are being managed away from major paediatric centres, it is important for general dental practitioners to have access to this knowledge. It is not the role of the specialist paediatric dentist to manage every medically compromised or difficult child. Indeed, it is our belief that the majority of these children can be safely and successfully managed in most general dental practices. On the other hand, the general practitioner must also know when it is appropriate to refer those children who require acute care and the facilities provided by modern children's hospitals.

This *Handbook* has been a collaborative effort by members of the Australasian Academy of Paediatric Dentistry and a wide range of specialists involved in paediatric care. It has been designed for dental undergraduate students and is also intended as a chairside reference for general practitioners. It provides a unique compilation of modern diagnostic and treatment philosophies, not only from Australasian, but from diverse world opinions. It has also been written with our medical colleagues in mind to provide them with appropriate information on contemporary paediatric dental care and to aid in the diagnosis of orofacial pathology.

The response to our previous editions of the *Handbook* has been wonderfully encouraging and it is with much anticipation that we embarked on this, our third edition. The text has now been translated into Spanish, Italian, Portuguese, Russian, Polish and Korean. There is no doubt that technological and scientific advances have continued apace both in the treatment and diagnostic areas and there has been extensive rewriting in many of the chapters, together with the inclusion of many new illustrations. The broad concepts of child dental care that we embraced in the previous editions received strong support from a wide range of healthcare professionals and we have incorporated many of these suggestions in this revised text.

We hope that this edition goes some way to complementing those clinicians with good paediatric skills and encouraging those who feel less capable to venture forward and further their skills. Please keep the text at the chairside when in your surgery and on the bedside table at night! We wish you all the very best of reading and learning.

Angus Cameron and Richard Widmer
Westmead, Sydney, Australia
January 2008

Acknowledgements

The editors are extremely grateful for the support of all those involved in the teaching of paediatric dentistry throughout Australia and New Zealand and the members of the Australasian Academy of Paediatric Dentistry. The list of contributors reflects the depth of experience in child dental care that has been gathered to complete this publication and we would like to thank all those who have been intimately involved, or have offered advice. We would especially like to thank the staff and registrars at Westmead Hospital and the Children's Hospital at Westmead, and in particular Mrs Frances Porter and Mrs Maggie Melink for their invaluable secretarial efficiency and patience.

Our families and close friends must not go unmentioned for their quiet support and encouragement and finally, we would like to thank our child patients, the responsibility for whose care we are entrusted. They give us wonder as we watch them grow, the joy in our daily work and the motivation for our endeavours.

Contents

1 Child assessment

Contributors

Richard Widmer, Angus Cameron, Bernadette K Drummond

What is paediatric dentistry?

Paediatric dentistry is specialty based not on a particular skill set, but encompassing all of dentistry's technical skills against a philosophical background of understanding child development in health and disease. This new edition of the handbook again emphasizes the broader picture in treating children. A dental visit is no longer just a dental visit – it should be regarded as a 'health visit'. We are part of the team of health professionals who contribute to the wellbeing of children, both in an individual context and at the wider community level.

The pattern of childhood illness has changed and with it, clinical practice. Children presenting for treatment may have survived cancer, may have a well-managed chronic disease or may have significant behavioural and learning disorders. There are increasing, sometimes unrealistic, expectations, among parents/carers that the care of their children should be easily and readily accessible and pain free and result in flawless aesthetics. There is a perception that children have slipped through the joys of childhood in the blink of an eye and that family life is more pressured and demanding.

Caries and dental disease should be seen as reflective of the family's social condition and the dental team should be part of the community.

> Your [patients] don't have to become your friends, but they are part of your social context and that gives them a unique status in your life. Treat them with respect and take them seriously and your practice will become to feel part of the neighbourhood, part of the community.
> (Hugh McKay, social commentator, *Sydney Morning Herald*)

In the evolving dynamics of dental practice we feel that it is important to change, philosophically, the traditional 'adversarial nature' of the dental experience. It is well recognized that for too many the dental experience was traumatic. This has resulted in a significant proportion of the adult population accessing dental care only episodically, for the relief of pain. Thus, it is vital to see a community, and consumer, perspective in the provision of paediatric dental services. The successful practice of paediatric dentistry is not merely the completion of any operative procedure but also ensuring a positive dental outcome for the future oral health behaviour of that individual and family. To this end an understanding of child development – physical, cognitive and psychosocial – is paramount. The clinician must be comfortable and skilled in talking to children, and interpersonal skills are essential. It will not usually be the child's fault if the clinician cannot work with the child.

Patient assessment

History
A clinical history should be taken in a logical and systematic way for each patient and should be updated regularly. Thorough history taking is time consuming and requires practice. However, it is an opportunity to get to know the child and family. Furthermore, the history facilitates the diagnosis of many conditions even before the hands-on examination. Because there are often specific questions pertinent to a child's medical history that will be relevant to their management, it is desirable that parents be present. The understanding of medical conditions that can compromise treatment is essential.

The purpose of the examination is not merely to check for caries or periodontal disease, as paediatric dentistry encompasses all areas of growth and development. Having the opportunity to see the child regularly, the dentist can often be the first to recognize significant disease and anomalies.

Current complaints
The history of any current problems should be carefully documented. This includes the nature, onset or type of pain if present, relieving and exacerbating factors, or lack of eruption of permanent teeth.

Dental history
- Previous treatment – how the child has coped with other forms of treatment.
- Eruption times and dental development.
- What preventive treatment has been undertaken previously.
- Methods of pain control used previously.

Medical history
Medical history should be taken in a systematic fashion, covering all system areas of the body. The major areas include:
- Cardiovascular system (e.g. cardiac lesions, blood pressure, rheumatic fever).
- Central nervous system (e.g. seizures, cognitive delay).
- Endocrine system (e.g. diabetes).
- Gastrointestinal tract (e.g. hepatitis).
- Respiratory tract (e.g. asthma, bronchitis, upper respiratory tract infections).
- Bleeding tendencies (include family history of bleeding problems).
- Urogenital system (renal disease, ureteric reflux).
- Allergies.
- Past operations or treatment/medications.

Pregnancy history
- Length of confinement.
- Birth weight.
- Apgar scores.
- Antenatal and perinatal problems, especially during delivery.
- Prematurity and treatment in a special or neonatal intensive care nursery.

Growth and development

In many countries, an infant record book is issued to parents to record post-natal growth and development, childhood illness and visits to health providers. Areas of questioning should include:

- Developmental milestones.
- Speech and language development.
- Motor skills.
- Socialization.

Current medical treatment

- Medications, including complementary medications.
- Current treatments.
- Immunizations.

Family and social history

- Family history of serious illness.
- Family pedigree tree (see Appendix O).
- Schooling, performance in class.
- Speech and language problems.
- Pets/hobbies or other interests.

This last area is useful in beginning to establish a common interest and a rapport with the child. When asking questions and collecting information, it is important to use lay terminology. The distinction between rheumatic fever and rheumatism is often not understood and more specific questioning may be required. Furthermore, questions regarding family and social history must be neither offensive nor intrusive. An explanation of the need for this information is helpful and appropriate.

Examination

Extra-oral examination

The extra-oral examination should be one of general appraisal of the child's wellbeing. The dentist should observe the child's gait and the general interaction with the parents or peers in the surgery. An assessment of height and weight is useful, and dentists should routinely measure both height and weight, and plot these measurements on a growth chart.

A general physical examination should be conducted. In some circumstances this may require examination of the chest, abdomen and extremities. Although this is often not common practice in a general surgery setting, there may be situations where this is required (e.g. checking for other injuries after trauma, assessing manifestations of syndromes or medical conditions). Speech and language are also assessed at this stage (see Chapter 13).

The clinician should assess:

- Facial symmetry, dimensions and the basic orthodontic facial type.
- Eyes, including appearance of the globe, sclera, pupils and conjunctiva.
- Movements of the globe that may indicate squints or palsy.
- Skin colour and appearance.
- Temporomandibular joints.
- Cervical, submandibular and occipital lymph nodes.

Intra-oral examination
- Soft tissues including oropharynx, tonsils and uvula.
- Oral hygiene and periodontal status.
- Dental hard tissues.
- Occlusion and orthodontic relations.
- Quantity and quality of saliva.

Charting
Charting should be thorough and completed on a form similar to that illustrated in Appendix R.

Provisional diagnosis
A provisional diagnosis should be formulated for every patient. Whether this is caries, periodontal disease or, for example, aphthous stomatitis, it is important to make an assessment of the current conditions that are present. This will influence the ordering of special examinations and the final diagnosis and treatment planning.

Special examinations
Radiography
The guidelines for prescribing radiographs in dental practice are shown in Table 1.1. The overriding principle in taking radiographs of children must be to minimize exposure to ionizing radiation consistent with the provision of the most appropriate treatment. Radiographs are essential for accurate diagnosis. If, however, the information gained from such an investigation does not influence treatment decisions, both the timing and the need for the radiograph should be questioned. The following radiographs may be used:
- Bitewing radiographs.
- Periapical radiographs.
- Panoramic radiographs.
- Occlusal films.
- Extra-oral facial films.

   Note that digital radiography, or the use of intensifying screens in extra-oral films, significantly reduces radiation dosage. As such, the use of a panoramic film in children is often more valuable than a full-mouth series.

Other imaging
Many modern technologies are available to the clinician today, and their applications can be a most valuable adjunct not only in the diagnosis of orofacial pathology but also in the treatment of many conditions. These modalities include:
- Computed axial tomography (CAT) and cone-beam CT with three-dimensional reconstruction.
- Magnetic resonance imaging (MRI).
- Nuclear medicine.
- Ultrasonography.

Pulp sensibility (vitality) testing
- Thermal (i.e. carbon dioxide pencil).
- Electrical stimulation.

Table 1.1 Guidelines for prescribing radiographs*

Patient	Child		Adolescent
	Primary dentition	**Mixed dentition**	
New patients			
All new patients to assess disease and growth and development	Bitewings if closed contacts between posterior teeth Panoramic film to assess other pathology or for growth and development	Bitewings and individualized examinations such as panoramic film to assess development and eruption of permanent teeth	Individualized radiographic examinations with bitewings and panoramic film
Recall patients			
No clinical caries and low risk	If contacts can be visualized or probed, then bitewings may not be required, otherwise bitewings at 12–24-month intervals	One set of bitewings once the first permanent molars have erupted	Bitewings every 18–36 months after the eruption of the second permanent molars up to age 20
Clinical caries or high risk of disease	Bitewings at 6–12-month intervals or until no new caries is evident over 12 months		
Growth and development	Usually not required	Individualized examination based on anomaly or disease presence, with periapicals or panoramic film	Panoramic or periapical films to assess position of third molars and other orthodontic considerations

*Based on recommendations from the American Academy of Pediatric Dentistry.

- Percussion.
- Mobility.
- Transillumination.

Blood investigations (see Appendix A)
- Full blood count with differential white cell count.
- Clinical chemistry.

Microbiological investigations
- Culture of micro-organisms and antibiotic sensitivity.
- Cytology.
- Serology.
- Direct and indirect immunofluorescence.

Anatomical pathology
- Histological examination of biopsy specimens.
- Hard-tissue sectioning (e.g. diagnosis of enamel anomalies, see Figure 9.26).

- Scanning and transmission electron microscopy (e.g. hair from children with ecto-dermal dysplasia, see Figure 9.2B).

Photography
Extra-oral and intra-oral photography provides an invaluable record of growing children. It is important as a legal document in cases of abuse or trauma, or as an aid in the diagnosis of anomalies or syndromes. Consent will need to be obtained for photography.

Diagnostic casts
Casts are essential in orthodontic or complex restorative treatment planning, and for general record keeping.

Caries activity tests
Although these are not definitive for individuals, they may be useful as an indicator of caries risk. Furthermore, identification of defects in salivation in children with medical conditions may point to significant caries susceptibility. Such tests include assessment of:
- Diet history.
- Salivary flow rates.
- Salivary buffering capacity.
- *Streptococcus mutans* and *Lactobacillus* colony counts.

Definitive diagnosis

The final diagnosis is based on examination and history and determines the final treatment plan.

Assessment of disease risk (see Chapters 3 and 4)

All children should have an 'assessment of disease risk' before the final treatment plan is determined. This is particularly important in the planning of preventive care for children with caries. This assessment should be based on:
- Past disease experience.
- Current dental status.
- Family history and carer status.
- Diet considerations.
- Oral hygiene.
- Concomitant medical conditions.
- Future expectations of disease activity.
   Social factors including recent migration, language barriers, and ethnic and cultural diversities, can impact on access to dental care and will therefore influence caries risk.

Low risk of disease
- No caries present.
- Favourable family history (appropriate diet, dentally healthy siblings, motivated parents and caregivers).

- Good oral hygiene.
- Access to community water fluoridation.

Moderate risk
- One or two new lesions per year.

High risk or future high risk
- Three or more new lesions per year.
- Orthodontic treatment.
- Chronic illness or hospitalization.
- Medically compromised children.
- Social risk factors.

Treatment plan

1. Emergency care and relief of pain.
2. Preventive care.
3. Surgical treatment.
4. Restorative treatment.
5. Orthodontic treatment.
6. Extensive restorative or further surgical management.
7. Recall and review.

Clinical conduct

Infection control
It is now considered that '**universal precautions**' are the expected standard of care in current paediatric dental practice. The principles of universal precautions are:
- Prevention of contamination by strictly limiting and clearly identifying a 'zone of contamination'.
- The need for elimination of contamination should be minimal if this zone of contamination is observed.

Universal precautions regard every patient as being potentially infectious. Although it is possible to identify some patients who are known to be infectious, there are many others who have an unknown infectious state. It is impossible to totally eliminate infection; thus, observing universal precautions is a sensible approach to minimizing the risk of cross-infection.

All children must be protected with safety glasses and clinicians must also wear protective clothing, eyeware, masks and gloves when treating patients.

Recording of clinical notes
Care must be taken when recording clinical information. Notes are legal documents and must be legible. Clinical notes should be succinct. The treatment plan should be reassessed at each session so that at each subsequent appointment the clinician knows what work is planned. Furthermore, at the completion of the treatment for the day, a note should be made regarding the work to be done at the next visit.

Use of rubber dam

Wherever possible, rubber dam should be used for children. This may necessitate the use of local anaesthesia for the gingival tissues. When topical anaesthetics are used they must be given adequate time to work (i.e. at least 3 minutes). All rubber-dam clamps must have a tie of dental floss around the arch of the clamp to prevent accidental ingestion or aspiration.

Consent for treatment (see Chapter 2)

There is often little provision in a dental file for a signed consent for dental treatment. The consent for a dentist to carry out treatment, be it cleaning of teeth or surgical extraction, is implied when the parent or guardian and child attend the surgery. It is incumbent on the practitioner, however, to provide all the necessary information and detail in such a way as to enable 'informed consent'. This includes explaining the treatment using appropriate language to facilitate a complete understanding of proposed treatment plans.

It is important to record that the treatment plan has been discussed and that consent has been given for treatment. This consent would cover the period required to complete the work outlined. If there is any significant alteration to the original treatment plan (e.g. an extraction that was not previously anticipated) then consent should be obtained again from the parent or guardian and recorded in the file.

Generally, when undertaking clinical work on a child patient, it is good practice to advise the parent or guardian briefly at the commencement of the appointment what is proposed for that appointment. Also it is helpful to give the parent or guardian and child some idea of the treatment anticipated for the next appointment. This is especially relevant if a more invasive procedure such as the use of local anaesthesia or removal of teeth is contemplated.

2 Child management

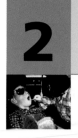

Contributors

Richard Widmer, Daniel W McNeil, Cheryl B McNeil, Jane McDonald, Eduardo A Alcaino, Michael G Cooper

Behaviour management

Promoting positive behaviour among children and adolescents in the dental surgery

This section is a practical guide for specific modes of interacting in the dental environment, which can help produce positive and compliant behaviours in child and adolescent patients. These guidelines are based on research findings and principles from behavioural dentistry, as well as behavioural, developmental, child and paediatric psychology.

Much has been written about management of problem behaviour with a focus on the use of various techniques. This guide, however, emphasizes specific and mostly simple techniques that can be used with almost all children and adolescents to enhance their comfort and cooperation in the dental surgery. The general idea is to use finesse instead of absolute control. As a sense of lack of control is one of the major components of anxiety and fear (along with lack of predictability), using methods that are encouraging rather than demanding can go a long way in enhancing comfort in the dental situation.

The perspective is that dentists, as integral members of the healthcare team for children and adolescents, must have awareness of practical methods that they can use, based on knowledge of psychological principles and issues of growth and development. The adage that 'children are not small adults' promotes the idea of special knowledge and behaviours that are important in caring for young dental patients. Dentists must have a knowledge base in child and adolescent medicine as well as in social and cultural factors affecting the health and behaviour of young people.

It is of the utmost importance that dental appointments in childhood and adolescence be positive, because research clearly shows that these early experiences have a strong effect on attendance in adulthood. Consequently, this section emphasizes the importance of the relationship between dentist and infant or child or adolescent patient. Interactions between dentist and parents or caregiver are also important because they are typically the most influential part of the child's life outside the surgery.

Developmental issues

Working with children is of course different from working with adults. Children are not all alike, and are in the process of developing language, intellect, motor skills, personalities and undergoing new experiences of life. The ages at which specific abilities develop vary. To provide quality dental services to children it is necessary to have some basic knowledge of child development, and for the dentist to work with a child or an adolescent on their particular developmental level.

9

Child behaviour in relation to development

As all children are different it is reasonable to expect their behaviour in the dental environment to also vary. Children's behaviour is a function of learning and development. The types of behaviour that represent the 'norm' for a particular chronological age group offer a convenient means to classify the expected level of cooperation. There will of course be much individual variation.

Under 2 years

The child has little ability to understand dental procedures and effective communication is impossible. Nevertheless, even without cooperation, an oral examination and some treatment can be accomplished without sedation.

Two years old

The ability to communicate varies according to the level of vocabulary development, which is expected to be limited. Thus, the difficulty in communication puts the child in a 'pre-cooperative' stage. They prefer solitary play and rarely share with others. They are too young to be reached by words alone, and are shy of new people (including the dentist) and places. Thus, the child must be allowed to handle and touch objects to understand their meaning. Children of this age should be accompanied by a parent.

Three years old

These children are less egocentric and like to please adults. They have very active imaginations, like stories and can usually be communicated and reasoned with. In times of stress they will turn to a parent and not accept a stranger's explanation. These children feel more secure if a parent is allowed to remain with them until they have become familiar with the dentist and the assistant. Then a positive approach can be adopted.

Four years old

These children listen with interest and respond well to verbal directions. They have lively minds and may be great talkers who are prone to exaggeration. In addition, they will participate well in small social groups. They can be cooperative patients, but some may be defiant and try to impose their views and opinions. They are familiar with and respond well to 'thank you' and 'please'.

Five years old

These children play cooperatively with their peers and usually have no fear of leaving their parents for a dental appointment because they have no fear of new experiences. They take pride in their possessions, and comments about clothing can be effectively used to establish communication and develop a rapport. By this age children should have relinquished comfort objects such as thumbs and 'security blankets'.

Six years old

By 6 years, children are established at school and are moving away from the security of the family so they are increasingly independent of parents. However, for some children this transition may cause considerable anxiety with outbursts of screaming, temper tantrums and even striking parents. Furthermore, some will exhibit marked increase in fear responses.

Piaget's four stages of intellectual development

Child development encompasses much more than a child's physical changes. It refers to a sequential unfolding of various abilities. Piaget hypothesized that:

- All children progress through the same sequence of cognitive stages.
- Children cannot reach a higher level of reasoning ability until they have mastered experiences in the previous stage (see Appendix K).

Understanding child temperament

There has been a longstanding debate in the literature on child development about the degree to which a child's development is influenced by 'nature' versus 'nurture'. Studies suggest that children do indeed enter the world with a characteristic temperament or personality that stays with them to some degree for the rest of their life. Thomas and Chess (1977) suggested that there are three basic temperaments that influence later personality:

- Easy temperament – These children are viewed as being generally positive in mood. Their body functions are regular and they are considered adaptable and flexible. When problems occur they tend to have reactions of low or moderate intensity. Rather than withdrawing from new situations, the easy temperament child typically displays a positive approach.
- Difficult temperament – These children tend to have irregular body functions, such that they are slow to develop a daily pattern for sleeping, eating and having bowel movements. In contrast with the easy temperament child, these infants often have an intense reaction to problems, have a tendency to withdraw from new situations and have difficulty adapting to changes in their environment.
- Slow to warm-up temperament – These children have a shy disposition. They tend to have a low activity level. Change is difficult for these children as they are slow to adapt and respond negatively to new situations. Their natural response to novelty is to withdraw and they respond to problems with a low-intensity reaction.

Approximately 65% of infants can be categorized into one of these three categories. The remainder have a mixture of traits (Thomas & Chess, 1977).

Implications for dentists

Dentists working with children must use different approaches and techniques depending on the personality type of the child. Whereas an easy temperament child may be flexible enough to handle a quick change in plan, a slow to warm-up child may need to be given a longer time to adjust. Difficult children respond best to a dentist who provides a great deal of structure in a confident manner. The slow to warm-up child needs the dentist to be patient, calm and sensitive.

Developmental milestones

A dentist who is aware of children's abilities at various ages can use that information to communicate at the child's level and to have appropriate expectations for a particular child in the dental surgery. Therefore, it is helpful to become acquainted with certain developmental milestones in the life of the child and to realize that there is a great deal of variability regarding the ages at which children meet these milestones. As such, age ranges are used to describe the time when most children develop a certain ability.

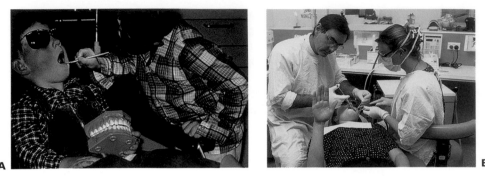

A   B

Figure 2.1 A Giving children control in the dental surgery. **B** It is essential to listen to your patient. A prearranged signal of a hand raised tells the clinician that the procedure is uncomfortable. This gives the child some control over what is happening without interfering with the procedure.

Use of verbal and non-verbal communication to promote positive behaviour in children

- Respect.
- Show interest in the child as an individual.
- Share 'free information'.
- Give well-stated instructions.
- Communicate at the child's level (Figure 2.1).
- Focus on the positive.
- Show ethnic, cultural and gender sensitivity.

Physical structuring and timing during the dental visit
Setting the stage for positive behaviour
In addition to communications from the dentist and dental staff, many aspects of the dental situation can be arranged in such a way that promote positive reactions in infants, children and adolescents. The following PRIDE skills are a useful conceptualization that can help prompt members of the dental team to structure their behaviour with children and youth. This is not to discourage spontaneity with youngsters, which can be so important in working positively with 'kids', but may provide a way for adults to think about including skills as part of their repertoire with children. In fact, the final point of the PRIDE skills is Enthusiasm, which speaks to communicating joy and spontaneous and fun action to youth.

PRIDE
- **Praise**: This can be either 'labelled' or 'unlabelled'. Labelled praises (e.g. 'That's a great job keeping your mouth open, Jane!') typically are more effective at managing behaviour than unlabelled praises (e.g. 'Well done, Jane!').
- **Reflection**: This is a demonstration of the dentist listening to the child, and can involve a simple repeating of some of the child's words, perhaps with embellishment.

- **Enquire**: This involves asking a question of a child, or otherwise prompting him or her to reply ('I'm wondering how you feel about coming to see me today'). Open-ended questions typically produce more information and promote a positive interview atmosphere, relative to closed-ended questions that can be answered with a yes or no, or a simple fact.
- **Describe**: This focuses on behaviour, and portraying the child's actions, typically in a positive light (e.g. 'Now you're keeping your mouth open so nicely, and keeping your feet and legs still').
- **Enthusiasm**: There is a time for animation and play on the part of the dentist and dental team, and a time for more reserved professionalism. With children in a dental environment, enthusiasm on the part of the dentist and team often is needed to combat the negative images of dental care portrayed in the media, by peers, and sometimes by parents and other caregivers.

Use of these PRIDE skills will be well received by children and youth, and can help make the dental appointment reinforcing and enjoyable. However, PRIDE skills should not be used in some automaton fashion, but rather flexibly and in concert with the dentist's own personality and the procedures at hand. Not only are these interpersonal communication skills essential, but the physical and structural aspects of the dental appointment are also crucial. Listed below are suggested practical guidelines for these physical and social aspects, as well as considerations of timing.

- Everyone in the surgery (dentist, auxiliary, parent) should be transmitting positive, comforting expectations to the patient.
- Use stimulating visual distracters in the surgery (child- and adolescent-oriented posters).
- Have age-appropriate materials (safe toys, magazines) in the waiting room. Include materials for parents.
- Have toys available for younger children as distracters or tangible rewards.
- Greet child in the waiting room without a mask and not wearing surgical garb.
- Pace procedures during the appointment, based on how the patient is coping, so that they are neither rushed nor bored. Ask them 'Is that OK?'
- Inform and discuss with parent at conclusion of appointment.
- Provide information in advance about the procedures to be performed at the next appointment so that the child is prepared.

Presence or absence of family members in the surgery
- It is appropriate that parents are able to support their children during treatment.
- If parents are unable to or are unwilling to provide appropriate support, then it may be more desirable for them to wait outside the surgery. It is important to note that parental access to their children should never be denied.
- When there are other siblings, who enjoy or readily cope with dental treatment, it is often helpful to use them as a model.

Transmission of emotion to the child or adolescent
- Children acquire some of their parents' fear and anxiety about the dental treatment both in the dental environment and in the long term.

Figure 2.2 Involving children in their treatment. It is important to feel that the dental environment is non-threatening and safe, and can be a place for enjoyment.

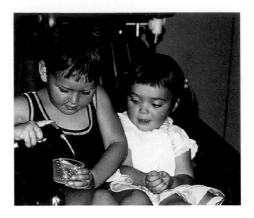

- Emotion is transferred from parents, siblings, dentist and auxiliaries to the child, whose emotional state also impacts on all of those persons. Dental staff who are calm and confident and use humour will promote positive experiences for their patients.

Physical proximity
- Initially work from the front, at eye level.
- Be aware of the child's 'intimate zone'. This zone is approximately 45 cm, but varies in different cultures. By necessity, the dentist must 'invade' this space, but frequent stopping between procedures allows the child some time for coping.

Timing
- It is best to introduce new procedures at an appropriate rate to avoid either rushing or boring the patient.
- Conducting less invasive procedures first will usually be more tolerable for the patient.

Stimulating and distracting objects and situations (Figure 2.2)
- Be aware of popular culture. In some settings, it is possible to have different areas of the surgery orientated to particular patient age ranges.
- An area might include puppets and pictures of colourful cartoon characters for children up to 8 years.
- For older children have wall posters of pop groups.
- Adolescents, like adults, are best treated in a modern, friendly environment.

Surgical clothing and instruments
- Never greet a child wearing a face mask and gloves.
- Explain the need for protective clothing.
- Familiarize children with appropriate instruments.

Greetings in the waiting room
- It is ideal, particularly in initial meetings, for the dentist to greet the child and parent in the waiting area.

- An interview room or non-surgical environment is useful for new patients (Figures 2.3–2.5).

Talking with parents
It is helpful for the dentist to have a positive relationship with both children and their parents. Keep parents well informed. While asking personal information always

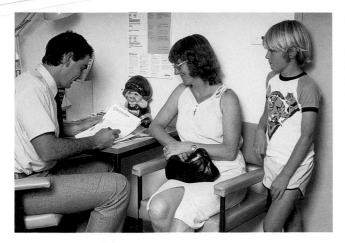

Figure 2.3 At the first visit, it is often good to see the child and parent away from the surgery. It provides an opportunity to talk with the child and establish rapport.

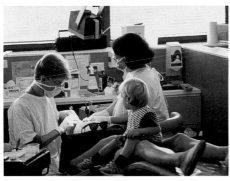

Figure 2.4 Introducing a child to the dental environment – part of familiarization.

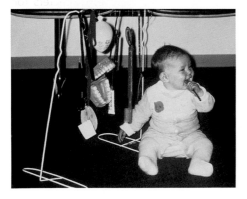

Figure 2.5 A dental mobile – every child should have one!

remember to involve the child in the discussion when appropriate. Be prepared to separate the child from the parent to discuss more sensitive issues. The chairside assistant can be asked to occupy the child, for example with a visit to the fish tank.

Talking with children and youth

Children, like adults, typically respond best if they are treated as individuals, somehow known and special to the provider. Consequently, using the child's name to refer to him or her, and repeating it in conversation periodically during the dental appointment, is helpful in producing a positive environment and in capturing and maintaining the child's attention. It usually helpful for the dentist and members of the dental team to speak with (not to) the child at the child's level, both physically and psychologically.

Dental jargon typically is best avoided with most patients, but particularly with children. Table 2.1 suggests terminology that might be used with younger patients. Of course, use of these terms should be at a developmentally appropriate level for the

Table 2.1 Dental terminology and lay language equivalents for use with youth (age levels are approximate, and should be based on the cognitive developmental level of the child)

Ages 1–5	
Dental terminology	**Lay language**
Air syringe	Wind blower
Water syringe	Water pistol
High evacuation suction	Vacuum cleaner
Saliva ejector	Straw
Radiograph	Picture of your tooth
Prophylaxis	Electric toothbrush
Explorer	Tooth counter
Rubber dam	Raincoat for your tooth
Local anaesthesia	Putting the tooth to sleep
High-speed handpiece	Tooth whistle
Low-speed handpiece	Tooth tickler
Extraction	Wiggle your tooth
Stainless steel crown	Silver hat
Ages 6–10	
Anaesthetize	Numb
Extract	Take out or wiggle
Caries, carious lesion	Hole
Pain	Tickle or pressure
Drill	Electric motor
Dental surgery	Treatment room

Table 2.2 Behavioural methods for removing anxiety (Herschell et al 2003)

Tell–show–do	Informing, then demonstrating, and finally performing part of a procedure
Playful humour	Using fun labels and suggesting use of imagination
Distraction	Ignoring and then directing attention away from a behaviour, thought, or feeling to something else
Positive reinforcement	Tangible or social reward in response to a desired behaviour
Modelling	Providing an example or demonstration about how to do
Shaping	Successive approximations to a desired behaviour
Fading	Providing external means to promote positive behaviour and then gradually removing the external control
Systematic desensitization	Reducing anxiety by first presenting an object or situation that evokes little fear, then progressively introducing stimuli that are more fear-provoking

child. Some mid and older adolescents, for example, actually may respond well to learning dental jargon, as it would give them a sense of being cognitively advanced and more like an adult, which is what they typically aspire to be.

Special arrangements for first-time dental visits
Certain steps are appropriate for an initial visit. In general, the pace of a first appointment is much slower.
- Use pre-appointment letters.
- Use an interview room for the initial contact.

The emphasis is on educating the child, promoting comfort, and allowing the visit to be exciting and fun. Relatively simple and less invasive procedures are preferred. Introducing the child to the office, staff and equipment and pointing out posters and other materials of interest in the treatment room can also be helpful.

Behavioural methods for reducing fear and pain sensitivity
Table 2.2 gives eight methods that can be used across a variety of situations with children and adolescents of all ages. The particular uses depend on the patient's developmental age and personality, as well as on a variety of other factors such as the quality and depth of the dentist's relationship with the child or adolescent.

Referring for possible mental health evaluation and care

When to refer
It is a role of the dentist to refer a child or family when there seem to be significant emotional or psychological issues. Even when such problems do not interfere with dental treatment it is the dentist's role, as a member of the healthcare team, to identify possible psychopathologies and to refer for proper care.

Common reasons for referring a child or adolescent for mental health concerns

- Evidence of abuse or neglect (e.g. bruises, broken teeth, cigarette burns, inappropriate clothing for weather, severe hygiene problems, untreated breaks or sprains, etc.).
- Extremes of behaviour or emotion (i.e. dental phobia).
- Neurological signs or symptoms (i.e. possible seizure activity, tics).
- Severe developmental or cognitive delay (e.g. possible learning disabilities, motor problems, feeding problems).
- Extremely poor parenting (i.e. sole use of excessive physical restraint and punishment).

Whom to refer the patient

Referrals for mental health concerns should be made to psychologists, psychiatrists or social workers. In a hospital setting, it is possible to refer to one of the available departmental services. In a dentist's private surgery, referrals can be made to professionals in private practice, community agencies or hospitals. The following guidelines are suggested when selecting a specialty for referral.

Psychologists

Refer in the case of abuse or neglect, extremes of behaviour, developmental or cognitive delay, or extremely poor parenting. When there is a need for sophisticated cognitive, personality, neuropsychological and/or behavioural assessment, referral to a psychologist is best as standardized psychometric tests can be used. Psychologists can also provide individual child/adolescent, parent/child, and/or family therapy to address problems in the child/adolescent and family system.

Psychiatrists

Refer when there are neurological signs or symptoms. When psychoactive medications may be needed, such as when a child demonstrates signs of psychosis, referral to a psychiatrist is most appropriate, similar to cases in which there are complicating medical factors.

Social workers

Refer for social problems, abuse or neglect. Referral to social workers is appropriate when there are existing social problems in the parents or family that require mobilization of community resources. Social workers know about, and help patients to use, available services in the community.

How to refer

It is acknowledged that suggesting mental healthcare to parents can be an anxiety-provoking task for the dentist. Nevertheless, it is essential that such referrals are made, because the dentist is in a unique role as a healthcare provider. If referrals are not made in a timely fashion then a condition can progress and worsen.

- Speak to the parents in a private setting, informing them of the signs or symptoms that are a cause for concern, without blaming or ascribing responsibility. When the parents understand the problems and your concern, referral to a specific professional or service can be made. It is often helpful to emphasize the good of the child and the need to address the problem for their proper development.

- Ensure that the parent and child or adolescent are aware of the referral and know the specialty of the referral. (It is not appropriate merely to describe the referral as 'to a doctor who will help your child').
- Refer first to only one of the mental health specialties. If additional referral is necessary it can be arranged by the first referral source. In making the referral one can ask for feedback from the mental health professional after the appointment. If there is behavioural disruption in the surgery the mental health professional may have recommendations for management once the child or family has been evaluated.
- Mental health concerns are considered private by many individuals. Given this desire for privacy, releases to exchange relevant information, signed by a parent or guardian and the child if of an age to understand it, are required. Such a form can be signed in the dental surgery and sent to the mental health professional along with a request for feedback.

Pain management for children

The proper treatment of pain in children is often inadequate and involves misconceptions such as:

- Children experience less pain than adults.
- Neonates do not feel or remember pain.
- Pain is character-building for children.
- Opioids are addictive and too dangerous in terms of respiratory distress.
- Children cannot localize or describe their pain.

Development of pain pathways

Even premature neonates have the physiological pathways and mediators to feel pain. The statement that infants and children do not experience pain, either partially or completely, is not physiologically valid.

Measurement of pain in children

There are individual circumstances for each child that affect how they respond to pain and, subsequently, how that pain will be assessed. These include:

- Age and developmental level.
- Social and medical factors.
- Previous pain experience.

Observation of non-verbal cues and behaviour is important. A quiet, withdrawn child may be in severe pain. Simple measures are there to measure pain in children of all ages. Methods for paediatric pain assessment include:

- Observer-based techniques which are useful in pre-verbal children, i.e. psychological scales that measure blood pressure, crying, movement, agitation and verbal expression/body language.
- Self-reporting of pain is valid in children over 4–5 years of age. A visual analogue scale using faces is useful in younger children.

- Older children and teenagers can use a normal visual analogue scale of 1–10.
- Scales with a 1–10 basis are more accurate than simpler ones that may only use a scale of 0–3 or 1–5.
- Children with severe developmental delay can be extremely difficult to assess regarding pain, even by their regular carers. Unusual changes in behaviour from normal may represent an expression of pain.

Analgesia prior to procedures (pre-emptive analgesia)

- Poor analgesia for an initial procedure in children can diminish the efficacy of analgesia for subsequent similar procedures.
- Consideration should be given to ensure adequate systemic and/or local analgesia prior to the commencement of a procedure. Appropriate time for absorption and effect should be allowed.
- A stronger analgesic may be required for the procedure with regular simple analgesics for the postoperative period.

Routes of administration

- Oral analgesia is the preferred route of administration in children. Absorption for most analgesics is generally rapid – within 30 minutes.
- Attention to formulation suitable to the individual child can help greatly with compliance, i.e. liquid versus tablets in younger children, taste.
- The rectal route of administration is valuable in a child who is fasting or not tolerating oral fluids. Doses and time to peak levels may vary compared with oral preparations and are usually much longer. Peak levels after rectal paracetamol may take 90–120 minutes. Adequate explanation should be given and consent should be obtained for the rectal administration of a drug. This route is not used in the immunocompromised child due to the risk of infection or fissure formation.
- Intranasal or sublingual administration of opioids has been described as an alternative to injection which avoids first pass metabolism by the liver.
- Repeated intramuscular injection should be avoided in children, they will often tolerate pain rather than have a painful injection. A subcutaneous cannula, inserted after using topical local anaesthetic cream (EMLA) can be used for repeat parenteral opioid analgesia.
- In obese children, the dosage given should be based on ideal body weight, which can be estimates as the 50th centile on an appropriate weight-for-age percentile chart.

Analgesics
See Table 2.3.

Paracetamol

- Dosage 20 mg/kg orally then 15 mg/kg every 4 hours.
- 30 mg/kg rectally as a single dose.
- Maximum 24-hour dosage of 90 mg/kg (or 4 g) for 2 days, then 60 mg/kg/day by any route of administration.

Table 2.3 Analgesic agents for children

Drug	Oral dose	IMI, SCI, IVI dose	Notes
Paracetamol	20 mg/kg orally 15 mg/kg every 4 hours		Maximum 90 mg/kg/ day (or 4 g) for 2 days then 60 mg/kg/day
Ibuprofen	5–10 mg/kg every 8 hours		Maximum 40 mg/kg/ day or 2 g/day
Naproxen	5 mg/kg every 12 hours		Maximum 10–20 mg/ kg/day or 1 g/day
Diclofenac	1 mg/kg every 8 hours 1 mg/kg every 12 hours (rectally)		Maximum 3 mg/kg/ day or 150 mg/day
Codeine	0.5–1 mg/kg every 4 hours	0.5–1 mg/kg every 3 hours Not for IV use	Maximum 3 mg/kg/day
Oxycodone	0.1–0.15 mg/kg/day		
Morphine	0.2–0.3 mg/kg every 4 hours	0.1–0.15 mg/kg every 3 hours	
Tramadol	1–1.5 mg/kg every 6 hours	1 mg/kg every 6 hours	Maximum 6 mg/kg/ day or 400 mg/day

IMI, intramuscular injection; IVI, intravenous injection; SCI, subcutaneous injection.

- Ensure adequate hydration.
- Useful as a pre-emptive analgesic.
- No effect on bleeding.
- Intravenous paracetamol is available (10 mg/mL). The same dose is used and administered over 15 minutes.
- Take care with dosing as many different strengths and preparations are available.

Non-steroidal anti-inflammatory drugs (NSAIDs)
- Effective alone after oral and dental procedures.
- Can be used in conjunction with paracetamol.
- Have an opioid-sparing effect.
- Increase bleeding time due to inhibition of platelet aggregation.
- Useful analgesic once haemostasis has occurred.
- Best given if tolerating food and drink.
- Can be used in infants over 6 months of age.
  NSAIDs are contraindicated in children with:
- Bleeding or coagulopathies.
- Renal disease.
- Haematological malignancies, who may have or develop thrombocytopenia.
- Asthma, especially if they are sensitive to asthma, steroid-dependent or have coexisting nasal polyps.

Aspirin

- Rarely used in children for mild pain due to the risk of Reye's syndrome.
- However, aspirin is commonly used in the management of juvenile rheumatoid arthritis.

Codeine

- Repeated administration causes constipation.
- Main action is due to metabolism to morphine (approximately 15%).
- 10% of Caucasians and up to 30% of Hong Kong Chinese cannot metabolize codeine and find it an ineffective analgesic.
- Intravenous use may cause profound hypotension.

Oxycodone

- Oral bioavailability.
- No pharmacological differences in metabolism.
- Available as a liquid.
- Useful alternative to codeine.

Morphine

- About 30% oral bioavailability as morphine sulphate.
- May cause nausea and constipation similar to all opioids.
- There is no risk of addiction for analgesic use in children.

Tramadol

- Can be used for moderate pain in children over 12 years of age.
- A weak μ-opioid agonist and has two other analgesic mechanisms (increasing neuronal synaptic 5-hydroxytryptamine and inhibition of noradrenaline uptake).
- 70% oral bioavailability.
- No effect on clotting.
- Avoid use in children with seizure disorders and those taking tricyclic or selective serotonin reuptake inhibitor (SSRI) antidepressants.

Scenario

A compliant 8-year-old boy is having several teeth extracted under local infiltration and inhalation sedation with nitrous oxide. Consider:
- Paracetamol 20 mg/kg orally, 30 minutes preoperatively.
- Postoperatively – ibuprofen 10 mg/kg and paracetamol 15 mg/kg every 6 hours or give these 30 minutes before bedtime that night.
- Consider an oral opioid if analgesia is inadequate when local anaesthesia wears off, i.e. oxycodone syrup 0.1 mg/kg every 4–6 hours for 2–3 doses.

Discharge criteria

Many drugs that are used for combination sedation and analgesia in children have reasonably a long half-life, exceeding several hours. Discharge criteria should be used to assess that the child is well enough prior to discharge from a free-standing facility. Criteria should include:

- Self-maintenance of airway.
- Easily rousable and able to converse.
- No ataxia, can walk properly.
- Tolerating oral fluids.
- Discharge in the care of a responsible adult with appropriate information about after-hours contact if a problem arises.

Local anaesthesia

The use of local anaesthesia in paediatric dentistry varies significantly between countries and there are individual preferences as well. Every clinician must be proficient at administering painless local anaesthesia. While it is the mainstay of our pain control for operative treatment, it also represents one of the greatest fears in our patients. Use of many of the non-pharmacological techniques described above will enable the dentist to deliver an injection without the child being aware. There are few patients, old or young, who are genuinely unafraid of injections, and there are obvious disadvantages in the physical size of the dental cartridge syringe. It makes sense **not** to hold the syringe in front of a young child to see. While it is essential not to lie to the child, tricks such as having the dental assistant or nurse talk, or use the low velocity suction are useful distractions.

The use of topical anaesthetics is essential to create the optimal experience for the child. While a multitude of agents are available with different flavours and properties, newer anaesthetics such as EMLA penetrate deeper through mucosa. Newer products such as electronic devices for slow injection techniques may replace more conventional techniques.

The use of infiltration versus block injections in the mandible is also the subject of debate, and clinicians differ in their choice of technique. The approach of the needle to the mandibular foramen differs in younger children as the angle of the mandible is more obtuse and a shorter needle (25 mm) may be sufficient. However, even with the best technique, a mandibular block injection may still be uncomfortable. Infiltration injections supplemented with intra-periodontal injection may be useful. Palatal anaesthesia is best achieved by slowly infiltrating through the interdental papilla after adequate labial or buccal anaesthesia to minimize discomfort to the child.

Need for local anaesthesia under sedation and general anaesthesia

Some form of pain control is required when invasive procedures are performed under any form of sedation (including inhalation sedation, oral sedation etc.). However, the need for local anaesthetic under general anaesthesia is controversial. It is well recognized that a patient's vital signs may change in response to painful stimuli (e.g. extraction), depending on the depth of anaesthesia. We do not routinely use local anaesthesia for extractions of primary teeth under general anaesthesia. We have observed that the child's postoperative recovery is usually independent of the procedure performed, and preschool children waking after having a general anaesthetic can be more distressed by the sensation of numbness in the mouth.

> **Clinical Hint**
>
> Successful local anaesthesia depends on:
> - Communication with the child and parent.
> - Routine use of topical anaesthesia, and leaving adequate time for it to act.
> - Slow injection of warm solution.
> - Avoid direct palatal injections.
> - Adequate anaesthesia for procedure being performed.

Table 2.4 Maximum dosages for local anaesthetic solutions

Anaesthetic agent	Maximum dose
2% Lidocaine without vasoconstrictor	3 mg/kg
2% Lidocaine with 1:100000 adrenaline	7 mg/kg
4% Prilocaine plain	6 mg/kg
4% Prilocaine with felypressin	9 mg/kg
0.5% Bupivacaine with 1:200000 adrenaline	2 mg/kg
4% Articaine with adrenaline 1:100000 (approximately 1.5 cartridge of 2.2 mL in 20 kg child)	7 mg/kg

Calculation of local anaesthetic dosage:
2% lidocaine = 20 mg/mL
2.2 mL/carpule = 44 mg/carpule
A 20 kg child (approximately 5 years old) can tolerate a maximum dose of 2% lidocaine with vasoconstrictor of:
7 mg/kg × 20 kg = 140 mg   Equivalent of 3 carpules (6.6 mL)

Complications with local anaesthesia

The most significant complication encountered is overdosage. Consequently, maximum doses (Table 2.4) need to be calculated according to weight and preferably written in the notes if more than just a short procedure is being performed. This clinical complication is highlighted in a paper that reviewed significant negative outcomes (death or neurological damage) in children due to local anaesthetic overdose (Goodson & Moore 1983).

Other complications are:
- Failure to adequately anaesthetise the area.
- Intravascular injection (inferior alveolar nerve blocks or, infiltration in the posterior maxillae, directly into the pterygoid venous plexus).
- Biting of the lower lip or tongue.

Consequently, adequate postoperative instructions to both children and parents are necessary to minimize these complications. In addition, inadequate local anaesthetic technique (inexperienced operator, fast delivery of solution, and inadequate behaviour management) may jeopardize a successful outcome in an otherwise cooperative child.

Allergic reactions to local anaesthetic solutions and needle breakage are rare in children.

The use of articaine with adrenaline has gained popularity recently. However, its safety and effectiveness in children under the age of 4 years has not been established. Finally, it is worth noting that there is significant evidence that inadequate local anaesthesia for initial procedures in young children may diminish the effect of adequate analgesia in subsequent procedures (Weisman et al 1998).

Sedation in paediatric dentistry

The decision to sedate a child requires careful consideration by an experienced team. The choice of a particular technique, sedative agent and route of delivery should be made at a consultation appointment to determine the suitability of a particular child (and their parents) to a specific technique.

The use of any form of sedation in children presents added challenges to the clinician. During sedation, children's responses are more unpredictable than adults, their smaller bodies are less tolerant to sedative agents and they may be easily over-sedated. Anatomical differences between the adult and the paediatric airways include:

- The paediatric airway has increased airway resistance (e.g. upper respiratory tract infections).
- Vocal cords positioned higher and more anterior.
- The smallest portion of paediatric airway is at the level of the subglottis (below cords) at the level of the cricoid ring.
- Children have a relatively larger tongue and epiglottis.
- Possible presence of large tonsillar/adenoid mass (Figure 2.6).
- Larger head to body size ratio in children.
- The mandible is less developed and retrognathic in children.
- Children have smaller lung capacity and reserve.

Patient assessment

The preoperative assessment is among the most important factors when choosing a particular form of sedation. This assessment must include:

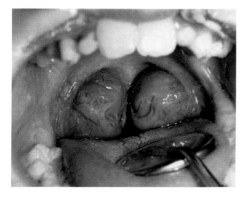

Figure 2.6 Large tonsils cause a significant risk of airway obstruction.

- Medical and dental history (including medications taken).
- Patient medical status (American Society of Anaesthesiologists (ASA) classification).
- History of recent respiratory symptoms or infections.
- Assessment of the airway to determine suitability for conscious sedation or general anaesthesia.
- Fasting status.
- Procedure being performed.
- Age.
- Weight.
- Parent factors.

The tonsil size is an important consideration when assessing the airway in children as the it may be a contributing factor to desaturation under sedation. Therefore, a thorough airway assessment is required preoperatively. The clinician should also be aware that in children the resting vital signs differ according to their age (Table 2.5).

The use of monitoring devices such as pulse oximetry is desirable for lighter sedation techniques and mandatory for moderate and deep sedation. Although the use of pulse oximetry has not been mandated for children undergoing dental treatment under inhalation sedation (nitrous oxide sedation, Figure 2.7) this may change in years to come as current research in paediatric sedation points to the application of more stricter guidelines requiring certified standards for all paediatric sedation across different medical specialties. Sedation and anaesthesia is a continuum and any dentist who sedates a children must be capable of resuscitating the patient or rescuing a patient from a deeper level of sedation than the one intended (Cote & Wilson 2006).

Table 2.5 Vital signs at different ages			
Age	Heart rate (beats/min)	BP (mm Hg)	Respiratory rate (breaths/min)
12 months	100–170	90/60	30–40
5 years	70–115	95/60	16
10 years	60–105	105/65	16
15 years	60–100	115/65	16

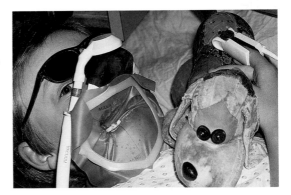

Figure 2.7 The use of nitrous oxide with rubber dam. Placement of dam ensures that there is no mouth breathing and children are usually more settled. Note the pulse oximeter on the finger. While the use of pulse oximetry is not mandatory it is a convenient measure of oxygen saturation and provides added safety. A disadvantage of the shape of the nasal mask is that it may make placement of protective glasses difficult.

Parental attitudes will often dictate the use of a particular approach. Regulations in particular countries, as well as cultural and socioeconomic factors will also determine whether sedation is used at all and which techniques are used.

Inhalation sedation (relative analgesia or nitrous oxide sedation)

Inhalation sedation is of great benefit in relieving anxiety. It is effective for children who are anxious but cooperative. An uncooperative child will often not allow a mask or nasal hood to be placed over the nose. Sedation also requires a child of sufficient maturity, age or understanding to be helpful during the dental procedure. The acceptance of the mask is usually the biggest hurdle clinically, and often it is useful in practice to lend the mask to the child so they can practise putting it on and familiarize themselves with it prior to their treatment visit. Alternatively, a trial appointment using inhalation sedation may be beneficial and help the dentist assess the correct concentrations that will be used. The use of nitrous oxide undoubtedly offers the clinician a safe and relatively easy technique to use as an adjunct to clinical care. It can provide a gentle introduction to operative dentistry for the very anxious patient, or ongoing help for those who take time to accept routine operative dental care.

Advantages
- Very safe and relatively easy technique.
- When only light sedation is required.
- Rapid induction and easily reversible with short recovery time.
- Can be titrated to required level.
- Only clinical monitoring required.

Contraindications
The only specific contraindication to inhalation sedation in children is a blocked nose. The following conditions may significantly affect the efficacy of this technique and it is best avoided in:
- Children with severe psychiatric disorders.
- Obstructive pulmonary disease.
- Chronic obstructive airway disease.
- Communication problems.
- Unwilling patients.
- Pregnancy.
- Acute respiratory tract infections (malignant hyperthermia is not a contraindication to the use of nitrous oxide).

Precautions in the use of nitrous oxide
Although nausea and vomiting may be a problem in some children, this can be usually minimized with the routine use of rubber dam during restorative dentistry. Nausea in children is often brought about by fluctuating concentrations of nitrous oxide due to alternate breathing through the mouth and nose.

Environmental concerns
Scavenging of nitrous oxide means minimizing trace amounts of the gas before, during, or after use by the patient. This can be achieved by monitoring the environment for

nitrous oxide concentrations (infrared spectrophotometry or time-weighted average dosimetry), preventing leakage from the delivery system through proper maintenance and periodic inspection of the equipment, control of waste gas with evacuation systems, and assessment of the adequacy of room ventilation and air exchange.

Nitrous oxide interferes with methionine synthase, which is required in vitamin B_{12} metabolism and DNA synthesis. It has been shown that chronic exposure at levels of 1800 ppm has no detectable biological effect, and 400 ppm is considered a safe and reasonable exposure level to trace gas. But exposure to nitrous oxide during pregnancy, especially in the first trimester, should be minimized. Currently, scavenging mask systems have become standard for all available designs. An evacuation flow rate has been established as optimal at 45 L/min. Therefore, exposure to nitrous oxide in the dental environment should be of more concern to staff who work with this technique routinely.

Although sterilization protocols are modified constantly, the use of disposable nasal hoods is recommended as well as the use of autoclavable conducting tubing and other equipment. The use of surface disinfection (e.g. glutaraldehyde) for nasal hoods is discouraged, as it may cause significant skin irritation. Surface disinfection and the use of barriers to cover equipment is also recommended.

Through careful and thoughtful behaviour management the use of relative analgesia can eventually cease, leaving a cooperative child patient coping well with their dental care.

Conscious sedation

The term 'conscious sedation' has been used in the past to imply a patient who is awake, responsive and able to communicate. This verbal communication with the child is an indicator of an adequate level of consciousness and maintenance of protective reflexes. In clinical practice however, sedation (conscious sedation, deep sedation and/or general anaesthesia) is a continuum. Any technique which depresses the central nervous system may result in a deeper sedation state than intended, and consequently clinicians who sedate children require a much higher level of skill with a particular technique, the relevant training and experience and the proper qualifications with the relevant regulating authority.

Sedation of children for diagnostic and therapeutic procedures remains an area of rapid change and considerable controversy. Recent publications identified several features associated with adverse sedation-related events and poor outcomes in studies, namely:

- Adverse outcomes occurred more frequently in a non-hospital-based facility.
- Inadequate resuscitation was more often associated with a non-hospital-based setting.
- Inadequate and inconsistent physiological monitoring contributed to poor outcome in all venues.
- Adverse events were associated with drug overdoses and interactions, especially when three or more drugs were used.
- Inadequate preoperative assessment.
- Lack of an independent observer.
- Errors in medication.
- Inadequate recovery procedures.

Considerations for paediatric sedation in the dental setting
- Uniform, specialty-independent guidelines for monitoring children during sedation are essential.
- The same level of care should apply to hospital-based and non-hospital-based facilities.
- Pulse oximetry should be mandatory whenever a child receives sedating medications for a procedure, irrespective of the route of drug administration or the dosage.
- Age and size-appropriate equipment and medications for resuscitation should be immediately available in a designated crash cart, regardless of the location where the child is sedated.
- All healthcare providers who sedate children, regardless of practice venue, should have advanced airway management and resuscitation skills.
- Practitioners must carefully weigh the risks and the benefits of sedating children beyond the safety net of a hospital or hospital-like environment.
- Practitioners must understand that the absence of skilled back-up personnel pose significant risks in the event of a medical emergency (Cote et al 2000, Cote & Wilson 2006, Cravero & Blike 2004).

Oral sedation
Oral sedation is the most popular route used by paediatric dentists, due to the ease of administration for most children. Several agents are used for this technique, including:
- Benzodiazepines (e.g. midazolam).
- Chloral hydrate.
- Hydroxyzine.
- Promethazine.
- Ketamine.

Midazolam
Midazolam has increased in popularity in the past decade due to its safety profile and short-acting nature, allowing quick recovery and discharge of the patient. Dosage varies from 0.3 mg/kg to 0.7 mg/kg, however a maximum ceiling dose (e.g. 10 mg) is usually determined for the older age groups. Several studies have reported on the use of oral midazolam, and this appears to be a successful technique for children, with following selection criteria:
- Children of ages 24 months to 6–8 years of age (depending on individual characteristics).
- Children ASA stage I or II.
- Short or simple procedures (under 30 minutes).
- Parents who are 'fit' for the technique.

Although the technique is successful in the older age groups, it may be more difficult to deal with children of larger size once sedated. Children over 6 years may become disinhibited and difficult to control. In addition, obese children may present added airway complications and depending on the drug used, redistribution of active drug components may increase the length of sedation. Appropriate fasting for elective procedures and a balance between depth of sedation and risk for those who are unable to fast because of the urgent nature should be made on an individual basis.

The main disadvantage of this technique is that drugs given orally cannot be titrated accurately. As most drugs undergo hepatic metabolism and only a fraction of the original dose is active, titration of the drug is difficult and may be unreliable, unlike other techniques such as inhalation or intravenous sedation. Equally, an overdose cannot be easily reversed. Furthermore, oral sedation requires cooperation from the child to ingest the medication, which is not always possible or some of the medication may be spat out. Never re-dose as is impossible to accurately determine how much of the drug was ingested.

In the preschool age group, a knee-to-knee position offers good access for the delivery of the medication if assistance in restraint is required. This technique is also used to treat young children as it allows good control of the patient, easy restraint by the parent/carer and good intra-oral vision for the clinician.

Rectal sedation
Absorption is excellent by rectal administration. Although routinely performed in Scandinavia and certain parts of Europe, rectal sedation is less commonly used in Australasia, the UK and the USA because of cultural sensitivities. It is, however, an excellent route for drug administration and provides a more reliable and controllable absorption than the oral route.

Nasal sedation
This implies delivery of medication directly to the nasal mucosa. However, due to reported complications and a poorly understood mechanism of action (the literature is divided as to whether the drug is absorbed directly from the blood stream or there is direct uptake to the central nervous system), this route is considered as an intravenous route, and consequently requires a higher level of training and monitoring.

Intravenous sedation
This technique requires a highly trained team, including an experienced and duly qualified sedationist or specialist anaesthetist, medical nurses trained in this technique, but also, most importantly, a dentist who understands that the conditions are different from clinical dentistry with no sedation. Appropriate monitoring, adequate facilities and recovery options are mandatory for the safe delivery of intravenous drugs. This is dictated by the relevant regulating body in each country.

Intravenous sedation has the advantage of the procedure being controllable and may be readily reversible, but as most children are frightened of needles it might seem an inappropriate form of drug administration in extremely anxious children. Although different drug combinations may be used intravenously, in Australia, a combination of a midazolam and a opioid analgesic (fentanyl) is often used. These drugs are readily reversible by flumazenil and naloxone, respectively.

Patients suitable for intravenous sedation
- Child patients 8 years of age or older.
- Child is ASA stage I or II.

- Child is cooperative and has a cooperative parent.
- Adequate venous access (dorsum of hand or antecubital fossa).

Suitable procedures for intravenous sedation
- Short procedures that require approximately 30 minutes duration.
- Primary teeth extractions or up to two permanent molars.
- 1–2 quadrants of restorative dentistry.
- Short surgical procedures with good access in the mouth.

Procedures usually *not* suitable for intravenous sedation
- 3–4 quadrants of restorative dentistry (unless minor restorative).
- Extractions of permanent molars in each quadrant (invasive procedure and bleeding from all four quadrants make airway management more difficult).
- Obese children (in whom resuscitation procedures may be difficult and the airway more unpredictable).
- Parents who may not provide adequate care to the child postoperatively.

Intravenous sedation is usually performed in a hospital environment or dental surgeries which have been duly accredited for the use of these more advanced sedation techniques.

General anaesthesia

The need for general anaesthesia represents the clinician's final solution to treating a child's dental problem. In most instances, a caring attitude in association with a period of familiarization will allow the child to be treated conservatively. The decision to arrange general anaesthesia should not be taken lightly as there is always a small risk of serious complications from the anaesthetic. The clinician must make a decision balancing the need with the risk. Economic factors and access to anaesthetic facilities may also be an issue. When deciding to place the child under general anaesthesia, the clinician must look at the whole picture.
- What is the dental condition?
  - Is there gross dental caries?
  - Does the child have a facial swelling?
  - Is the child in pain?
- Is the treatment absolutely necessary?
  - Could the patient be managed more conservatively?
  - Has the child undergone a period of familiarization?
  - Has there been a history of emotional trauma associated with the dental environment?

Certain clinical situations automatically indicate the need for general anaesthesia:
- Multiple carious and abscessed teeth in multiple quadrants in very young children.
- Severe facial cellulitis.
- Facial trauma.

Often it is necessary for the patient to have several routine visits before the clinician can be sure dental work needs to be done; such visits also allow assessment of whether the child's behaviour precludes satisfactory completion of the work. The child must have a sensible treatment plan arranged. It should include home-care instruction (for the parents to help clean the child's teeth), dietician's referral, use of home fluorides and return visits. If, after seeing the child several times, the clinician feels the child needs dental work, but is unmanageable, a general anaesthetic should be considered.

Consent for treatment
Consent for children younger than 14 years old
In children under 14 years of age, a specific 'Consent for Minor' form is usually required. The parent or guardian must sign the form and a third party, usually the dentist, must witness the signature.

Consent of children 14–16 years of age
Children aged 14–16 years must give their consent for the treatment to be performed. Although a 'responsible informed child' can give this consent, the parent or guardian should also give consent and sign the form. The dentist should explain the procedure and witness the signatures.

Although there is no authoritative statement in statue law regarding consent for children younger than 16 years, common law (Australasia and the UK) dictates that:

> as a matter of law the parents' right to determine whether or not their minor child below the age of 16 will have medical treatment terminates if and when their child achieves a sufficient understanding to enable him to understand fully what is proposed.
>
> (*Gillick* v *West Norfolk Area Health Authority* [1986] AC 112, UK)

Consent over 16 years
A patient 16 years and over must consent for their own treatment.

Emergency treatment
In emergency situations, dental treatment may be performed without the consent of the child or parent or guardian if, in the opinion of the practitioner, the treatment is necessary and a matter of urgency in order to save the child's life, or to prevent serious damage to the child's health (Section 20B of the Children [Care and Protection] Act [1987] NSW, Australia). Fortunately there are few situations where this will occur in the dental environment, although situations do arise for those working in hospital settings. The overriding point is to 'do no harm'.

It is important that 'informed consent' be obtained. The clinician must carefully explain all the procedures planned using lay language as appropriate. All potential risks need to be mentioned, discussed and documented. When completing the sections on standard forms on the nature of the operation, be specific, do not use abbreviations and include all the procedures planned. Where appropriate use simple terminology to describe the operation.

Pre-anaesthetic assessment for general anaesthesia
A medical history and examination by the anaesthetist is required prior to the procedure. If a patient has complex medical problems a preoperative anaesthetic assessment

may need to be made during a separate consultation with the anaesthetist prior to the day of surgery.

The anaesthetist will particularly want to be aware of:

- Behavioural issues, e.g. autism, developmental delay, extreme anxiety and needle phobia.
- Syndromes, e.g. Down's syndrome, velocardiofacial syndrome.
- Cardiac disease heart murmurs, previous surgery for congenital defects.
- Respiratory disease, e.g. asthma.
- Airway problems, e.g. history of croup, cleft palate, micrognathia, previous tracheostomy, known history of intubation difficulties, sleep apnoea.
- Neurological disease, e.g. epilepsy, previous brain injuries, cerebral palsy.
- Endocrine and metabolic disorders, e.g. diabetes, genetic metabolic disorders.
- Gastrointestinal problems, e.g. reflux, difficulty swallowing or feeding.
- Haematological, e.g. haemophilia, thrombocytopenia, haemoglobinopathies.
- Neuromuscular disorders, e.g. muscular dystrophy.

Allergies must be noted including latex allergy.

Medications must be documented. Most medications should be continued until the time of anaesthesia unless there is a clear reason to withhold (e.g. with anticoagulants or insulin). Consultation with the original prescriber should be made before warfarin or aspirin is ceased to make an assessment of the risk or benefit of ceasing these drugs. Management of diabetic patients will require consultation with the patient's endocrinologist.

Upper respiratory tract infection

If a child presents with an upper respiratory tract infection on the day of surgery it may be appropriate to delay elective anaesthesia for 2–3 weeks. This decision can be balanced against economic and social issues and patient factors such as the child's age, urgency of treatment, severity of the infection and any other medical problems the child may have. Ultimately the decision to cancel or proceed is up to the anaesthetist.

Fasting

Normally, the stomach is empty of clear fluids two hours after ingestion. Accepted practice for fasting for anaesthesia is:

- 6 hours from solids and milk.
- 4 hours from breast milk.
- 2 hours from clear fluids.

Keeping fasting instructions close to these guidelines will cause the least distress for the patient. Unfortunately difficulties with organizational factors often results in longer fasting times. There is no evidence that oral medications taken during the time of fasting increases the risk of aspiration during anaesthesia.

Operating theatre environment

To reduce the child's fear and anxiety strategies should be used to help them to cope with the operating theatre environment. For example:

- Minimizing the waiting time prior to the procedure.
- Leaving them in their own clothes. It is not necessary to change into theatre attire for routine restorative procedures.

- Allowing a parent to stay with the child during induction of anaesthesia.
- Using topical local anaesthetic cream such as EMLA if an intravenous induction is planned.
- Allowing a parent into the recovery area to be with the child as soon as they are awake and stable.
- Reassuring parents at all stages about what to expect.

Premedication
Some children may require oral premedication prior to anaesthesia. Suggested regimens are paracetamol 15 mg/kg and midazolam 0.2–0.5 mg/kg.

Induction
Anxiety is minimized by allowing a parent to be with the child during induction. Anaesthesia induction may be intravenous or gaseous. The use of topical local anaesthetic cream prior to insertion into a vein alleviates some of the pain of obtaining intravenous access. Some extremely uncooperative children may require induction with intramuscular ketamine 2–3 mg/kg. These are usually larger autistic children or children with developmental delay.

Sharing the airway (Figure 2.8)
- The anaesthetist and dentist must share the airway, so teamwork, and mutual understanding of each other's needs, is necessary.
- Nasotracheal intubation with a nasal RAE (Ring, Adair & Elwyn) tube provides good access for the dentist and a secure airway for the anaesthetist. A throat pack is usually used and it is extremely important to ensure the removal of a throat pack at the end of the case.
- The throat pack should not be so bulky that the tongue is forced anteriorly limiting the access to the mouth for the dentist. In young children, reduce the size of an adult-sized pack to one third (ribbon gauze of about 30 cm moistened with saline).
- An oral laryngeal mask airway or endotracheal tube provides a satisfactory airway for the anaesthetist but may or may not give the dentist the access they require, as it encroaches on the work area. However, this is a useful technique for less extensive dental work, such as extractions of primary teeth after trauma.
- A face-mask-only technique may be used for simple extractions. The mask is removed for a short time while the extraction is performed.
- During anaesthesia it is important to protect the eyes from injury by taping them shut and possibly covering them with padding.
- Before waking the patient all foreign material such as rolls, gauze and throat packs must be removed and accounted for.

Analgesia
Analgesia as is appropriate should be given while the patient is asleep. The use of intravenous opioids may be required but can cause an increase in postoperative vomiting. As mentioned earlier, local anaesthetics may be used, but often the feeling of numbness around the mouth causes even more distress than the discomfort of the procedure. NSAIDs such as ibuprofen 10 mg/kg 6-hourly, may be prescribed.

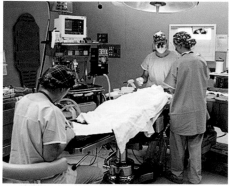

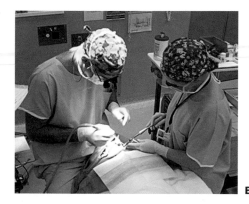

A

B

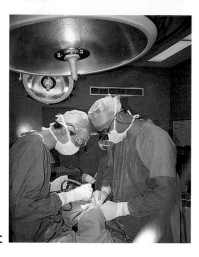

C

Figure 2.8 Management under general anaesthesia. **A**, **B** Treatment under general anaesthesia must be conducted in a comfortable atmosphere. There must be cooperation between the anaesthetist and the operating dentist, both of whom need access to the oral cavity and the airway. Nasal intubation is invaluable. Note that the anaesthetic machine in close proximity but out of the way of the operating surgeon and the dental assistant also has all required equipment close at hand. Individual institutions' protocols vary however, and it is not usually necessary to scrub for restorative procedures as these are considered to be 'non-sterile'. **C** Surgical procedures should be performed under sterile conditions.

Paracetamol 15 mg/kg 4-hourly may also be used. Occasionally oral morphine or codeine phosphate may be required.

Emergence
Ideally, parents should be able to come into the recovery area once the child is awake and in a stable condition. Distress on waking is not uncommon, and can be partly due to emergence delirium. The child is quite likely to be upset by the unfamiliar environment, an unpleasant taste in the mouth, or because their mouth feels different because of missing teeth or new crowns. Usually the pain is not severe.

Categories of anaesthetic risk
American Society of Anesthesiologists (ASA)
- Class 1– Healthy patient.
- Class 2 – Mild to moderate systemic disease without significant limitations.
- Class 3 – Severe systemic disturbance without limitations.
- Class 4 – Life-threatening systemic disorder.

Figure 2.9 A day-stay recovery ward with one-to-one nursing care after general anaesthesia. Normal day-stay recovery is a minimum of 1.5 hours after the operation.

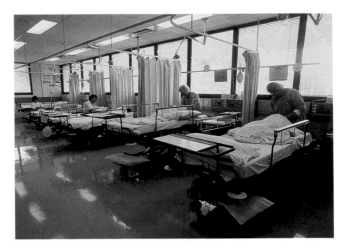

- Class 5 – Moribund patient not expected to survive >24 hours.
- Class E – Emergency patient.

Suitability for day-stay anaesthesia
Most children who are ASA 1 or 2 will be suitable for day-stay anaesthesia (Figure 2.9). However, children with more severe systemic disease may need overnight hospital care to ensure that they are maintaining their airway, tolerating oral food and fluids, that any pain is satisfactorily managed and that there is no ongoing bleeding.

Ward instructions
Postoperative instructions and consultation notes in the medical file must be clear and legible. It is important for nursing staff to understand what procedures have been performed and by whom. They should also know whom to contact if complications arise.

References and further reading

Pain control for children
Analgesic Expert Group 2007 Therapeutic Guidelines: Analgesic Version 5. Melbourne, Therapeutic Guidelines Ltd
Australian and New Zealand College of Anaesthetists and Faculty of Pain Medicine 2005 The paediatric patient. In: Acute Pain Management: Scientific Evidence, 2nd edn. Australian and New Zealand College of Anaesthetists and Faculty of Pain Medicine, NHMRC. Available at: www.anzca.edu.au/publications/acutepain.htm (accessed 24 October 2007)
Herschell AD, Calzada E, Eyberg SM et al 2003 Clinical issues with parent–child interaction therapy. Cognitive and Behavioral Practice 9:16–27
Lamacraft G, Cooper MG, Cavalletto BP 1997 Subcutaneous cannulae for morphine boluses in children: assessment of a technique. Journal of Pain Symptoms and Management 13:43–49
NSW Health Paracetamol Use 2006 PD2006_004 [policy directive] Sydney (www.health.nsw.gov.au/policies/pd/2006/PD2006_004.html) (accessed 24 October 2007)

Paediatrics and Child Health Division, Royal Australasian College of Physicians. Guideline Statement: management of procedure related pain in children and adolescents, 2005. Available at www.health.nsw.gov.au/policies/pd/2006/PD2006_004.html

Thomas A, Chess S 1977 Temperament and development. Brunner/Mazel, New York

Weisman SJ, Berstein B, Schechter NL 1998 Consequences of inadequate analgesia during painful procedures in children. Archives of Pediatrics and Adolescent Medicine 152:147–149

Williams DG, Hatch DJ, Howard RF 2001 Codeine phosphate in paediatric medicine. British Journal of Anaesthesia 86:413–421

Sedation

Cote CH, Wilson S 2006 Guidelines for monitoring and management of pediatric patients during and after sedation for diagnostic and therapeutic procedures: an update. Pediatrics 118:2587–2602

Cote CJ, Notterman DA, Karl HW et al 2000a Adverse sedation events in pediatrics: a critical incident analysis of contributing factors. Pediatrics 105:805–814

Cote CJ, Notterman DA, Karl HW et al 2000b Adverse sedation events in pediatrics: analysis of medications used for sedation. Pediatrics 106:633–644

Cravero JP, Blike GT 2004 Review of pediatric sedation. Anesthesia and Analgesia 99:1355–1364

Goodson JM, Moore PA 1983 Life-threatening reactions after pedodontic sedation: an assessment of narcotic, local anesthetic, and antiemetic drug interaction. Journal of the American Dental Association 107:239–245

Hosey MT 2002 UK National Clinical Guidelines in Paediatric Dentistry. Managing anxious children: the use of conscious sedation in paediatric dentistry. International Journal of Paediatric Dentistry 12:359–372

Houpt M 2002 Project USAP 2000 – use of sedative agents by pediatric dentists: a 15-year follow-up survey. Pediatric Dentistry 24:289–294

Kupietzky A, Houpt MI 1993 Midazolam: a review of its use for conscious sedation of children. Pediatric Dentistry 15:237–241

Lee JY, Vann WF, Roberts MW 2000 A cost analysis of treating pediatric dental patients using general anesthesia versus conscious sedation. Pediatric Dentistry 22:27–32

Primosch RE, Buzzi IM, Jerrell G 1999 Effect of nitrous oxide-oxygen inhalation with scavenging on behavioral and physiological parameters during routine pediatric dental treatment. Pediatric Dentistry 21:417–420

Wilson S 2004 Pharmacological management of the pediatric dental patient. Pediatric Dentistry 26:131–136

Yagiela JA, Cote CJ, Notterman DA et al 2001 Adverse sedation events in pediatrics. Pediatrics 107:1494

3 Dental caries

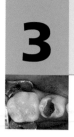

Contributors
David Manton, Bernadette K Drummond, Nicky Kilpatrick

Factors influencing dental caries

It can be said that the major work of the dental profession is controlled by this disease process and yet many clinicians have a poor understanding of the mechanisms by which caries is initiated, how to identify patients at risk and how to put management plans in place to ensure that the disease does not progress. Too often only the outcomes of the carious process are treated and not the cause of the disease itself.

Dental caries should be regarded as a transmissible disease. It involves a complex process of enamel demineralization and remineralization that occurs due the action of organic acids produced by micro-organisms within the dental plaque. Dental caries is a multifactorial disease, resulting from the interplay between environmental, behavioural and genetic factors. The four factors that influence its progression are shown in Figure 3.1.

Dental plaque biofilm

Increasingly dental plaque is viewed as a dynamic biofilm (Figure 3.2). This implies that plaque maintains its own microenvironment and has actions that influence oral health. While the plaque biofilm is usually viewed as undesirable, its presence may be positive, e.g. in acting as a fluoride reservoir or as a protective barrier to erosion.

Dental plaque contains bacteria that are both acidogenic and aciduric. Although many bacterial subspecies have been shown to be associated with caries, *Streptococcus mutans* is still believed to be the most important bacterium in the initiation and progress of this disease. Later, following enamel cavitation, lactobacilli become increasingly important. In the caries process, once the pH of the plaque drops below a critical level (around 5.5), the acid produced begins to demineralize the enamel. This will last for 20 minutes or longer depending on the availability of substrate and effect of the saliva.

The mutans streptococci (*S. mutans* and *S. sobrinus*) is the major group of bacteria involved in the initiation of enamel demineralization. Normally, an infant is inoculated with *S. mutans* by the mother or primary caregiver. The initial inoculation was thought to be dependent on the presence of a hard surface, and therefore the eruption of the first tooth, however recent research has shown the presence of this organism in newborns. In general, the earlier the inoculation with mutans streptococci, the greater the caries risk of an infant. Repeated consumption of fermentable carbohydrates leads to the proportional overgrowth of mutans streptococci, and the subsequent production of organic acids (lactic, formic, acetic), an increase in the extracellular polysaccharide matrix and a change in the relative components of the microflora leading to increased risk of dental caries.

Figure 3.1 The multifactorial nature of caries involves the Host, Substrate, Bacteria and Time.

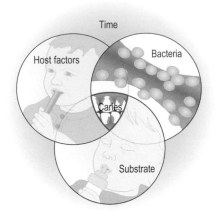

Figure 3.2 Scanning electron micrograph of dental plaque (4555× magnification). This image shows the typical 'corncob' arrangement of streptococci held by an extracellular polysaccharide matrix on a web of central filamentous micro-organisms. (Courtesy, Institute of Dental Research, SEM Unit, Westmead.)

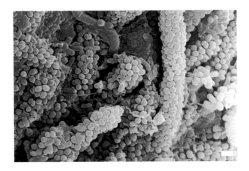

Substrates

Bacteria use fermentable carbohydrates for energy and the end-products of the glycolytic pathway in bacterial metabolism are acids. Sucrose is the fermentable carbohydrate most frequently implicated, but it is important to remember that the bacteria can use all fermentable carbohydrates, including cooked starches. Although any carbohydrate may cause the production of acid, it is the availability of glucose that drives bacterial metabolism to produce lactic acid rather than weaker byproducts such as formate, acetoacetate and alcohols. Furthermore, the amount of fermentable carbohydrate is relatively unimportant, as even minute amounts of fermentable carbohydrate will be used immediately.

Host factors

The traditional triad of host factors – the teeth, the microbes and their diet – is a simplistic representation of the complex inter-relationships in the oral cavity. With regard to the caries process, the quality of tooth structure and the saliva are the major host factors that should be considered. Poor tooth quality, such as hypomineralized enamel, is associated with increased rates of caries, and changes in salivary quantity and/or quality has a profound effect on the whole oral environment, affecting caries rates, oral comfort, periodontal health and resistance to infection.

Saliva

The importance of saliva is often overlooked, however, it has several critical roles in the caries process. Saliva is excreted at different rates and with different constituents depending on the presence or absence of stimulatory factors. Saliva stimulated by chewing has increased calcium and phosphate ion concentrations. A gustatory effect, such as that induced by some food acids, has been shown to stimulate a higher flow rate of saliva than stimulation by mechanical chewing. By removing substrate and buffering plaque acid, saliva helps to balance the caries process and has a critical role in remineralization as it provides a stabilized supersaturated solution of calcium and phosphate ions as well as fluoride ions from extrinsic sources. The major constituent of saliva is water (~99.5%), with a wide range of other inorganic and organic components, the most relevant being the salivary proteins, especially the histatins, mucins and statherins, which provide:

- Antibacterial and antifungal and antiviral activity.
- Lubrication, which also assists in bolus formation.
- Inhibition of demineralization and stabilization of calcium and phosphate ions, which assists remineralization.

Therefore, a decrease in the amount or quality of saliva can increase significantly the caries risk.

Time

When acid challenges occur repeatedly, the eventual collapse of enough enamel crystals and subsequently rods will result in surface breakdown. This may take from months to years depending on the intensity and frequency of the acid attack. This means that in all mouths (as most mouths will contain some cariogenic bacteria) there is continual demineralization and remineralization of enamel; therefore, an individual is never free of dental caries. The process of enamel demineralization and remineralization is constantly cycling between net loss and gain of mineral. It is only when the balance leans towards net loss that clinically identifiable signs of the process become apparent. The long-term outcome of this cycling is determined by:

- The composition and amount of plaque.
- Sugar consumption (frequency and timing).
- Fluoride exposure.
- Salivary flow and quality.
- Enamel quality.
- Immune response.

Thus the term 'caries free' often used to describe a child with no visible decay is best changed to the term 'caries inactive' to more accurately reflect this clinical reality. For the balance to be maintained there should be sufficient time between cariogenic challenges for the remineralization process to take place. When these challenges become too frequent, or occur when salivary flow is reduced, the rate of demineralization and subsequent tooth breakdown will increase.

The caries process

Dental enamel demineralization is a chemical process. The dissolution of hydroxyapatite can be described simply:

$$Ca_{10}(PO_4)_6(OH)_2 + 10H^+ \rightarrow 10Ca_2 + 6H(PO_4)^{3-} + 2H_2O$$

with enamel demineralization summarized as a net loss of enamel mineral due to the action of either intrinsic or extrinsic acids, leading to dental caries or erosion. Dental caries is primarily caused by lactic and acetic acids which diffuse through the plaque and into the enamel pores between the rods as neutral-ion species, where they dissociate and decrease the pH of the fluid surrounding the enamel crystals. Once dissociated, the protons dissolve the hydroxyapatite crystal surface depending on the degree of saturation of the specific apatite and the inter-rod fluid calcium and phosphate ion concentration increases.

The buffering of calcium and phosphate at the enamel surface and in the plaque biofilm leads to the development of a subsurface (or white spot lesion) with a proportionately hypermineralized surface layer. The optical changes occur due to the increased pore spaces between the thinned rods and the effect this has on the refractive qualities of the enamel. The continuation of this process eventually undermines the support for the surface layer and surface breakdown occurs – the development of a physical cavity.

Caries detection

With the significant reduction in the prevalence, incidence and severity of caries in a great proportion of Western society over the past three decades, notwithstanding some disadvantaged communities and individuals who remain at high risk, the sensitivity of many diagnostic tests for caries has been reduced. Occlusal caries detection is complicated clinically by surface morphology, fluoride exposure, anatomical fissure topography and the presence of plaque and stain. The current methods used for caries detection are:

- Visual and tactile inspection.
- Radiography.
- Transillumination.

Clinical Hint

The traditional use of a probe or explorer in pits and fissures and on demineralized smooth surfaces may damage demineralized enamel and transfer cariogenic bacteria from one site to another, increasing the likelihood of restorative intervention. This invasive method provides little additional information, therefore, the probe should only be used to clean the fissures before examination, and the diagnostic criterion of 'sticky fissure' should be eliminated.

New methods of caries detection

In the past two decades, laser and light-induced fluorescence methods have been developed to detect and quantify enamel mineral content. These methods rely on the different fluorescence characteristics (loss of fluorescence) of demineralized enamel due to the scattering of light in the carious lesion. There is a strong correlation between mineral loss and fluorescence in white spot (demineralized) lesions of enamel.

The recent commercial development of a quantified light-induced fluorescence (QLF) system using light of wavelength 290–450 nm has the potential to increase the accuracy of measurement of mineralization levels of in vivo smooth surface enamel. This is because:

- Current clinical methods are limited to detecting enamel caries only at an advanced stage.
- QLF can detect small changes in mineralization microscopically.
- Mineral loss can be quantified.
- Serial changes in lesion characteristics can be recorded.

Preventing dental caries

Preventing, reversing or at least slowing down dental caries generally consists of altering one or more of the factors described above.

Diet modification

Although often given minimal attention by dental practitioners, diet is probably the single most important factor in caries risk. Although some dietary habits have changed, the overall consumption of sugar has not altered over the past 50 years in most Western countries. Many foods, although not obviously cariogenic, contain hidden sugars and fermentable carbohydrates. Dietary histories may be useful in identifying those children at high risk. Achieving changes in dietary habits is extremely difficult and therefore advice must be individual, practical and realistic.

- Frequency of intake is more important than overall quantity.
- 'Grazing' between meals should be discouraged.
- The frequent consumption of soft drinks (including fruit juices and sports drinks) should be avoided. Not only are they cariogenic but also extremely erosive and highly caloric.
- Sweets etc. are useful rewards, but should be limited to mealtimes.
- Many foods labelled 'No added sugar' contain high levels of natural sugars.
- Dietary advice should not be all negative. Positive alternatives should be identified.
- The chewing of pH-neutral sugar-free gum increases salivary flow and assists in remineralization and the prevention of demineralization.
- Probably the best dietary advice of all is to 'give teeth a rest' for at least 2 hours between every meal or snack.

Fluorides

The principal mode of action of all fluoridated modalities (toothpastes, rinses, gels and community water fluoridation) is the topical effect at the enamel surface. Even low concentrations of fluoride in the micro-environment around the teeth inhibit demineralization and promote remineralization of the tooth surface. The incorporation of fluorine (as fluoroapatite) into the enamel will decrease its solubility (and increase its resistance to caries). However, it is now recognized that the incorporation of systemically administered fluoride into developing (unerupted) enamel has a lesser role in increasing enamel resistance (see Chapter 4).

Calcium and phosphate

The ability for net remineralization to occur is limited by available calcium and phosphate ions, intrinsically provided by saliva; therefore remineralization is 'saliva limited'. Attempts have been made over past decades to provide supersaturated ionic calcium and phosphate solutions to increase remineralization. However, these attempts have been limited by the low solubility of these ions. Recently, it has been reported that milk-derived casein phosphopeptides stabilize calcium and phosphate in an amorphous form (casein phosphopeptide-amorphous calcium phosphate fluoride (CPP-ACP)), providing a supersaturated environment that drives remineralization and limits demineralization. CPP-ACP has been added to topical pastes, chewing gums and mouthrinses to increase remineralization and decrease demineralization, and to sports drinks to decrease erosivity.

Fissure sealants

Even in communities with a low incidence of caries, the pits and fissures are still susceptible to caries. The most effective way to prevent pit and fissure caries is by fissure sealing (see Chapter 5).

Plaque removal

Tooth brushing

In communities with water fluoridation, caries mostly occurs in pits and fissures and inter-proximally. If all plaque could be removed from the tooth surfaces, dental caries would not occur. However, this is not physically and behaviourally possible.

- Besides removing plaque, tooth brushing should be regarded also as vehicle for topical fluoride application.
- The mechanical action of tooth brushing alone will not prevent caries as it does not effectively remove plaque from the areas mentioned above.
- Children should be encouraged to adopt good brushing habits. Brushing should commence when teeth first erupt, as a part of everyday hygiene. Gauze or a face cloth on a finger, or a small very soft toothbrush may be used to remove the plaque in infants.
- It is beneficial for adults to continue to assist with tooth brushing until children are around 8–10 years old and have developed the dexterity to remove plaque effectively by themselves. Ideally, tooth brushing should be carried out twice a day with a fluoridated toothpaste but parents should understand that at least once a day is essential to decrease the risk of dental caries (see Chapter 4).

Flossing

In preschool years, and in early mixed dentition, the interproximal surfaces of the primary molars become more at risk of caries. Parents can be shown how to floss these areas when the teeth are in contact and especially if there are signs of demineralization. Older children should be taught to floss themselves. They may find it easier to use one of the commercial floss holders.

Disclosing of plaque

Children, their parents and older patients find it difficult to know when they have effectively removed plaque from their teeth. Disclosing solutions and tablets are very

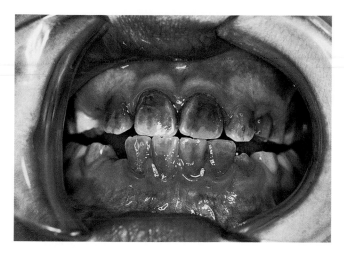

Figure 3.3 Disclosing plaque is an important part of teaching children about oral hygiene and educating parents.

useful for helping patients and parents to see and remove plaque more effectively (Figure 3.3).

Antimicrobials

Antibacterial mouthwashes have become part of the preventive dentistry regimen in the past few years. They do have a role for some patients in caries prevention. In particular, chlorhexidine- and triclosan-containing rinses, gels, toothpastes or varnishes may be used for patients with high risk of caries to help with plaque and microbial control. Their main role is as one part of the multifactorial management of high caries individuals and especially for those who are medically compromised. Systemic antimicrobials (antibiotics) cause significant alterations in oral microflora and have no use in caries prevention.

Determining patients at risk of dental caries

The development of a treatment strategy for a patient that is based on risk factors pertinent to that individual is the gold standard of minimally invasive treatment. That is, before deciding the appropriate methods and preventive products to advise, the patient's caries risk should be determined. This may be achieved by considering several aspects such as:

- Presence of white spot lesions.
- Individual and familial caries history.
- Socioeconomic status.
- Ethnicity.
- Diet.
- Fluoride exposure.
- Salivary flow and quality.
- Oral hygiene.
- Medical history.
- Presence of developmental defects of enamel.

These factors – especially the background factors – can only be a guide, but that they are important to consider when deciding what preventive measures to put in place for individual patients. When the risk has been determined a preventive programme, incorporating the appropriate methods, can be used. A suggested approach is shown in Table 3.1.

Patient background
- Water fluoride levels.
- Epidemiology of caries, the caries susceptibility of the group to which the patient belongs.
- Ethnicity.
- Socioeconomic variables.

Individual characteristics
Age
- Different teeth sites are at risk at different ages.
- Specific patient characteristics.
- Teeth may be at particular risk in association with orthodontic treatment (Figure 3.4) or in those with a medical co-morbidity.

Medical history
- Frequent medication?
- Does medication alter saliva?
- Is medication sweetened with a fermentable carbohydrate?
- Is oral hygiene a problem?
- Is the diet altered?
- In utero and perinatal history.

Diet
- Fermentable carbohydrate frequency?
- What is the parent's/patient's knowledge of foods with sugars?
- Protective foods (i.e. dairy foods)?
- Are there risk-associated habits?
- Nursing bottle in bed or at-will breastfeeding?
- Use of sipper bottles or feeding cups?
- Frequent snacking in sports training?

Family history of caries
Cariogenic bacteria are transmitted vertically from the parents and possibly horizontally from other caregivers and close associates.
- Are the parents caries active?

Intra-oral information
Caries history
- Past restorations or caries around existing restorations.
- Signs of demineralization (white spot lesions).

Table 3.1 Instituting preventive programmes

	No caries	Early caries	Active caries
Risk	Low risk	Medium risk Clinical/radiographic enamel demineralization	High risk New lesions at each recall, including risk behaviours
Question	How to keep teeth caries free?	How to heal existing lesions and prevent new lesions?	How to restore existing lesions and prevent new lesions?
Preventive plans			
Plaque	Check what the patient is doing Either reinforce the behaviour or improve efficacy	Disclose, have patient remove the disclosing agent and clean as appropriate Advise fluoridated floss or flossing with fluoride toothpaste	Disclose, have patient remove the disclosing agent and clean as appropriate Advise fluoridated floss or flossing with fluoride toothpaste
Diet	Reinforce and present good dietary habits Check for recent changes such as sports diets and give advice	Advise against frequent fermentable carbohydrate intake Check for recent changes such as sports diets	Check the dietary habits thoroughly with a 24-hour recording and/or a food frequency questionnaire Advise against frequent fermentable carbohydrate intake and check that the patient can identify these Check for recent changes such as sports diet
Fluoride	Check that it is being used appropriately	Check that it is being used appropriately Introduce daily mouthwashes if appropriate for age Consider high-concentration fluorides for demineralized areas	Check that it is being used appropriately Introduce daily mouthwashes if appropriate for age Apply concentrated fluoride treatments such as gels or varnishes Provide supplementary ionic calcium and phosphate
Fissure sealants	Apply to deep retentive fissures only	Apply to molars, especially those showing demineralization	Ensure all open lesions are restored permanently or temporarily to reduce bacterial numbers Apply fissure sealant to all molars and premolars
Recall	12-monthly if there have been two 6-month periods of no caries activity	6-monthly while there are signs of caries activity or risk remains	6-monthly or 3-monthly with medically compromised or very-high-risk children

Figure 3.4 It is important to note that risk can change. A child who was previously free of caries has developed cervical lesions during orthodontic treatment.

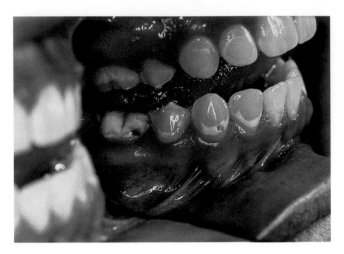

Eruption of teeth
- The early permanent dentition may be more at risk than the mature dentition.
- It takes time for caries to progress to a detectable stage. Risk may not be obvious for 3–4 years after eruption.

Oral health
- Presence of plaque.
- How effective is the oral hygiene?
- Is plaque accumulation associated with demineralization?
- Does the patient use floss?
- Is a fluoridated toothpaste used?

Tooth morphology
- Deep and uncleansable fissures.
- Enamel hypomineralization or hypocalcification (in utero, perinatal and infantile history).
- Have the teeth been fissure sealed?

Radiographic signs
- Are lesions increasing in size?
- How quickly are the lesions progressing?

Other diagnostic tests
- Use of light and laser fluorescence (e.g. QLF and DiagnoDent).
- DIFOTI (Digital Imaging Fiber-Optic Trans-Illumination).
- Electrical impedance.

Saliva
- Is the rate of flow and buffering capacity normal?
- Is there anything that may be affecting the composition of the saliva?

Early childhood caries

One of the causes of early childhood caries or rampant caries in young children is allowing infants and toddlers to sleep with a bottle. The reported prevalence ranges from 2.5% to 15%.

Characteristics of feeding bottle induced early childhood caries

- Rampant caries affecting the maxillary anterior teeth (Figure 3.5).
- Lesions appear later on posterior teeth, both the maxillary and mandibular first primary molars.
- Canines are affected less than first molars because of later eruption.
- Mandibular anterior teeth are unaffected. This is thought to be because of salivary flow and the position of the tongue.
- The bottle is often used as a pacifier to get the infant to sleep.
- Bottle caries occurs in all socioeconomic groups and as such often reflects the social dynamics of the family. Children who are difficult sleepers or have colic are often pacified with a bottle. The bottle can contain any liquid with fermentable carbohydrate, even milk. Commonly, drinks and juices containing vitamin C are used.
- This pattern of caries may also occur with prolonged at-will breastfeeding.

Aetiology of early childhood caries

- Long periods of exposure to cariogenic substrate. If this is from a feeding bottle, the teat is held next to the palatal surfaces of the upper anterior teeth for up to 8 hours. However, other habits such as 'grazing' (snacking on food constantly) also puts many children at risk as does the use of feeding cups and sipper bottles that toddlers walk around with.
- Low salivary flow rate at night, and reduced buffering.
- Parental history of active and untreated caries – particularly in the mother.

Management

- Cessation of habit.
- Dietary advice.
- Possible use of antimicrobial products.
- Fluoride application.
- Build-up of restorable teeth. This may consist of glass ionomer restorations, composite resin-strip crowns and/or stainless steel crowns.
- Extractions if required. Loss of the upper anterior teeth will not result in space loss if the canines have erupted. Speech will develop normally. If posterior teeth have to be extracted, the parents will need to be informed about possible space loss, and an assessment should be carried out to determine if a space maintainer is appropriate.

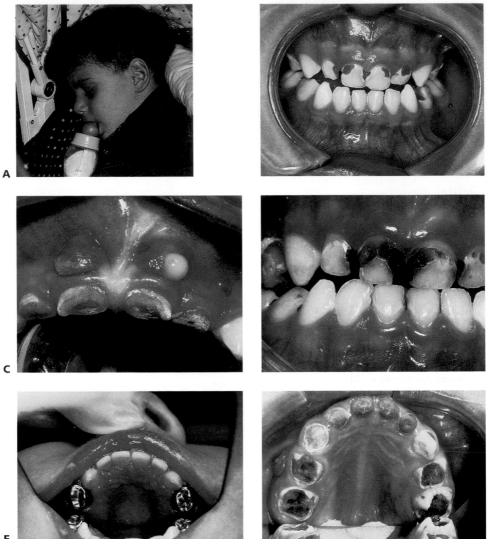

Figure 3.5 Early childhood caries. **A** Parents must be encouraged not to use the bottle as a pacifier. **B** Bottle caries showing the characteristic pattern of decay. The upper anterior teeth and the molars are affected but the lower anterior teeth are spared. **C** These upper anterior teeth are necrotic and require extraction. The abscesses will heal once the teeth are removed. **D** Bottle caries in an older child showing arrested caries. Removal of the cause of caries has allowed the process of demineralization to slow down. **E** Restoration of a case of bottle caries with composite strip crowns and stainless steel crowns on the first primary molars. **F** Gross caries in the primary dentition of a child with a cardiac defect living in a fluoridated community. Every tooth was carious and a full clearance was performed.

It is important to give appropriate advice to the family about early childhood caries. Blame should never be attributed; in many situations the condition has arisen out of ignorance, misinformation, or in frustration of coping with a sleepless infant. Elimination of a bottle habit can be achieved by gradually reducing the amount of sugar in the bottle by diluting with water. This can be done over several weeks. Alternatively, some parents find it easier to remove the bottle immediately.

Treatment under general anaesthesia is often required for small children.

References and further reading

Dental caries
Burt BA 1998 Prevention policies in the light of the changed distribution of dental caries. Acta Odontologica Scandinavica 56:179–186

Cai F, Manton DJ, Shen P et al 2007 Effect of addition of citric acid and casein phosphopeptide-amorphous calcium phosphate to a sugar-free chewing gum on enamel remineralization in situ. Caries Research 41:377–383

Armfield JW 2005 High caries children in Australia: a tail of caries distribution. Australian Dental Journal 50:204–206

Kidd EAM 2004 How 'clean' must a cavity be before restoration? Caries Research 38:305–313

Featherstone JDB 1999 Prevention and reversal of dental caries: role of low level fluoride. Community Dent Oral Epidemiol 27:31–40

Fejerskov O 2004 Changing paradigms in concepts on dental caries: consequences for oral healthcare. Caries Research 38:182–191

Kühnisch J, Dietz W, Stüsser L et al 2007 Effects of dental probing on occlusal surfaces – a scanning electron microscopy evaluation. Caries Research 41:43–48

Law V, Seow WK, Townsend G 2007 Factors influencing oral colonization of mutans streptococci in young children. Australian Dental Journal 52:93–100

Manton DJ, Messer LB 2007 The effect of pit and fissure sealants on the detection of occlusal caries in vitro. European Archives of Paediatric Dentistry 8:43–48

Petersen PE, Bourgeois D, Ogawa H et al 2005 The global burden of oral diseases and risks to oral health. Bulletin of the World Health Organization 83:661–669

Tranæus S, Shi XQ, Angmar-Månsson B 2005 Caries risk assessment: methods available to clinicians for caries detection. Community Dental and Oral Epidemiology 33:265–273

Ter Pelkwijk A, Van Palenstein Helderman WH, Van Dijk JWE 1990 Caries experience in the deciduous dentition as predictor for caries in the permanent dentition. Caries Research 24:65–71

Twetman S 2004 Antimicrobials in future caries control? Caries Research 38:223–229

Van Nieuw Amerongen A, Bolscher JGM, Veerman ECI 2004 Salivary proteins: protective and diagnostic value in cariology? Caries Research 38:247–253

Early childhood caries
Acs G, Shulman R, Ng MW et al 1999 The effect of dental rehabilitation on the body weight of children with early childhood caries. Pediatric Dentistry 21:109–113

Berkowitz RJ 2003 Causes, treatment and prevention of early childhood caries: a microbiologic perspective. Journal of the Canadian Dental Association 69:304–307

Johnston T, Brearley Messer L 1994 Nursing caries: literature review and report of a case managed under local anaesthesia. Australian Dental Journal 39:373–381

Habibian M, Roberts G, Lawson M et al 2001 Dietary habits and dental health over the first 18 months of life. Community Dental and Oral Epidemiology 29:239–246

Hallonsten AL, Wendt LK, Mejare I et al 1995 Dental caries and prolonged breast-feeding in 18-month-old Swedish children. International Journal of Paediatric Dentistry 5:149–155

Lopez L, Berkowitz R, Zlotnik H et al 1999 Topical antimicrobial therapy in the prevention of early childhood caries. Pediatric Dentistry 21:9–11

Marchant S, Brailsford SR, Twomey AC et al 2001 The predominant microflora of nursing caries lesions. Caries Research 35:397–406

Tinnanoff N, O'Sullivan BS 1997 Early childhood caries: overview and recent findings. Pediatric Dentistry 19:12–16

4 Fluoride modalities

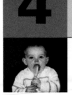

Contributors
Louise Brearley Messer, Kareen Mekertichian

Introduction

Fluoride is used widely to prevent dental caries. The caries reduction that has been achieved by the use of fluoride has been a major public health accomplishment. Community water fluoridation is safe and cost effective, and it should be maintained in communities that have benefited from it and also extended to low-fluoride communities wherever feasible. There is now clear evidence, on a population basis, that caries reduction is most effective when a low concentration of fluoride is maintained consistently in the oral environment. (This is in contrast with earlier concepts of the mechanism of action of fluoride that attributed the major benefit of fluoride to pre-eruptive maturation of forming enamel.) Although any method of using fluoride that helps to maintain this low oral concentration is desirable, community fluoridated water and fluoride toothpaste rank first as public health measures in developed countries.

Fluoride is widespread in nature, occurring in fresh water, sea water, fish, vegetables, milk and organic compounds. Physiologically, fluoride is unique in that it does not behave like the other halogens and has been termed a seeker of mineralized tissues. When present in solution with calcium and phosphate, fluoroapatite will be formed preferentially. It is absorbed into the blood from the gastrointestinal tract and then is deposited in bones or excreted by the kidneys.

New guidelines for use of fluoride modalities

In late 2006, new guidelines for the use of fluoride modalities in Australia were published by the Australian Research Centre for Population Oral Health (ARCPOH). A total of 18 guidelines for the use of fluorides resulted from the deliberations of experts and stakeholders, considering systematic literature reviews and position papers on fluoride modalities at a 2-day consensus conference held in Adelaide, South Australia, in October 2005. The guidelines address the use of community water fluoridation, self-applied fluoride products, professionally applied fluoride products, and the development and monitoring of caries-preventive approaches.

The introduction to the guidelines reiterated that 'fluoride is the cornerstone in the prevention of dental caries', and that all fluoride modalities should be assessed with reference to their potential benefit (i.e. prevention of caries) and risk (i.e. dental fluorosis). At the levels recommended in the guidelines for the use of the various fluoride modalities, no adverse health effect is considered likely.

Mechanisms of action of fluoride

Concepts of how fluoride prevents caries have changed considerably over the past two decades, and as stated above it is now recognized that the predominant effect is topical rather than systemic.

- Fluoride acts for the most part, topically, promoting remineralization and reducing demineralization as a post-eruptive phenomenon. Calcium and phosphate need to be present in solution to effect remineralization.
- Fluoride can prevent mineral loss at crystal surfaces and enhance remineralization with calcium and phosphate ions. Because the mode of action of fluoride is predominantly post-eruptive, the prevention of caries requires lifelong exposure. When remineralization takes place in the presence of fluoride the remineralized enamel is more caries resistant than the original enamel mineral due to increased fluoroapatite and decreased carbonated apatite. This effect is evident with even very low fluoride concentrations (less than 0.1 ppm) across the liquid phase surrounding the enamel matrix.
- Fluoride has an effect on the glycolytic pathway of oral micro-organisms reducing acid production and interfering with the enzymatic regulation of carbohydrate metabolism. This reduces the accumulation of intracellular and extracellular polysaccharides (i.e. plaque).
- The continuous presence of low levels of fluoride at the plaque fluid–enamel interface provides the most effective mode of remineralization of demineralized enamel.
- There has been a general increase in availability of fluoride from foods, beverages, toothpastes and topical agents resulting in a so-called 'halo effect' in low-fluoridated communities, which can benefit from the widespread distribution of these products from fluoridated communities where they have been manufactured.

This topical effect explains the efficacy of fluoridated toothpastes, gels, fluoride rinses and fluoride in drinking water. With concentrated topical fluoride application such as from fluoride varnishes and gels, the formation of calcium fluoride is favoured, persisting in the pores of enamel for extended periods and acting as a fluoride reservoir during remineralization.

Community water fluoridation

The naturally occurring concentration of fluoride in drinking water in Australia is typically in the range of 0.1–0.4 ppm. Fluoride is added to reticulated community water supplies of most large urban populations to achieve a concentration of between 0.8 ppm and 1 ppm.

The ARCPOH guidelines (1–3) strongly support the continuation of community water fluoridation, which remains effective, efficient and socially equitable, and a safe population approach to caries prevention. Community water fluoridation should be extended to as many people as possible.

Caries reduction

The caries reduction of 20–40% now recorded in fluoridated communities is considerably less than was the case when water fluoridation was first introduced into contemporary Western populations because of the general increase in availability of fluoride from other sources.

- There is a reversal of protective benefits after removal of fluoride from water supply.
- Fluoride benefits adults as well as children.
- There is a decreased prevalence of root-surface caries in lifelong inhabitants of areas with fluoridated water.
- Considering the cost effectiveness and widespread community exposure, the preferred source of fluoride is from community water fluoridation.

In Western communities, the continuing existence of approximately 20% of children with a high caries experience indicates the need to maximize protection through the combined use of community water fluoridation and topical fluoride modalities.

Bottled and filtered waters

Bottled waters have shown rapid market growth, and for many individuals water consumption from this source may have fully replaced use of reticulated water. Since the fluoride content of bottled water may be very low (unless supplemented during manufacture), consumers of bottled water in fluoridated communities may be missing out on the benefits of fluoride.

Some water filters may remove fluoride, although this is mostly limited to those filters with reverse osmosis, bone or charcoal filters, distillation or ion exchange. The 'use by' date on these products should not be exceeded. Normal membrane filters will not remove a small ion such as fluoride. Ceramic and carbon filters retain fluoride in the filtered water.

Individuals should have choice in bottled and filtered waters, and manufacturers are encouraged to market bottled waters of 1.0 mg F^-/L (1 ppm F^-) and water filters that do not remove fluoride. Bottled waters and water filters should be labelled to indicate the fluoride content of water consumed or resulting from the use of such products.

The fluoride tablets previously marketed as oral supplements may now be used as water supplements as follows to supplement filtered water to the level of 1 ppm F^-:

- One 2.2 mg NaF tablet containing 1.0 mg F^- dissolved in 1 L of water.
- Two 1.1 mg NaF tablets each containing 0.5 mg F^- dissolved in 1 L of water.
- Four 0.55 mg NaF tablets each containing 0.25 mg F^- dissolved in 1 L of water.

Fluoride tablets dissolve readily in water at room temperature. The fluoridated water should then be refrigerated and used for drinking and food preparation for the entire family.

Home water fluoridation

Approximately 70% of the Australian population benefits from fluoridation of reticulated water. In areas that are non-fluoridated, there should be a choice of home fluoridation. It has been recommended that sodium fluoride tablets should be marketed as a water supplement for addition to non-fluoridated water to achieve 1 mg F⁻/L (1 ppm F⁻).

To achieve this, one 2.2 mg sodium fluoride tablet (contains 1 mg F⁻) or two 1.1 mg sodium fluoride tablets (each contains 0.5 mg F⁻), or four 0.55 mg sodium fluoride tablets (each contains 0.25 mg F⁻), is dissolved in 1 litre of water (dissolves readily at room temperature), and stored in the refrigerator for use in food preparation or drinking for the entire family.

Dental fluorosis (see Chapter 9)

Dental fluorosis is a qualitative defect of enamel (hypomineralization), resulting from an increase in fluoride concentration within the microenvironment of the ameloblasts during enamel formation. In more severe forms, fluorosis may also manifest as a quantitative defect (hypoplasia).

Reports from Australia, the USA and several other developed countries indicate a trend towards increasing levels of mild dental fluorosis. This trend has been apparent in both fluoridated (a 33% increase) and non-fluoridated communities and is caused by the additive effects of the following:

- Fluoride supplements (as tablets or drops).
- Fluoride in the individual's diet (baby foods and beverages produced in fluoridated areas).
- Fluoride toothpastes.
- Topical applications of high-concentration fluoride solutions during enamel formation.

The above levels may be sufficient to induce cosmetically noticeable fluorosis, even in areas without the fluoridation of community water supplies (Figure 4.1). Following a reduction in the use of fluoride supplements and the introduction of children's strength toothpaste in the past decade in Australia, there has been a marked reduction in mild fluorosis in children and adolescents.

Threshold dose
Unknown, but suggested to be around 0.1 mg/kg body weight.

Manifestations
The clinical appearance of enamel fluorosis can vary greatly, depending on severity:

- Questionable to very mild – loss of translucency of enamel at the incisal margin and proximal margins of the labial surface (snow capping).
- Very mild – white flecks.
- Mild – fine white lines or striations following the striae of Retzius.
- Moderate – very chalky, opaque enamel which fractures soon after tooth eruption.
- Severe – mottling and pitting with loss of portions of the outer layers of enamel, post-eruptive staining of the enamel.

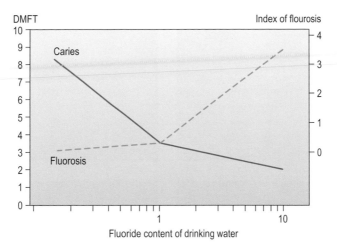

Figure 4.1 A comparison of decayed, missing and filled permanent teeth (DMFT) with Dean's index of fluorosis in relation to fluoride content of drinking water.

There are several ways of ranking the severity of fluorosis. Although attempts have been made to classify the severity according to the histopathology and to the degree of fluoride exposure, the appearance of the tooth will change over time. Indeed, in moderate to severe cases in which the entire surface of the tooth is opaque at the time of eruption, with time this layer will be abraded and pits will form with staining, and the tooth appearance will change remarkably. As the fluoride content of water increases beyond 1 ppm (Figure 4.1) the increase in severity of fluorosis is greater than the corresponding decrease in caries (Figure 4.2).

Actions of high-dose fluoride on enamel formation

Dental fluorosis primarily affects permanent teeth and is a dose-related condition. Diagnosis of dental fluorosis requires a detailed history of fluoride exposure. Fluoride has several detrimental actions on enamel formation including:

- Alteration of the production or composition of enamel matrix during ameloblastic secretory phase.
- Interference in the initial mineralization process caused by changes in ion-transport mechanisms.
- Disruption of ameloblast function affecting the withdrawal of protein and water from initial mineralization of enamel during the maturation phase.
- Disruption of nucleation and crystal growth in all stages of enamel formation, resulting in various degrees of enamel porosity (hypomineralization).

Enamel mineralization appears uniquely sensitive to fluoride, and high doses of fluoride can affect breakdown and withdrawal of enamel matrix proteins (e.g. enamelins,

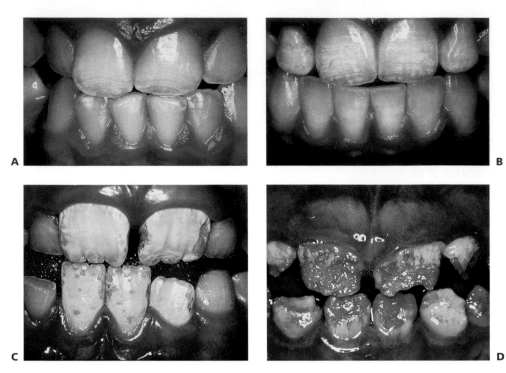

Figure 4.2 The clinical range of fluorosis. **A** Very mild fluorosis with opacities following the outline of the perikymata. **B** Mild fluorosis with white flecking through the crowns of the incisors. Note that the lower incisors are only minimally affected. **C** Moderate opacity affecting the whole crown. Note that the pits and brown mottling is secondary to tooth-surface wear and the acquisition of stains. **D** Severe fluorosis and mottling of the enamel.

amelogenins), resulting in permanent hypomineralization of enamel (subsurface and surface porosity). High doses of fluoride also seem to affect the activity of the ameloblasts. Consequently, excessive fluoride intake is of particular concern, especially during the first 36 months of life when crowns of the maxillary permanent incisors are undergoing mineralization or enamel maturation.

Toothpaste ingestion has been identified as a significant source of excess fluoride in young children. In National Health and Medical Research Council reviews, toothpastes account for a large proportion of ingested fluoride in young children, irrespective of the level of fluoride in the reticulated water system. Another source of excess fluoride is infant formula. However, marked variations exist in the concentration of fluoride in infant formulas before reconstitution with water: a range of 0.9–2.8 ppm.

Clinical management of dental fluorosis
Clinically, dental fluorosis can be managed by remineralization, microabrasion or restorative replacement of the affected discoloured enamel. Still in the experimental stages, mildly fluorosed enamel can be remineralized by casein phosphopeptide-

amorphous calcium phosphate (CPP-ACP) or casein phosphopeptide-amorphous calcium phosphate fluoride (CPP-ACPF), which clinically reduces the whiteness (opacity) and promotes remineralization of mild fluorotic lesions, resulting in improved aesthetics. The effect is enhanced by pretreatment with sodium hypochlorite as a deproteinizing agent.

The defective surface enamel of fluorotic lesions can be judiciously removed with microabrasion (using commercially available kits, or dilute hydrochloric acid or 35% phosphoric acid and pumice paste) followed by remineralization with topical fluoride, CPP-ACP or CPP-ACPF. More extensive lesions can be restored with labial veneers of composite resin or porcelain once the tooth is fully erupted and the height of the marginal gingivae is established.

Topical fluorides

Lifetime protection against dental caries results from the continuous use of low-concentration fluoride. In addition to the role of topical fluorides in caries prevention, they may be used to enhance the remineralization of white spot lesions, control initial invasive carious lesions and limit lesions occurring around existing restorations. This is effective for both adults and children.

An optimal concentration of fluoride is required each day which, if present at both the tooth surface and in saliva, will help minimize caries risk. Factors that should be considered before committing to a fluoride regimen include:

- Caries risk – high, medium, low.
- Cariogenicity of the diet/oral clearance rate.
- Patient age and compliance.
- Use of systemic and topical fluoride modalities.
- Community water fluoridation levels.
- Existing medical conditions.

Fluoridated toothpastes
Fluoridated toothpastes provide the most feasible way of maintaining elevated fluoride concentrations at the plaque–enamel interface. Fluoride is added to toothpastes as sodium fluoride, sodium monofluorophosphate (MFP), stannous or amine fluoride.

The use of fluoridated toothpastes has led to a 25% reduction in the prevalence of caries in developed countries, with the greatest benefit being observed on interproximal and smooth surfaces as well as newly erupted teeth.

Children's toothpastes
Low concentration fluoridated toothpastes containing 250 ppm, 400 ppm, 500 ppm F$^-$ are available for children. Recent meta-analyses have reported that 250 ppm F$^-$ toothpaste is less effective in caries prevention than the standard 1000 ppm F$^-$ toothpastes.

As up to 30% of the fluoridated toothpaste delivered on a child's toothbrush can be swallowed, parents are advised to:

- Use a pea-sized amount of toothpaste, smeared across (rather than along) the brush head.
- Brush and floss for the child until they can capably do these procedures for themselves.

- Supervise all 'play brushing'.
- Use a low-fluoride children's toothpaste in optimally fluoridated areas.

Recent studies and meta-analyses on the use of fluoridated toothpastes by children have shown the value of good oral hygiene habits:

- Tooth brushing twice per day in children younger than 2 years significantly reduced caries.
- This benefit increased with higher frequency of use and with supervised brushing.
- The action of 'swishing and pumping' a fluoride toothpaste between the teeth significantly reduced caries in preschool aged children.
- Commencing tooth cleaning before one year of age was associated with reduced caries prevalence compared with delayed tooth cleaning.
- Starting fluoridated toothpaste at younger ages may be more important for children not receiving the benefit of water fluoridation.
- The risk of fluorosis increased for children using fluoridated toothpaste before 30 months of age in a fluoridated community.

The ARCPOH guidelines (7, 8) state that from the time teeth first erupt (about 6 months of age) to the age of 17 months, children's teeth should be cleaned by a responsible adult, but toothpaste should not be used. For children aged 18 months to 5 years (inclusive), teeth should be cleaned twice a day with toothpaste containing 0.4–0.5 mg F^-/g (400–500 ppm F^-). Toothpaste should always be used under supervision of a responsible adult, a pea-sized amount should be applied to a child-sized soft tooth brush and children should spit out, not swallow, and not rinse.

The ARCPOH Guidelines (9,10) state that for individuals aged 6 years or more, the teeth should be cleaned twice a day or more frequently with standard fluoridated toothpaste (1 mg F^-/g, 1000 ppm F^-). They should spit out, not swallow, and not rinse. For children who do not consume fluoridated water or who are at higher risk of developing caries for any other reason, guidelines about toothpaste should be varied, as needed, based on professional advice. Variations could include more frequent use of a fluoridated toothpaste, commencing fluoridated toothpaste at a younger age, or earlier commencement of use of a standard toothpaste (1 mg F^-/g).

Standard fluoridated toothpastes

Fluoridated toothpastes are very effective in caries prevention and a successful population strategy. Clinical trials have shown that the absolute level of caries protection with fluoride toothpastes is less than a lifetime exposure to community water fluoridation, but the preventive effects are additive to those of fluoridated water.

Standard fluoride toothpastes contain 1000–1100 ppm F^- (1–1.1 mg F^-/g paste).

High-concentration fluoridated toothpastes

Also known as treatment toothpastes, high-concentration fluoridated toothpastes represent one-step topical fluoride treatment in conjunction with fluoridated toothpaste. High concentration fluoridated toothpastes contain 1500–5000 ppm F^- (1.5–5.0 mg F^-/g paste).

The ARCPOH guideline (11) states that for teenagers, adults and older adults who are at higher risk of developing caries, dental professional advice should be sought to determine if they should use toothpaste containing a higher fluoride concentration (>1 mg F^-/g).

Fluoride mouth rinses

Supervised fluoridated-rinse programmes can reduce caries by 20–50%. Weekly 0.2% sodium fluoride and daily 0.05% sodium fluoride rinses are considered to be ideal public health measures. The use of such rinses is now recommended, principally for individuals with high caries risk or during times of increased caries susceptibility.

The ARCPOH guidelines (13, 14) state that fluoridated home rinses should not be used for children under 6 years of age, but may be used for people aged 6 years or more who have a higher risk of developing caries. A fluoridated mouth rinse should not substitute for tooth brushing with fluoridated toothpaste if feasible and should be used at a time of day when fluoride toothpaste is not used. A fluoridated mouth rinse should be spat out and not swallowed.

Daily rinses

- 0.05% w/v neutral sodium fluoride (220–227 ppm F^-).
- Partly acidulated solution of sodium fluoride, phosphoric acid and sodium phosphate monobasic (200 ppm F^-).

Weekly or fortnightly rinses

- 0.2% w/v neutral sodium fluoride (900–910 ppm F^-).

Indications

- Children undergoing orthodontic treatment.
- Children with post-irradiation hyposalivation.
- Children unable to perform adequate tooth brushing.
- Children at high risk of dental caries.

Contraindications

Fluoride mouth rinses are not recommended for children before the eruption of the permanent incisors.

Fluoridated varnishes

Fluoridated varnishes were originally developed to prolong contact times between fluoride and enamel with a view to increasing the formation of fluorapatite. Fluoridated varnishes bind fluoride to enamel for longer periods than other topical fluoride preparations. However, the reduction of caries has been of the same order (approximately 30%).

Fluoridated varnishes are effective in both primary and permanent dentitions. No fluorosis has been seen following twice-yearly applications. The slow release of fluoride from the resin vehicle results in lower peak plasma fluoride levels than from swallowed fluoridated gels.

Indications

- Hypersensitive areas.
- Newly erupted teeth.
- Local remineralization of white spot lesions.
- Individuals at high caries risk.
- Individuals in high caries risk groups.

Duraphat (Colgate Oral Care) is an alcoholic solution of natural varnishes containing 50 mg NaF/mL (5% NaF, 2.26% F⁻, 22 6000 ppm F⁻, 22.6 mg F⁻/mL)). This varnish resin remains on the teeth for up to 12–48 hours after application, slowly releasing fluoride from the wax-like film.

Fluor Protector (Ivoclar Vivadent) is a silane fluoride varnish with a lower concentration of fluoride (0.8%) in a polyurethane lacquer.

Application of fluoride varnish

Prophylaxis of the teeth is not required routinely before topical fluoride application, however, gross plaque and stains should be removed. Fluoride uptake is not reduced by surface plaque and caries reduction can be achieved without cleaning the teeth before fluoride application. In fact, plaque can serve as a recycling reservoir for fluoride and allow access to enamel – unfortunately the plaque is also the source of the organic acids leading to demineralization. Drying of the teeth before application facilitates adhesion and may also be beneficial for fluoride uptake.

With such highly concentrated fluoridated products, great care must be taken to avoid ingestion and overdose swallowing. The manufacturer of Duraphat (Colgate Oral Care) recommends application of the following amounts of varnish which should not be exceeded:

- Primary dentition: 0.25 mL (6 mg F⁻).
- Mixed dentition: 0.40 mL (9 mg F⁻).
- Permanent dentition: 0.75 mL (17 mg F⁻).

The ARCPOH guideline (15) states that fluoridated varnish should be used for people with higher risk of developing caries, including children under age 10 years, in situations where other professionally applied fluoridated vehicles are unavailable or impractical.

Concentrated fluoridated gels, foams, solutions and cremes

Concentrated fluoridated gels are marketed as caries-preventive gels and treatment gels. There is recent clinical evidence that concentrated fluoridated gels are more effective in the permanent dentition than the primary dentition, benefiting particularly the first permanent molars. Variable dosage during application, followed by inadvertent swallowing, can result in ingestion of large amounts of fluoride, which may contribute to mild fluorosis of mineralizing permanent teeth.

High concentration fluoridated gels (e.g. 9000–12 300 ppm F⁻) should be limited to professional use in the dental practice and not dispensed for home use. Lower concentration gels (e.g. 1000 ppm F⁻) can be used at home following careful professional instruction and demonstration of proper product use.

The ARCPOH guideline (16) states that high concentration fluoride gels and foams (>1.5 mg/g F⁻, 1500 ppm F⁻) may be used for people aged 10 years or more who are at a higher risk of developing caries in situations where other fluoride vehicles may be unavailable or impractical.

Acidulated phosphate fluoride gels

Acidulated phosphate fluoride (APF) gels, containing 12 300 ppm F⁻ (1.23% APF, 1.23% w/v F⁻) are used for professional applications and consist of a mixture of sodium fluoride, hydrofluoric acid and orthophosphoric acid. Gels containing 5000 ppm F⁻ are also limited to professional use and contain sodium fluoride, phosphoric acid and sodium phosphate monobasic.

- Such highly concentrated fluoridated gels should be limited to professional use and should not be dispensed for home use in children.
- The incorporation of a water-soluble polymer (sodium carboxymethyl cellulose) into aqueous APF produces a viscous solution that improves the ease of application using custom-made trays.
- Thixotropic gels in trays flow under pressure, facilitating gel penetration between teeth.
- APF gels are used primarily for the prevention of caries development.

Neutral sodium fluoride gels

A neutral pH gel (e.g. 2% w/v neutral NaF gel, 9000 ppm F^-) can be used for cases of enamel erosion, exposed dentine, carious dentine or where very porous enamel surfaces (such as hypomineralization) exist.

- Sodium fluoride is chemically very stable, has an acceptable taste and is non-irritating to the gingivae. It does not discolour teeth, composite resin or porcelain restorations, in contrast to APF or stannous fluoride, which may cause discoloration.
- A neutral pH fluoridated gel or solution is preferred where restorations of glass ionomer cement, composite resin or porcelain are present as acidic preparations may etch these restorations.

Stannous fluoride gel

A stannous fluoride (SnF_2) treatment gel in a methylcellulose and glycerine carrier (marketed as Gel Kam by Colgate Oral Care) can be used for remineralization of white spot and hypomineralization lesions of enamel (e.g. molar or incisor hypomineralization). Anecdotal clinical reports support the efficacy of this product, for example, where localized remineralization is desirable prior to placement of definitive restorations. The 0.4% stannous fluoride gel has also proved effective in arresting root caries and has been incorporated into a synthetic saliva solution to reduce caries in post-irradiation cancer patients.

- Contains 1000 ppm F^- and 3000 ppm Sn^{2+}.
- A very small amount is placed on a cotton bud and applied to dried tooth surfaces by adult patient or for a child by the parent at home.
- In applying to children's teeth, the parent must be fully compliant in following professional instructions.

Stannous fluoride solution

- 10% stannous fluoride may be used to target local 'at-risk' surfaces of teeth such as deep fissures and pits or white spot lesions on accessible proximal surfaces.
- Rapid penetration of tin and fluoride into enamel and the formation of a highly insoluble tin–fluorophosphate complex coating on the enamel are the main mechanisms of its action. The stannous ion may cause discoloration of teeth and staining on margins of restorations, particularly in hypocalcified areas.

Casein phosphopeptide-amorphous calcium phosphate crèmes

CPP-ACP and CPP-ACPF are available as crèmes for topical application at home (Tooth Mousse; Tooth Mousse Plus, GC Corp, Japan). Applied to surfaces at risk for caries or erosion or with white spot lesions, CPP-ACPF releases fluoride, calcium and phosphate ions for local remineralization of enamel.

- Contains 900 ppm F⁻ (Tooth Mousse Plus).
- Fluoridated product for use by people over age 6 years.
- Applied to teeth after brushing and flossing by smearing across tooth surfaces with a clean finger or cotton-tipped applicator. The crème is not rinsed out.
- Should not be used by people with a milk protein allergy.

Systemic fluorides

Evidence from studies in several countries over the past two decades has indicated the following with reference to the use of fluoride supplements (as drops or tablets):

- Fluoride supplements have limited application as a public health measure but may be of benefit to individuals with a high risk of caries.
- Fluoride supplements are beneficial in reducing dental caries only among children in non-fluoridated communities, but this benefit is small.
- There are limited clinical data demonstrating the caries preventive effects of prenatal fluoride supplements.
- Overzealous use of supplements has been associated with dental fluorosis.
- The period between 2 and 3 years is when the permanent incisor teeth are most susceptible to fluorosis.

In view of the dubious efficacy of fluoride supplements in caries prevention, the risk of fluorosis and the variability in compliance, it is recommended that fluoride supplements in the form of drops or tablets to be chewed and/or swallowed, should not be used. Previously published dose schedules are therefore no longer followed in Australia.

The fluoride tablets previously marketed as oral supplements may now be used as water supplements (see section on 'Bottled and filtered waters' above).

Considerations in fluoride therapy for infants and children

There is increasing recognition that young children may acquire fluoride from a wide variety of dietary sources, toothpastes, supplements and topical fluoride applications. This can result in mild or very mild dental fluorosis. There is evidence to show that mild fluorosis will occur with ingestion of 2 mg or more of fluoride per day.

Minimizing risk

- Parents should supervise tooth brushing closely, performing tooth brushing and flossing themselves for children up to about 8 years of age and should supervise these children in 'play' brushing.

- Because clinical studies indicate that infants and children under 6 years of age ingest approximately 30% of toothpastes used, only use a 'pea-size' amount of toothpaste (smeared across the head of a child's toothbrush).
- Toothpaste should not be swallowed.
- Parents should use low-fluoride toothpastes (400 ppm or 500 ppm fluoride) for infants and young children (before the eruption of the permanent central incisors) living in optimally fluoridated areas.
- Application of the new guidelines is likely to result in greater professional use of fluoridated varnishes, and reduced use of fluoridated gels, for children aged under 10 years.

With these points in mind, given that all other sources are constant and low, the total fluoride intake should not exceed the recommended upper limit of 0.07 mg F⁻/kg of body weight for a child between 2 and 7 years of age.

Recommended schedules for topical fluoridation

Despite the changing caries distribution in developed nations over the past 20 years and a tendency to target solely preventive strategies on high-risk populations, the baseline frequency of twice-daily tooth brushing with a fluoridated toothpaste beginning before 2 years of age remains the cornerstone of preventive advice for the whole population. Review of epidemiological data for Australia and overseas indicates that the twice-daily use of a toothpaste containing fluoride will prevent new caries development in approximately 80% of children, and an estimated 60–70% of adults.

Implementation of appropriate preventive therapies should be in accordance with an assessment of caries risk. As the aetiological factors leading to the development of caries are multifactorial, risk assessment should involve all likely key factors. Such assessment is a dynamic and evolving art, which will continue to improve with the advent of emerging sciences and technologies. However, social, behavioural, microbiological, environmental and clinical factors still remain essential in the determination of the likelihood of caries risk during specific time periods. The Caries-risk Assessment Tool (CAT) as proposed by the American Association of Pediatric Dentistry provides an appropriate set of physical, environmental and general health related factors in such evaluation.

Low risk
- No new carious lesions within 12 months.
- Twice-daily use of an appropriate strength toothpaste containing fluoride.
- Spot application of topical fluoride to newly erupting permanent posterior teeth.

Increased risk
Use of low-level fluoride supplementation in cases of:
- Adolescent patients without access to fluoridated water.
- Patients temporarily at higher risk of caries (i.e. orthodontic patients before and during treatment, children undergoing chemo or radiotherapy).

Schedule
- 0.02% NaF or APF daily mouthrinse.
- Spot application of topical fluoride to newly erupting permanent posterior teeth.

Moderate caries rate
- One to two new lesions per year and/or development of cervical white spot lesions.

Schedule
- 0.05% neutral NaF mouthrinse daily or 0.2% neutral NaF mouthrinse weekly.
- Spot application of fluoride varnish to susceptible areas *and* professional 1.23% APF topical applications every 3 months or professional 10% SnF$_2$ topical applications every 3 months.

High caries rate
- More than two new lesions per year.

Schedule
- Initial use of 0.2% neutral NaF mouthrinse daily *and* professional 1.23% APF topical applications every 3 months or professional 10% SnF$_2$ topical applications every 3 months.
- Spot application of fluoride varnish to susceptible areas.
  All fluoride regimens should be seen in the context of salivary quality and quantity, as fluoride is not completely effective in the absence of calcium and phosphate ions. If it is believed that there is insufficient saliva or that the caries risk is great enough to overwhelm the salivary capability, supplementary bioavailable calcium and phosphate should be provided.

Fluoride toxicity

Overwhelming evidence exists for the safety of fluorides at low concentration but high concentrations increase the possibility of toxic overdose. The first signs of chronic fluoride overdose are enamel mottling. Crippling bone fluorosis and acute toxicity occur at much higher doses. Reviews of fluoride benefits and risks by the US Public Health Service, based on more than 50 human studies, concluded that no evidence exists to show an association between fluoride intake and cancer.

Estimated probable toxic dose
- 5 mg F$^-$/kg of body weight.
- Gastrointestinal symptoms have been noted following ingestion of 3–5 mg F$^-$/kg by young children and very frail adults.
- For a 10 kg child this corresponds to all the contents of a 45 g tube of toothpaste. Therefore, young children should not be allowed unsupervised access to fluoride toothpastes or fluoride supplements.

Probable toxic dose
- 32–60 mg F⁻/kg of body weight.
- Fatalities in children have been reported at doses of 16 mg F⁻/kg of body weight. A number of concentrated topical preparations could provide such levels for young children if used in a single dose.

The inappropriate prescription of home-fluoride treatments with high concentration fluoridated gels for very young children (for example, in the management of early childhood caries), is of concern. Concentrated fluoride products in excess of 1000 ppm F⁻ should not be prescribed for home use.

Acute poisoning
- Cellular metabolism blocked.
- Inhibition of enolase in the glycolytic pathway.
- Interference with calcium metabolism.
- Nerve-impulse and conduction disorders.

Signs and symptoms
- The clinical course in acute fluoride toxicity develops with alarming rapidity.
- Generalized signs and symptoms include:
  - nausea and epigastric distress, often accompanied by vomiting
  - excessive salivation, tear production, mucous discharges from the nose and mouth, and sweating
  - headache
  - diarrhoea
  - generalized weakness.

Potentially lethal doses
- Myopathological signs including spasm of the extremities, tetany and convulsions.
- Progressive failure of the cardiovascular system with a barely detectable pulse, hypotension and cardiac arrhythmias.
- Disturbances in electrolyte balance, particularly hypocalcaemia and hyperkalaemia.
- As respiration is depressed an accompanying respiratory acidosis progressively develops.
- Patient may become extremely disoriented before lapsing into unconsciousness.

Management
The management of acute fluoride toxicity consists of:
- Estimating the amount of fluoride ingested.
- Minimizing further absorption.
- Removing fluoride from the body fluids.
- Supporting the vital signs.
  If vomiting has not occurred spontaneously:
- Give as much milk as can be ingested, or
- Administer orally 5% calcium gluconate or calcium lactate or milk of magnesia.

While this immediate action is being taken, the hospital should be advised that a case of acute fluoride poisoning is in progress so that preparation for appropriate therapeutic intervention can be made.

Note that while previous protocols advocated the use of an emetic such as syrup of Ipecac, there has been a move away from encouraging vomiting because of the risk of aspiration of vomitus and the risk of burning the oesophagus by the hydrofluoric acid formed in the stomach (by the interaction of fluoride with hydrochloric acid). Modern emergency department protocols advocate the use of activated charcoal or gastric lavage in most poisonings.

Management by dosage
<5 mg/kg
- Give calcium orally (milk) and observe for up to 4 hours.

5–15 mg/kg
- Admit to hospital, support vital signs and observe.
- Empty stomach by gastric lavage.
- Give calcium orally (milk, 5% calcium gluconate, calcium lactate).

>15 mg/kg
- Admit to hospital immediately.
- Administer activated charcoal and begin gastric lavage.
- Cardiac monitoring and life support.
- Intravenous calcium gluconate.

Calculation of fluoride ingestion (see Table 4.1)
- A 1000 ppm toothpaste contains 1 mg F$^-$/g toothpaste.
- A 400 ppm toothpaste contains 0.4 mg F$^-$/g toothpaste.

Example
- A 2-year-old child weighing 10 kg swallows one tube of toothpaste (i.e. 90 g of a 0.76% MFP toothpaste).
- Amount of fluoride in ingested: 1 mg/g × 90 g toothpaste = 90 mg.

Table 4.1 Amount of toothpaste ingested to receive a probable toxic fluoride dose*

Age of child	Average weight	Probable toxic dose F$^-$	Amount of 1000 ppm toothpaste (90 g tube = 90 mg F$^-$)		Amount of 400 ppm toothpaste (45 g tube = 18 mg F$^-$)	
			Weight	Tube	Weight	Tubes
2 years	12 kg	60 mg	60 g	66%	150 g	3
4 years	15 kg	75 mg	75 g	85%	188 g	4
6 years	20 kg	100 mg	100 g	Over 1 tube	250 g	5½

*Probable toxic dose: 5 mg F$^-$/kg.

- Weight of child = 10 kg.
- Fluoride dosage ingested 90 mg/10 kg = 9 mg F$^-$/kg body weight.
- Treatment must be commenced as described above.

It is often difficult to determine the exact amount of toothpaste that has been swallowed and it would be prudent for any suspected overdose to be taken seriously and immediate specialist medical advice should be sought. Most children's hospitals have a poisons information service.

Refer to Appendix P for sample calculations of fluoride values for dental products.

References and further reading

Adair SM 2006 Evidence-based use of fluoride in contemporary pediatric dental practice. Pediatric Dentistry 28:133–142

American Dental Association Council on Scientific Affairs 2006 Professionally applied topical fluoride: evidence-based clinical recommendations. Journal of the American Dental Association 137:1151–1159

Aoba T, Fejerskov O 2002 Dental fluorosis: chemistry and biology. Critical Reviews in Oral Biology and Medicine 13:155–170

Australian Research Centre for Population Oral Health 2006 The use of fluorides in Australia: guidelines. Australian Dental Journal 51:195–199

Burt BA, Keels MA, Heller KE 2000 The effects of a break in water fluoridation on the development of dental caries and fluorosis. Journal of Dental Research 79:761–769

Den Besten PK 1999 Biological mechanisms of dental fluorosis relevant to the use of fluoride supplements. Community Dentistry and Oral Epidemiology 27:41–47

Franzman MR, Levy SM, Warren JJ et al 2006 Fluoride dentifrice ingestion and fluorosis of the permanent incisors. Journal of the American Dental Association 137:645–652

Ismail AI, Bandekar RR 1999 Fluoride supplements and fluorosis: a meta-analysis. Community Dentistry and Oral Epidemiology 27:48–56

Reynolds EC 1997 Remineralisation of enamel subsurface lesions by casein-phosphopeptide-stabilised calcium phosphate solution. Journal of Dental Research 76:1587–1595

Warren JJ, LevY SM 1999 A review of fluoride dentifrice related to dental fluorosis. Pediatric Dentistry 21:265–271

Young A, Thrane PS, Saxegaard E et al 2006 Effect of stannous fluoride toothpaste on erosion-like lesions: an in vivo study. European Journal of Oral Sciences 114:180–183

Useful websites

Journal of the American Dental Association: http://jada.ada.org

US Food and Drug Administration. Health claim notification for fluoridated water and reduced risk of dental caries: www.cfsan.fda.gov/~dms/flfluoro.html

Fdiworlddental.org: www.fdiworlddental.org/public_health/3_7fluoride.html

Australian Dental Association. Your Oral Health. Water Fluoridation in Australia – the official position: www.ada.org.au/oralhealth/flinaust.aspx

(All websites accessed in October 2007.)

5 Restorative paediatric dentistry

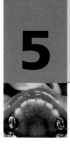

Contributors
Erin Mahoney, Nicky Kilpatrick, Timothy Johnston

Primary teeth

Why restore primary teeth?
Our child patients deserve the best dental treatment that clinicians can provide as any treatment – preventive or restorative – will shape their dental future. The objective of any restorative treatment is to:

- Repair or limit the damage of dental caries.
- Protect and preserve remaining the pulp and remaining tooth structure.
- Ensure adequate function.
- Restore aesthetics (where applicable).
- Provide ease in maintaining good oral hygiene.

In addition restoring primary teeth ensures that the natural spaces in the child's primary dentition are retained for the developing permanent dentition.

Choice of materials
The choice of material to use in a given situation is not always simple and should not be based merely on technical considerations. Factors other than durability may be equally important in the choice of material, particularly in children.

Age
The age of a child will influence their ability to cooperate with procedures such as rubber dam application and local anaesthesia. The age of the child will also dictate for how long a restoration is required to remain satisfactory. A restoration in a first primary molar in a 9-year-old child does not require the same durability as a restoration in a first permanent molar in a 6-year-old child or a second primary molar in a 4-year-old child.

Caries risk
Restorations in a child considered to be at high risk of caries may need to fulfil different objectives from restorations in a low-risk child. Although the use of a fluoride-releasing material has obvious preventive advantages, glass ionomer cements (GICs) may not be the most appropriate choice in a mouth that is at high risk of further acid attack. Stainless steel crowns may involve a significant amount of tooth destruction, but this will be appropriate if it eliminates the need to re-treat in the future. Alternatively, GICs have a useful role in initial caries control in cases of rampant caries.

71

Cooperation of the child

Many young children have behaviour that is not conducive to perfect, textbook, cavity preparation and restoration. In these cases highly technique-sensitive procedures are inappropriate. A more forgiving restoration such as an amalgam that can tolerate a certain amount of moisture contamination, without detriment to its longevity, may be suitable. The use of GICs in the management of caries in anterior primary teeth may be an excellent method of slowing the carious process and temporarily restoring aesthetics in a 2-year-old child, without recourse to general anaesthesia. By the age of 3 or 4 years, the child may be able to cope with more definitive treatment with composite resin and strip crowns.

Restorative situation

Unfortunately not all children are able to cooperate with respect to dental treatment under local anaesthesia. This may be because of their age or due to physical or intellectual disabilities necessitating the completion of treatment under sedation or general anaesthesia. When treatment is provided this way, the highest standard of dentistry possible should be provided to reduce future dental treatment for these high-need children. Use of materials and techniques that are known to have longevity, such as stainless steel crowns, is mandatory.

Restorative materials

Owing to the variety of restorative materials available today, many appropriate materials can be used to restore carious lesions in the primary dentition. Given the large number of techniques and products available on the market, and the unavoidable experimentation that clinicians undertake, the mixing and matching of materials is common place. When replacing any lost dental tissue, whatever the procedure favoured, it is important for clinicians to understand exactly the nature of the system they are using and to be aware that all systems are operator and technique sensitive.

Table 5.1 summarizes the main advantages and disadvantages of the various dental restorative materials.

Amalgam

Historically, owing to the simplicity of its use dental amalgam is the most popular restorative material. Amalgam possesses excellent physical properties and its use in primary molars has resulted in highly successful long-term restorations. However, there are many disadvantages to the use of amalgam. Amalgam is not adhesive and therefore cavity design needs to include some form of mechanical retention resulting in larger restorations which are inevitably closer to the pulp. Possibly the biggest problem associated with its use is the recent upsurge in public opinion concerning its safety. In many countries the use of amalgam in children's teeth has been restricted. The rationale for these restrictions is based on environmental concerns rather than concerns over amalgam toxicity. Nevertheless, the dental profession may be forced to use alternatives to amalgam by a combination of public opinion and legislation.

Table 5.1 Advantages and disadvantages of restorative materials used in paediatric dentistry

	Advantages	Disadvantages
Amalgam	Simple Quick Cheap Technique insensitive Durable	Not adhesive Requires mechanical retention in cavity Environmental and occupational hazards Public concerns
Composite	Adhesive Aesthetic Reasonable wear properties Command set	Technique sensitive Rubber dam required Expensive
Glass ionomer cement (packable)	Adhesive Aesthetic Fluoride leaching	Brittle Susceptible to erosion and wear
Resin-modified glass ionomer	Adhesive Aesthetic Command set Simple to handle Fluoride release	Water absorption Significant wear
High-viscosity glass ionomer	Adhesive Aesthetic Simple to handle Fluoride release High compressive strength and wear resistance	Water absorption Colour not as good a match as composite resins, compomers and other GICs Poorer mechanical properties than compomer and composites
Polyacid-modified composite resin	Adhesive Aesthetic Command set Simple to handle Radiopaque	Technique sensitive Less fluoride release than GICs
Stainless steel crowns	Durable Protect and support remaining tooth structure	Extensive tooth preparation Patient cooperation required Unaesthetic

Glass ionomers

One of the most significant advances in contemporary paediatric dental practice has been the development of GICs. A glass ionomer consists of a basic glass and an acidic water-soluble powder that sets by acid–base reaction between the two components. A principal benefit of GIC is that it will adhere to dental hard tissues. A number of GICs are available on the market today, each having its advantages and disadvantages.

Conventional GICs

Conventional GICs are chemical-set glass ionomers with the weakest mechanical properties. The setting reaction is complete within minutes but continues to 'mature' over the following months. It is important to protect these materials from salivary contamination in the hours following placement or the material may shrink, crack and even debond.

Adhesion of all GICs is enhanced by the use of enamel and dentine conditioning agents before placement.

Resin-modified glass ionomers

Resin-modified glass ionomers were developed to overcome the problems of moisture sensitivity and low initial mechanical strength. They consist of a GIC along with a water-based resin system which allows curing with light before the acid–base reaction of the glass ionomer takes place. This reaction then occurs within the light polymerized resin framework. The resin increases the fracture strength and wear resistance of the GIC.

Another type of resin-modified glass ionomer is a 'tri-cured' material. It has three setting reactions:

1. The acid–base reaction between glass and polyacid.
2. A light-activated, free-radical polymerization of methacrylate groups of the polymer.
3. A dark-cure, free-radical polymerization of methacrylate groups.

The potential advantage of this material is that it will continue to cure in the depth of the cavity after the light source has been removed. Only one proprietary example of this type of GIC is currently available.

High-viscosity GIC

High-viscosity GICs were developed for the atraumatic restorative technique (ART). These chemically cured GICs have significantly better mechanical properties than the other materials. They do not command set as with the resin-modified glass ionomers, but they are fast setting. Although no GIC yet has the ideal physical properties of a restorative material, the high-viscosity GIC have the best physical properties and there-fore should be used in posterior primary teeth when a GIC is contemplated.

Composite resins

Resin-based composites (along with photopolymerization) have revolutionized clinical dentistry, although problems related to wear resistance, water absorption and polym-erization contraction can limit their use in larger restorations in the posterior per-manent dentition. In the primary dentition, composite resins are being increasingly used in combination with GICs in a 'sandwich'-style aesthetic restoration. Placement of these materials is highly technique sensitive, and patient compliance and adequate moisture isolation can prove difficult in the younger, more challenging child patient.

Compomers (polyacid-modified composite resin)

Polyacid-modified resin composite resins or compomers are materials that contain a calcium aluminium fluorosilicate glass filler and polyacid components. They contain either or both essential components of a GIC. However, they are not water-based and therefore no acid–base reaction can occur. As such, they cannot strictly be described as glass ionomers. They set by resin photopolymerization. The acid–base reaction does occur in the moist intra-oral environment and allows fluoride release from the material. Successful adhesion requires the use of dentine-bonding primers before placement.

Stainless steel crowns

Stainless steel crowns are preformed extra-coronal restorations that are particularly useful in the restoration of grossly broken down teeth, primary molars that have undergone pulp therapy, and hypoplastic primary or permanent teeth. They are also indicated when restoring the dentition of children at high risk of caries, particularly those having treatment under general anaesthesia. Stainless steel crowns are a very durable restoration and should be the technique of choice in the high-caries mouth.

Recently stainless steel crowns have been shown to provide such a good seal to external cariogenic stimuli that researchers in the UK have attempted to cement stainless steel crown without any caries removal or tooth preparation, directly over the carious tooth. The results to date show that this simple technique can provide successful restorations in the short term. Although this technique of stainless steel crown placement, now called the 'Hall' technique, is not advocated at present, the findings of ongoing studies using this technique may change the recommendations for its use in the coming years.

Restoration of primary anterior teeth

Composite resin strip crowns (Figure 5.1)

Composite is the material of choice for the restoration of primary anterior teeth. An anterior strip crowns with composite resin provides an aesthetic and durable restoration.

Method

1. Local anaesthesia and rubber-dam isolation should be used if possible. Alternatively, because of age and poor cooperation of younger children, the restorative work may be completed under general anaesthesia.
2. Select the correct celluloid crown form depending on the mesiodistal width of the teeth.
3. Remove the caries using a slow-speed round bur.
4. Using a high-speed tapered diamond or tungsten carbide bur, reduce the incisal height by around 2 mm, prepare interproximal slices and place a labial groove at the level of gingival and middle thirds of the crown.
5. Protect the exposed dentine with a glass ionomer lining cement.
6. Trim the crown form and make two holes in the incisal corners by piercing with a sharp explorer.
7. Etch the enamel for 20 seconds, and wash and dry.
8. Apply a thin layer of bonding resin and cure for 20 seconds, ensuring all surfaces are covered equally.
9. Fill the crown form with the appropriate shade of composite and seat with gentle, even pressure, allowing the excess to exit freely. The use of small wedges may be helpful in avoiding interproximal excess.
10. Light cure each aspect (labially, incisally and palatally) equally.

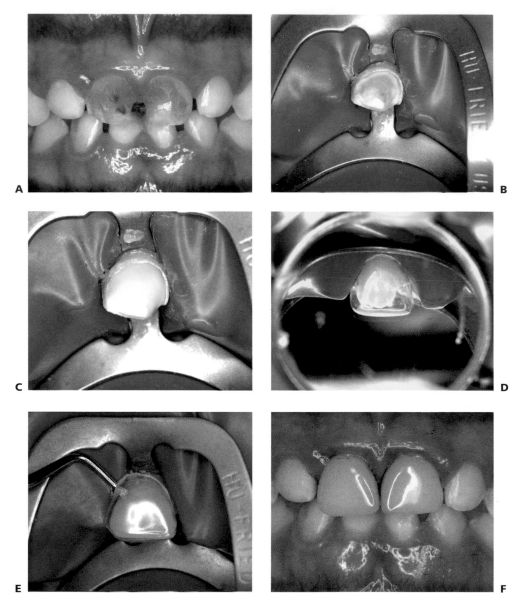

Figure 5.1 Placement of anterior strip crowns on the primary incisors. **A** Bottle caries affecting the upper anterior teeth. **B** Initial reduction of incisal edge and caries removal under rubber dam (butterfly clamp). Proximal reduction is achieved using a high-speed tapering diamond bur. **C** Placement of a glass ionomer cement base over the dentine. **D** Trial fitting of the cellulose acetate strip crown which is then filled with composite resin. **E** Removal of the strip crown with a small excavator. **F** Final restoration after polishing. (Courtesy of Dr E Alcaino.)

11. Remove the celluloid crown gently, and adjust the form and finish with either composite finishing burs or abrasive discs.
12. Check the occlusion after removing the rubber dam.

Interproximal stripping

Stripping of interproximal enamel may be used occasionally for minimal caries in the anterior primary teeth. Opening of the contact points allows saliva and fluoride to arrest the carious process, even when the caries involves the dentine. This is often, however, an unaesthetic alternative. It goes without saying that the initiating cause, such as a nursing-bottle habit, must be eliminated.

Method

The contact points are removed with a long tapering diamond or tungsten carbide bur and a topical fluoride is applied to the enamel and dentine. Placement of a fluoride varnish is useful for these cases. Regular follow-up is required.

GICs, resin-modified GICs, compomers

All of these materials have a place for one-surface restorations in primary anterior teeth. They provide aesthetically acceptable results and provide a degree of prevention as a result of fluoride release. It is important that the preparations must be caries-free for optimum results.

Restoration of primary posterior teeth

Amalgam

The use of dental amalgam to restore primary molars is common and supported by evidence from clinical trials. Clinical studies, evaluating the durability of dental amalgam in primary molars, have laid down the benchmarks against which other restorations should be judged.

Indications

- Amalgam may be useful in children who are at moderate caries risk or who are not totally cooperative, i.e. when moisture control is a problem.
- There is limited indication for the use of amalgam in Class I cavities in children as a high-viscosity GI, compomer or composite resin will provide a comparably successful restoration while preserving the tooth tissue.

Success

The success rate for Class II amalgam restorations in primary molars has been reported to be between 70% and 80%.

Method for interproximal (Class II) amalgam restoration

1. Use local anaesthesia and rubber-dam isolation.
2. Use a small round or pear-shaped diamond bur in a high-speed handpiece to gain access to the caries. The occlusal outline should not extend into all the fissures but needs to incorporate a small isthmus and a dovetail for retention (Figure 5.2).

Figure 5.2 The modified outline form of a Class II amalgam for primary molars.

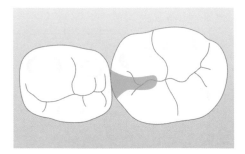

3. Extend the cavity into the proximal area by gently proceeding gingivally until the contact point is broken. Buccolingually, the cavity should extend so that just a tip of an explorer can reach the margins of the restoration.
4. Deeper caries should be removed using a slow-speed round bur.
5. Bevel the floor of the cavity at the junction of the axial wall and occlusal floor to increase the strength of the restoration. One of the most common sites of failure of the class II amalgam is at the isthmus, which probably results from insufficient bulk of amalgam to withstand occlusal forces.
6. In deep lesions a calcium hydroxide or Ledermix liner should be placed whereas in moderately deep lesions a light-cured glass ionomer liner is appropriate over the whole area of dentine.
7. Adapt a matrix band to the circumference of the tooth. A narrow curved brass T-band is useful for this procedure, particularly if back-to-back restorations are being placed. Both the Siqveland and Tofflemire matrix bands are adequate for single restorations. Wedging is essential for creating a good contact point.
8. Insert the amalgam incrementally, starting with the proximal box, using a small plugger to ensure good condensation in all the line angles.
9. Slightly overfill the cavity and carve the occlusal form using a small ball-ended burnisher and cleoid-discoid carver. An explorer is useful for creating the form of the marginal ridge.
10. Remove the matrix band carefully and pass a length of floss between the contact point to remove any debris.
11. Check the occlusion after removing the rubber dam.

GICs, resin-modified GICs and compomers
These materials have an increasingly important role in the management of carious lesions in primary molars because of their adhesive and fluoride-leaching properties.

Indications
- Because of their lack of strength GICs should not be used in large restorations that are to be subject to significant occlusal load in teeth that need to be retained for more than 3 years.
- Small occlusal and interproximal cavities.
- Where possible, use the stronger, high-viscosity GIC and avoid using resin-modified GICs for posterior restorations, as wear resistance is better.

Success

- The failure rate of GICs is higher than amalgam (33% over 5 years compared with 20% for amalgam).
- The average survival time for a GIC has been reported as 33 months.
- The incidence of secondary caries is reduced around fluoride-releasing materials.
- The use of polyacid-modified composite resins/compomers show considerable potential, particularly in terms of handling characteristics and radio-opacity. However, they have limited fluoride-leaching ability.
- Four-year results available now suggest that they are adequately durable for use in the primary dentition.

Method for glass ionomer restorations

1. Local anaesthesia and rubber-dam isolation should be used where needed (Figure 5.3).
2. The outline of the cavity should follow the extent of the carious lesion. There is no need for extension for prevention. A small occlusal dovetail is not usually necessary for interproximal restorations, however, additional retention form for minimal proximal cavities can be achieved by placing grooves into the dentine using very small (size ½) round burs (Figure 5.4).
3. Remove all soft caries using a slow round bur or with hand instruments. Be aware of the large pulp chamber as it is easy to expose the pulp of a primary molar.
4. Precondition the dentine using 10% polyacrylic acid for 10 seconds, and wash and dry.
5. When using encapsulated materials, ensure that the capsules are compressed for at least 3 seconds to facilitate adequate mixing of the powder and liquid components. After mixing for 10 seconds in the amalgamator, discard the first 3–4 mm of the mixed material as this is often unsatisfactory. Place the remainder directly in to the cavity.

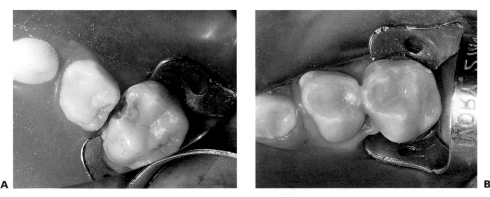

A   B

Figure 5.3 Two methods for using rubber dam in children. **A** Traditional isolation of single teeth. **B** Split-dam technique, isolating the teeth from the canine to second primary molar with one large hole in the dam.

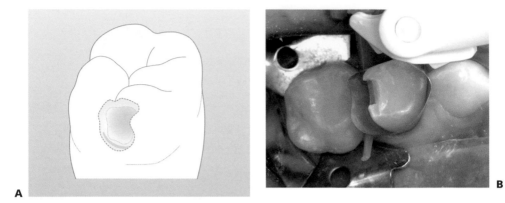

A   B

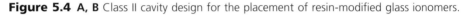

Figure 5.4 A, B Class II cavity design for the placement of resin-modified glass ionomers.

6. Once the relatively thick material has been placed in to the cavity it is compressed with a ball burnisher – dipping the tip in a small amount of bonding agent or unfilled resin prevents the material sticking to the instrument.
7. The final restoration must be protected from moisture contamination. This is best achieved by the placement of a thin layer of unfilled resin over the surface and polymerizing for 20 seconds. In young children with behaviour management problems, Vaseline rather than unfilled resin, may be appropriate.
8. The occlusion should be checked on removal of the rubber dam.

Composite resins
In primary molars composite is a satisfactory restorative material provided that the child is cooperative.

Indications
Small to moderately sized occlusal and proximal cavities.

Success
Clinical studies suggest that Class II composite restorations in primary molars are only moderately durable, with one study reporting less than 40% success after 6 years. However, recent studies have shown greatly improved success rates with the newer resin-based composites.

Method
For interproximal lesions the cavity design needs to be modified slightly from that described for amalgam – a bevel should be prepared around the occlusal margins for additional adhesion to enamel. The biggest problem encountered with composite restorations is the integrity of the bond at the depth of the proximal box. Placement of composite is technically difficult and highly sensitive to moisture contamination. Placement of a glass ionomer liner over the dentine not only ensures a good bond at the base of the cavity, reducing microleakage, but also provides fluoride release locally. The use of rubber dam and incremental placement of composite in the proximal box may reduce handling and polymerization contraction problems.

Increasingly, parents are requesting tooth-coloured restorations. It should be recognized, however, that use of these materials is associated with increased technical demands and expense.

Stainless steel crowns
Indications
Stainless steel crowns are preformed extra-coronal restorations that are particularly useful in the restoration of:
- Grossly broken down teeth.
- Primary molars that have undergone pulp therapy.
- Hypoplastic primary or permanent teeth.
- Dentitions of children at high risk of caries, particularly children having treatment under general anaesthesia.

Success
- Stainless steel crowns undoubtedly provide the most durable restoration for the primary dentition with survival times in excess of 40 months.
- They are relatively expensive in relation to both time and money in the short term. However, the rate of replacement of these restorations is low (3% compared with 15% for class II amalgam restorations). This makes them economically more attractive over the long term.
- They may be considered unaesthetic and require a significant amount of tooth preparation, and invariably local anaesthesia.

Method (Figure 5.5)
Irrespective of whether the tooth to be restored is vital or non-vital, local anaesthesia should be used when placing a stainless steel crown because of the soft-tissue manipulation. Rubber dam, although sometimes difficult to place in the broken down dentition, should be used where possible.
1. Restore the tooth using a GIC or compomer prior to preparation for the stainless steel crown.
2. Reduce the occlusal surface by about 1.5 mm using a flame-shaped or tapered diamond bur. Uniform occlusal reduction will facilitate placement of the crown without interfering with the occlusion.
3. Using a fine, long, tapered diamond bur, held slightly convergent to the long-axis of the tooth, and cut interproximal slices mesially and distally. The reduction should allow a probe to be passed through the contact area (Figure 5.6).
4. Little buccolingual reduction is needed unless there is a prominent Carabelli's cusp etc. However, such reduction should be kept to a minimum as these surfaces are important for retention.
5. An appropriate size of a precontoured crown is chosen by measuring the mesiodistal width.
6. A trial fit is carried out before cementation. It is important that the crown should sit no more than 1 mm subgingivally. If there is excessive blanching of the gingival tissues the length of the crown should be reduced. The margins should be smoothed with a white stone.

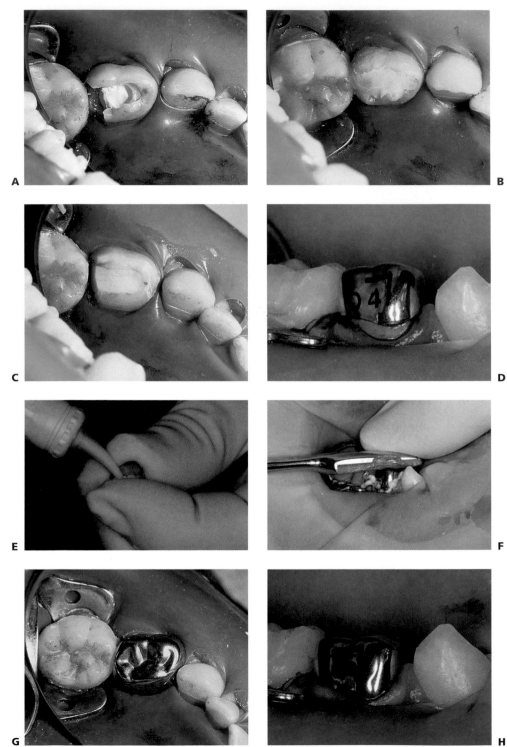

Figure 5.5 Placement of a stainless steel crown after a pulpotomy. **A** The intermediate restorative material (IRM) base has been covered with a glass ionomer cement **B**. **C** Interproximal reduction has been completed with a fine tapering diamond bur in addition to occlusal reduction of 1.5 mm. **D** Trial fit of the crown, by sealing from the lingual onto the buccal surface. **E** The crown is filled with a glass ionomer cement for luting and **F** the crown placed with finger pressure and a seating tool. **G, H** The completed restoration should last the lifetime of the tooth. (Courtesy of Dr J Winters.)

◄——

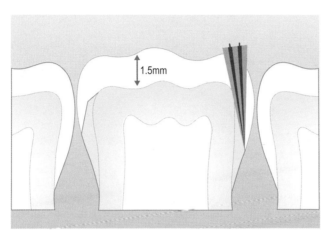

1.5mm

Figure 5.6 Coronal and proximal preparation required for the placement of a stainless steel crown. Note that in the proximal areas there is a smooth contour without any ledge or step. Any such step will cause great difficulty in seating the crown.

7. Cement the crown with a GIC or polycarboxylate cement. If the crown has been built up before the placement of the crown, a glass ionomer luting cement may be used, otherwise a restorative GIC should be used. Care should be taken while holding the crown as it can be easily dropped during placement. Excess cement should be wiped away and a layer of Vaseline placed around the margins while the cement is setting.

Minimal intervention dentistry

The philosophy of minimal intervention

Minimal intervention is based on an increasing body of evidence that the traditional approach to cavity design involved excessive removal of tooth structure. Traditionally, all discoloured dentine was removed. However, it is now accepted, that beneath the infected, soft and discoloured carious dentine lies a layer of 'affected' demineralized, and often discoloured, but not 'infected' dentine. Using the adhesive technology of

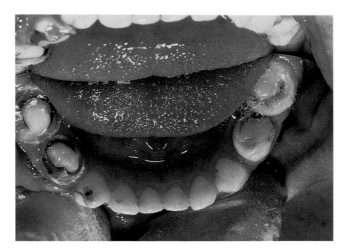

Figure 5.7 Breakdown of GIC restorations from conservative (minimal intervention) dentistry. Note however, that there has been a substantial slowing of the caries rate such that all the lesions are inactive and the teeth have been preserved in the mouth. While it is easy to criticize the quality of these restorations, these had been placed in a child whose behaviour was extremely difficult, without the access to general anaesthesia or other forms of sedation. Although some arch length has been lost, as the crowns have not been restored to their natural contour the majority of the space occupied by the teeth has been preserved. This still permits the placement of stainless steel crowns in the future, when the child is better able to cope with more extensive treatment procedures in the event of an improvement in behaviour. The question should be asked whether these restorations have 'successfully' retained the teeth. Is this treatment better than having no treatment or having all these primary teeth extracted?

materials such as GICs with their innate ability to release fluoride and other minerals, it is possible to remineralize this affected layer. This enables us to minimize the amount of tooth tissue that is removed, which is of potential advantage in restoring primary molars with their thin enamel and dentine, and relatively large dental pulps.

Atraumatic restorative technique

ART was designed for use by dentists and dental auxiliaries working in remote areas of underdeveloped countries with no access to modern dental equipment (such as turbine handpieces). Essentially ART involves the use of hand instruments for removal of the carious infected dentine and severely weakened enamel followed by restoration with a chemically cured, high-viscosity GIC. In general, in Australasia and elsewhere, access to modern dental equipment and facilities enables the provision of superior dental treatment. Therefore ART is not regularly used in most Australasian clinics, although the ART technique is of particular use as an interim treatment modality in children with behaviour management problems (Figure 5.7). Clinicians should be aware, however, that this form of treatment is only appropriate when the child can be regularly reviewed and any deficiencies in the restoration can be remedied. Thus, this type of restoration must only be considered as an interim measure prior to the placement of a definitive restoration.

Management of occlusal caries in permanent teeth

Of great importance is the preservation of tooth structure. Over the past decade, papers by Elderton and others have highlighted the deficiencies of the use of accepted concepts such as 'extension for prevention'. The placement of unnecessarily large amalgam restorations undermines the marginal ridges and weakens the cusps which will eventually fracture. The tooth then will require even larger restorations with the risk of pulp disease, root canal treatment and finally full coverage restoration. There must be a different approach to the management of permanent teeth that have not been previously restored compared with those teeth which require replacement of restorations.

Amalgam is an inappropriate material for the restoration of early lesions on the occlusal surfaces of permanent teeth. Here, the preventive resin restoration is more desirable. Minimal tooth structure is lost in cavity preparation and has the advantage that the occlusal table is protected by a fissure sealant (Figure 5.8).

Fissure sealants

In fluoridated communities throughout Australasia, where the average DMFT (decayed, missing and filled permanent teeth) is less than 1.0, the majority of caries occurs in the pits and fissures of the first permanent molar teeth. A simple and economical way of preventing pit and fissure caries is by the use of fissure sealants.

The indications for a fissure sealant are controversial. On a population basis it has been suggested that only those children who are at moderate risk of caries should have sealants placed, but because nearly 90% of children up to 18 years have some caries (mainly in the first permanent molars) all children should be assessed for fissure sealants throughout the eruption of the permanent dentition. Treatment should be prescribed according to the individual patient's need (Figure 5.9).

As fissure sealants should not be thought of as permanent restorations, diligent diagnosis and technique should be followed when one is contemplated. All teeth should be checked radiographically immediately prior to placement of the fissure sealant. Other options to aid diagnostic accuracy before sealing of fissures include the use of miniature burs to investigate staining, laser fluorescence, electronic caries

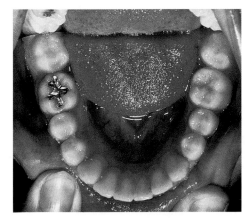

Figure 5.8 While this amalgam restoration has been well placed, it is an inappropriate restoration for a patient of 20 years whose only caries is an incipient lesion on the occlusal surface. This amalgam will weaken the marginal ridges and supporting cusps and compromise the tooth in the long term. A preventive resin restoration would have been a much better alternative.

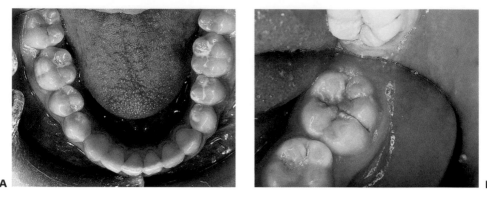

A   B

Figure 5.9 Fissure sealants. **A** An assessment must be made in the individual of caries risk. Not every tooth in every arch requires sealing, but it is important to remember that risk can change. **B** Caries-susceptible fissures. Sealing of the buccal pit in this child is essential.

detectors and micro abrasion. If caries is noted or suspected, a preventive resin restoration should be placed.

Indications
- All permanent molars in children at medium or high risk of caries (see Table 3.1). Premolars should be sealed in those children at high risk.
- In children at low risk, only the fissures that are deep and retentive need to be sealed.
- Primary posterior teeth in children at risk high of caries.

Risk assessment should continue throughout teenage years, even where caries risk was initially low. Risk status can change and fissure sealing continues to be protective into adulthood.

Sealant material
- Although some studies show differences, there seems to be no strong evidence to favour light-cured over chemically cured sealants or either opaque, clear or coloured fissure sealants at this time.
- Sealants should be opaque so that they can be detected by other clinicians. Use of clear sealants shows stains in the fissures, which are most probably inactive caries. However, another clinician, on seeing these stains, may choose to cut a cavity into a sound tooth, defeating the whole purpose of the sealant.
- Current studies support resin-based sealants over glass ionomer sealants, which do not have as good retention.
- Glass ionomers are useful in high caries-active individuals as temporary sealants until the teeth have erupted sufficiently to allow conventional fissure sealing.

The main problem with the use of GICs as fissure sealants is the brittleness of the material when used in thin section over the occlusal surface. However, it has been shown that despite very low retention rates, the incidence of caries under GIC sealants is low in long term similar to retained resin-based sealants. It has been suggested that either the GIC is retained in the depths of the fissures at a microscopic level or that fluoride, from the GIC, is taken up by the surrounding enamel so increasing the resistance of the fissure walls to demineralization.

Method (Figure 5.10)
1. Isolate the tooth with rubber dam. If the tooth cannot be isolated then a high-dose fluoride treatment such as a fluoride varnish or a GIC material should be applied. Review the eruption of the tooth in the following months and when the tooth has erupted sufficiently, place a fissure sealant.
2. Remove gross debris with a blunt probe and if necessary, clean the occlusal surface with oil-free pumice and water. In many instances, minimal widening of the occlusal fissure with a very, thin, small, tapered diamond fissure bur will facilitate the penetration of sealant material into the depth of the fissure. It also removes the more acid-resistant surface layer of enamel lining the walls of the occlusal fissure.
3. Etch the tooth with a gel etchant for 20 seconds and wash with copious water and dry with air irrigation for 20 seconds.
4. If the tooth is contaminated it should be re-etched for 15 seconds.
5. Apply a thin coat of sealant to the pits and fissures, making sure to include the buccal extension on lower molars and the palatal groove in upper molar teeth. Apply the polymerization light for 20 seconds.
6. Remove the rubber dam and check the occlusion.

Preventive resin restoration
Due to its superior wear resistance and superior mechanical properties, composite resin materials rather than glass ionomers are the material of choice for the treatment of early occlusal caries in permanent teeth. The development of preventive resin restorations has changed the management of occlusal caries dramatically in young patients.

Indications
- Enamel-only lesions.
- Incipient lesions just into dentine.
- Small class I lesions.

Success
The durability of preventive resin restoration has been proved to be as good as occlusal amalgam restorations and can be achieved with significantly less removal of sound tooth tissue.

Method for preventive resin restoration
1. Use local anaesthesia and rubber-dam isolation if caries extends into dentine.
2. With a small high-speed diamond bur obtain access into the questionable fissure.
3. Remove the carious dentine. Although it is important not to remove more enamel than necessary it is essential to have adequate access to the underlying dentine to be certain of complete caries removal. Unsupported enamel need not be

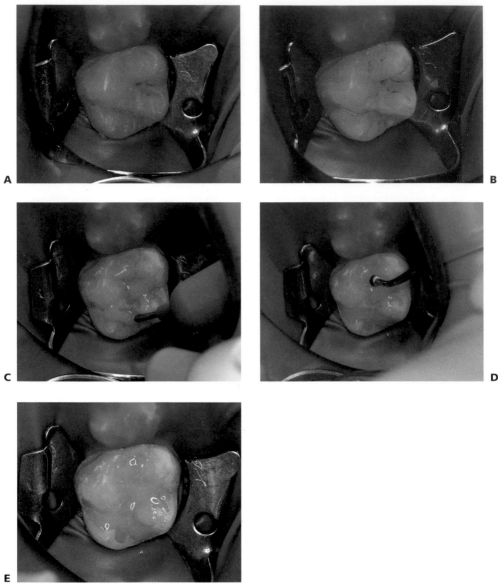

Figure 5.10 Placement of a fissure sealant. **A** Caries-susceptible fissure in an upper first permanent molar. The tooth is isolated with rubber dam. **B** Tooth surface etched. **C, D** A flowable composite resin has been used and is spread into the fissures with a ball-burnisher. **E** The completed sealant placement after curing.

removed if access and vision are clear. The cross-section most closely resembles a tear drop shape (Figures 5.11, 5.12).

4. Deeper dentinal caries should be removed using a slow-speed round bur.
5. Place a glass ionomer liner over the dentine extending it up to the amelodentinal junction and light cure for 40 seconds.
6. Gel etchant is placed for 20 seconds on the enamel margins and occlusal surface, and washed and dried. It is not necessary to etch the liner; sufficient roughening of the surface of the GIC will result from the washing process.
7. Place a thin layer of bonding resin into the cavity and cure for 20 seconds. An excess of resin will produce pooling and reduce the integrity of the bond.
8. Incrementally fill and polymerize the cavity with hybrid composite resin until it is level with the occlusal surface.
9. Flow opaque unfilled fissure sealant over the restoration and the entire occlusal fissure pattern and cure for 20 seconds. There is no need to re-etch the occlusal surface prior to placing the fissure sealant.
10. Remove the rubber dam and check the occlusion.

New techniques for tooth preparation

From the discussion above, clearly paediatric dentistry relies heavily on the use of standard high-speed and low-speed handpieces. Standard handpieces allow clinicians to remove carious dentine and shape a cavity. However, in recent years several hard-tissue removal techniques have been developed that also have a place in modern paediatric dentistry.

Air abrasion
Air abrasion is a technique that uses kinetic energy to remove carious tooth structure. When the aluminium oxide particles hit the tooth surface, without heat or noise of

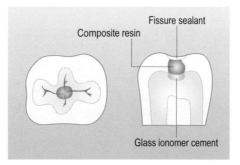

Figure 5.11 Preventive resin restoration.

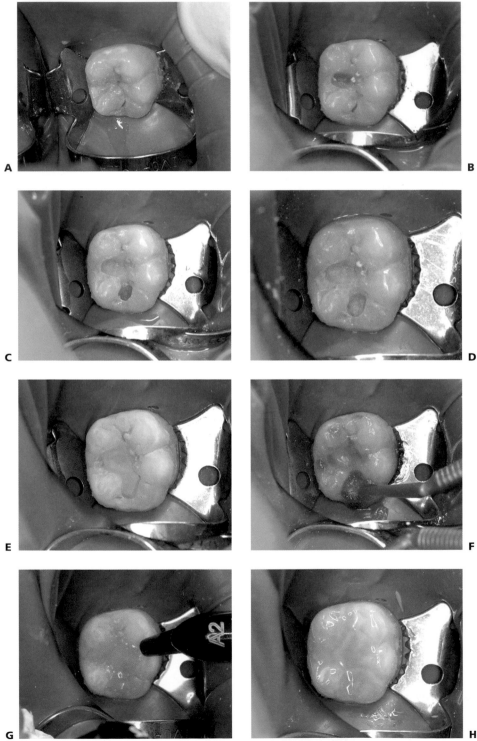

Figure 5.12 Technique for Class I composite restoration in a permanent molar. **A** The true extent of the caries may not be visible from the occlusal surface. **B–D** Progressive investigation of the fissures reveals further extension of dentinal caries. **E** Placement of a glass ionomer base. **F** Etching. **G** Incremental placement with nanofilled composite resin. **H** Final restoration with sealant placed over surface.

←

vibration, they remove tooth tissue. This technique requires additional equipment in the dental office for safe particle extraction and requires the use of rubber dam, but has been shown to be useful in some child patients who may be nervous of the noise or the feeling of conventional handpieces. Care should be taken due to the possibility of particle inhalation when using this method in children with severe dust allergy, open wounds and lung diseases such as asthma.

Laser-assisted dentistry

Laser is an acronym for *l*ight *a*mplification by *s*timulated *e*mission *r*adiation. Dental lasers are devices that use the energy generated by atomic electron shifts producing coherent monochromatic electromagnetic radiation between the ultraviolet and the far infrared section of the electromagnetic spectrum. The photo-biological effects of the lasers most commonly used in dentistry are:

- Laser-induced fluorescence (caries/calculus detection).
- Photo-acoustics causing disruption and ablation (soft- and hard-tissue treatments).
- Photo-thermal effect inducing coagulation and vaporization (soft-tissue treatments).

Bio-stimulation and photochemical effects induced by short-wavelength lasers for treatments including wound healing, analgesia and tissue growth will become more commonplace in time. Laser-assisted fluoride and bleaching treatments also show promising application.

Erbium lasers display bio-resonant properties on neural tissue causing Na^+/K^+ pump blockade and polarization of the A delta fibres and possibly C fibres. For many applications, local anaesthesia can be reduced and occasionally eliminated due to the analgesic properties of the lasers themselves.

Hard-tissue application

The two lasers most commonly used for dental hard-tissue treatments are in the 2790 nm (ErCr:YSGG (erbium-chromium:yttrium-scandium-gallium-garnet)) and 2940 nm (Er:YSG (erbium-doped yttrium aluminium garnet)) wavelengths. The tissue is removed by a non-contact beam that ablates based on the photo-acoustic affect on water molecules. The water content of the treated tissue and the power density of the laser beam affect the cutting efficiency. Hard-tissue applications include cavity preparation, caries and calculus removal, endodontic treatments, desensitization and bone surgery. The advantages of lasers include:

- Ability to selectively remove only carious dental tissue.
- Limited noise.
- No vibration.
- Ability to cut dental tissue without the need for local anaesthesia (in some cases).

Table 5.2 Guide to the use of restorative materials in paediatric dentistry

Primary dentition	
Occlusal (Class I)	Glass ionomer cement (GIC) Composite resin Compomer
Interproximal (Class II)	GIC Compomer Amalgam Composite resin/GIC sandwich Stainless steel crown
Gross carious breakdown or restoration after pulp therapy	Stainless steel crown
Permanent dentition	
Occlusal table	Fissure sealant
Occlusal enamel caries	Fissure sealant
Occlusal caries with minimal involvement of dentine	Preventive resin restoration
Occlusal caries with extension into dentine	Composite resin
Interproximal	Amalgam
Incisal edge	Composite resin
Cervical	GIC Composite resin

Therefore, lasers can be extremely useful for nervous patients; however, they are expensive and care must be taken during use to ensure that excess heat is not generated, which may be detrimental to the pulp tissue.

Indications for the use of restorative materials in paediatric dentistry

See Table 5.2.

References and further reading

Restoration of primary teeth

Attari N, Roberts JF 2006 Restoration of primary teeth with crowns: a systematic review of the literature. European Archives of Paediatric Dentistry 7:58–62

Chadwick BL, Evans DJ 2007 Restoration of class II cavities in primary molar teeth with conventional and resin modified glass ionomer cements: a systematic review of the literature. European Archives of Paediatric Dentistry 8:14–21

Gross LC, Griffen AL, Casamassimo PS 2001 Compomers as class II restorations in primary molars. Pediatric Dentistry 23:24–27

Innes NP, Ricketts DN, Evans DJ 2007 Preformed metal crowns for decayed primary molar teeth. Cochrane Database of Systematic Reviews 1:CD005512

Innes NP, Stirrups DR, Evans DJ et al 2006 A novel technique using preformed metal crowns for managing carious primary molars in general practice – a retrospective analysis. British Dental Journal 22;200: 451–454

Kilpatrick NM 1993 Durability of restorations in primary molars. Journal of Dentistry 21:67–73

Kilpatrick NM, Neumann A 2007 Durability of amalgam in the restoration of class II cavities in primary molars: a systematic review of the literature. European Archives of Paediatric Dentistry 8:5–13

Qvist V, Manscher E, Teglers PT 2004 Resin-modified and conventional glass ionomer restorations in primary teeth: 8-year results. Journal of Dentistry 32:285–294

Randall RC 2002 Preformed metal crowns for primary and permanent molar teeth: review of the literature. Pediatric Dentistry 24:489–500

Scott JM, Mahoney EK 2003 Restoring proximal lesions in the primary dentition: is glass ionomer cement the material of choice? New Zealand Dental Journal 99:65–71

Van't Hof MA, Frencken JE, Van Palenstein Helderman WH et al 2006 The atraumatic restorative treatment (ART) approach for managing dental caries: a meta-analysis. International Dental Journal 56:345–351

Restoration of permanent teeth

Manton DJ, Brearley Messer L 1995 Pit and fissure sealants: another major cornerstone in preventive dentistry. Australian Dental Journal 40:22–29

Mejare I, Mjor IA 1990 Glass ionomer and resin-based fissure sealants: a clinical study. Scandinavian Journal of Dental Research 98:345–350

Mjor IA, Jokstad A 1993 Five year study of class II restorations in permanent teeth using amalgam, glass polyalkenoate (ionomer) cement and resin-based composite materials. Journal of Dentistry 21:338–343

Murdoch-Kinch CA, McLean ME 2003 Minimally invasive dentistry. Journal of the American Dental Association 134:87–95

Simonsen RJ 2005 Preventive resin restorations and sealants in light of current evidence. Dental Clinics of North America 49:815–23

Vehkalahti MM, Solavaara L, Rytomaa I 1991 An eight year follow-up of the occlusal surfaces of first permanent molars. Journal of Dental Research 70:1964–1967

Welbury RR, Walls AWG, Murray JJ et al 1990 The management of occlusal caries in permanent molars. A 5-year clinical trial comparing a minimal composite restoration with an amalgam restoration. British Dental Journal 169:361–366

6

Pulp therapy for primary and immature permanent teeth

Contributors
John Winters, Angus Cameron, Richard Widmer

Introduction

Dental caries, trauma and the iatrogenic effects of conservative dental treatment, all provoke a biological response in the pulpodentinal complex. This chapter is concerned with the cascade of therapeutic interventions used to promote an adaptive biological response in the pulpodentinal complex of the treated tooth, and optimize subsequent growth and development. Therapeutic efforts are directed towards the retention of carious or traumatized teeth, maintaining normal function, with the resolution of, or freedom from, clinical symptoms.

Role of primary teeth

Primary teeth play an integral role in the development of the occlusion. Premature loss of a primary tooth through trauma or infection has the potential to destabilize the developing occlusion with space loss, arch collapse, and premature, delayed or ectopic eruption of the permanent successor teeth. In general, the effects of early extraction of primary teeth are more profound in the buccal segments than in the anterior dentition.

Effective pulpal therapy in the primary dentition must not only stabilize the affected primary tooth, but also create a favourable environment for normal exfoliation of the primary tooth, without harm to the developing enamel or interference with the normal eruption of its permanent successor. Where these outcomes cannot reasonably be achieved over the clinical life of the primary tooth, it is appropriate to extract the affected tooth and consider alternative strategies for occlusal guidance and maintenance of arch integrity (see Chapter 11).

Immature permanent teeth

Permanent teeth are still immature when they erupt. In addition to the important phase of post-eruptive enamel maturation, the roots of newly erupted permanent teeth will take up to 5 years before their growth is completed. During this period, the roots are short, the root apex is wide open, the dentine is relatively thin, and the dentine tubules are relatively wide increasing the permeability of dentine to bacteria. The open apex is associated with excellent pulpal vascularity and the potential for a favourable healing response.

Therapeutic efforts are directed towards preserving the vitality of the pulpodentinal complex to facilitate normal root development and maturation (Figure 6.1). If pulp necrosis occurs prior to root maturation, the affected tooth can still be preserved using non-vital endodontic strategies, but will be compromised with regard to strength, root length, and apical development. Retention of a compromised immature permanent

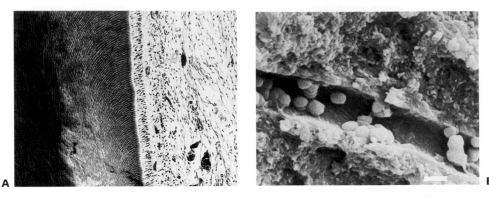

A

B

Figure 6.1 A Healthy pulp. The aim is preservation of this tissue. **B** Ingress of oral streptococci into dentine tubules. (Courtesy of the Institute of Dental Research, SEM Unit, Westmead.)

tooth with a poor long-term prognosis may still be beneficial for arch integrity and normal alveolar development during the period of dentofacial growth (see Chapter 11).

Evidence for current practice

The current evidence base for pulp therapy in the primary dentition is poor with a demonstrated paucity of prospective randomized controlled trials. The single biggest issue surrounding pulp therapy in the primary dentition is the lack of correlation between clinical symptoms and pulpal status. Hence, at present, there is no single recognized technique for pulp treatment in primary teeth, and a range of different protocols and medicaments are suggested for different combinations of symptoms and clinical findings.

The information in this chapter is based on established clinical practice, retrospective descriptive studies, clinical experience and expert opinion. In general, it is appropriate to use the least invasive intervention that is predictably associated with a healthy, adaptive healing response in the affected primary or permanent tooth. Obviously, effective primary prevention and early intervention will obviate the need for many of the procedures and techniques described later in this chapter.

Clinical assessment and general considerations

Diagnosis of pulpal status

Effective pulpal therapy requires the correct assessment and interpretation of clinical signs and symptoms, leading to an accurate diagnosis of the pulpal condition. Ineffective or inappropriate pulp therapy is associated with both acute and chronic clinical signs and symptoms. Unfortunately, there are no objective or definitive tests to determine the health of the pulpodential complex in the primary or immature permanent tooth.

Clinical signs and symptoms are poorly correlated with actual pulp histology. Acute signs and symptoms include:

- Pain.
- Mobility.
- Periapical abscess.
- Facial cellulitis or progression to spreading infections of the neck (Ludwig's angina).
  Chronic signs and symptoms include:
- Persistent infection.
- Discharging sinus.
- Enamel dysplasia (Turner's tooth).
- Infected follicular cyst.
- Failure of exfoliation of primary teeth.
- Apical fenestration.
- Ectopic permanent teeth (Figure 6.2).

Pulp sensibility tests

Standard techniques of pulp sensibility testing are of limited value in children. These techniques rely on patient feedback in response to thermal and electrical stimulation. In the primary dentition, it is likely that children will not have achieved the cognitive development necessary to respond reliably to a potentially painful stimulus and response challenge. In the immature permanent tooth, raised response thresholds to electrical stimuli are observed. These decrease to normal levels with root maturation and apical closure.

Pain (Figure 6.3)

Young patients frequently vary in their reporting of pain. It is often not until their pain is severe and prolonged when parents might become aware. Symptoms of severe, prolonged, spontaneous or nocturnal pain suggest irreversible pulpitis or a dental abscess (Figure 6.3B). A history of repeated need for analgesics is also suggestive of pulp necrosis. Dental pain will frequently resolve once a sinus tract establishes

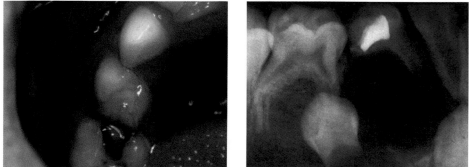

A   B

Figure 6.2 A Failure to diagnose pulp necrosis and persistent coronal microleakage has led to an acute facial cellulitis from the first primary molar. **B** Periapical radiograph showing site of coronal microleakage, radicular cyst, ectopic first premolar and previously undiagnosed congenital absence of second premolar.

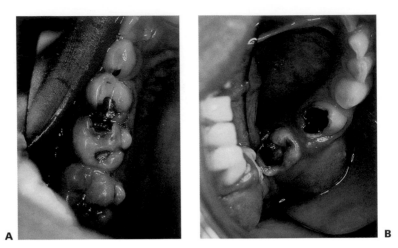

A   **B**

Figure 6.3 A Much of the pain that children experience may be caused by food impacting on to gingiva that has overgrown into a cavity. Even without radiographs it is important to recognize that the pulp will always be involved when the carious lesion is of this size.
B Buccal swelling not only indicates pulpal necrosis and pus formation but also the loss of bone and perforation of the cortical plate. It may also be difficult to initially determine which tooth is responsible for the swelling; in this case, both teeth should be removed.

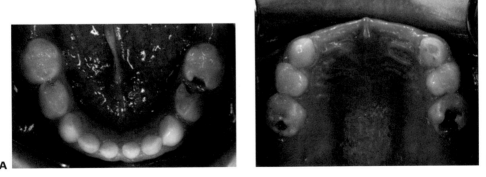

A   **B**

Figure 6.4 A Loss of marginal ridge of first primary molar suggests carious pulpal involvement. **B** Undermined triangular ridge or cusp suggests carious pulpal involvement.

drainage, and thus relieves pressure. In these cases, the underlying pathology is still present and must be resolved despite the lack of obvious discomfort.

Other clinical signs
Careful clinical examination of teeth can reveal useful diagnostic information.
- Coronal discoloration is suggestive of pulp necrosis.
- Clinical mobility is associated with abscess or imminent exfoliation.
- Marginal ridge fracture in a primary tooth is suggestive of carious pulpal involvement in contact point caries (Figure 6.4A),

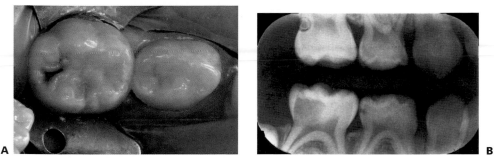

Figure 6.5 A Caries may be much more extensive than clinically visible. **B** The full extent of caries is only radiographically evident and shows pulpal involvement.

- Fracture of the occlusal triangular ridges or carious undermining of the cusps in pit and fissure caries also suggests carious involvement (Figure 6.4B).

Unfortunately, the external appearance of the carious lesion can in some cases be misleading (Figure 6.5). Persistent symptoms occurring soon after placement of a restoration indicate pulpal pathology. Lack of coronal seal will inevitably lead to pulpal pathology. Radiographic examination is essential to supplement clinical findings and enhance diagnostic accuracy.

Radiographs

Longitudinal radiographs showing normal dentine deposition within the pulp chamber and the roots, suggests pulpal health. Irregular pulp calcification or pulpal obliteration suggests pulpal dystrophy, while failure of physiological pulp regression or arrested root development suggests pulpal necrosis. In a single radiographic examination, individual teeth can be compared with their antimere to identify asymmetry.

Clinical signs or symptoms suggesting carious involvement of the pulp require radiographic investigation. Radiographs will show the extent of the carious lesion, the position and proximity of pulp horns, the presence and position of the permanent successor, the status of the roots and of their surrounding bone. Radiographic examination should be considered mandatory before undertaking endodontic procedures. The presence of caries in the furcation, internal or external root resorption including physiological root resorption, and periapical or furcation bone lesions, are all contraindications to endodontic treatment in the primary dentition. Primary teeth with these radiographic signs should be extracted.

Swelling

Alveolar swelling, particularly involving the vestibular reflection, facial swelling, coronal discoloration, and the presence of a sinus are indicators of pulp necrosis and abscess formation (see Figure 6.3B).

Mobility

Inappropriate tooth mobility, tenderness to palpation or a sensation of occlusal interference also suggests abscess formation.

Antibiotic usage to control acute infection (see Chapter 8, Odontogenic infection) may temporarily resolve some or all of these clinical signs, but will not resolve the underlying pathology. A primary tooth that cannot be saved requires extraction despite potential future orthodontic complications.

Factors in treatment planning

Medical history

A thorough medical assessment is essential prior to the commencement of any dental treatment. Medical issues may limit or change treatment options in a number of ways. As pulp therapy necessarily relies on the adaptive healing response after treatment, so patients with a significantly compromised immune system are considered poor candidates for endodontic therapy.

Contraindications

- Congenital cardiac disease (see Appendix E). Patients who are considered to be at risk of bacterial endocarditis should be free of oral infection. Any primary tooth with clinical signs of infection should be extracted. There is no evidence to suggest that a primary tooth with a large restoration is more or less likely to become infected if it has undergone endodontic treatment according to established guidelines.
- Immunosuppressed patients (see Chapter 10, Immunodeficiency).
- Children with poor healing potential (i.e. uncontrolled diabetes).

Generally, children with well-managed diabetes present no particular problem in relation to healing potential. The use of long-term corticosteroids for the management of asthma or asthma should not affect the decision to retain primary teeth. However, children who are severely immunosuppressed, such as oncology patients, must be treated more aggressively (e.g. extractions).

Indications

- Bleeding disorders and coagulopathies (see Chapter 10). Current management protocols for patients with a bleeding diathesis (such as haemophilia) may use regular, often home-based, factor replacement. Where patients have access to such medical treatment, the decision to extract or retain a pulpally involved primary tooth should not be determined by the bleeding diathesis, but should be based on the same criteria used for any other patient. Consultation with the child's haematologist is essential.
- Oligodontia (i.e. ectodermal dysplasia; see Chapter 9). In cases of oligodontia, the decision to extract or retain individual teeth will be influenced by the overall orthodontic strategy. In some cases, there is a requirement to extract primary teeth early to encourage occlusal drift and space closure. In these cases, timing of extractions can be critical, necessitating an interim restoration of the affected primary tooth. In other cases it is necessary to maintain a primary tooth without a successor. In the absence of acute symptoms, a formal orthodontic evaluation should be considered.

Behavioural factors

Effective endodontic treatment requires a high level of patient compliance. If a child is unable to cooperate with pretreatment diagnostic procedures including radiographs, they are unlikely to cope with complex endodontic and associated restorative procedures. Where cooperation cannot be obtained, or is fragile, it is reasonable to consider the elective use of general anaesthesia, or even elective extraction of the affected tooth rather than complex endodontic and restorative procedures.

Endodontics requires effective pain control. Even with usually effective doses of local anaesthetic, a child may experience breakthrough pain. This is particularly so on entry to the pulp chamber. The sedative effects of inhalation sedation used in conjunction with local analgesia can facilitate patient comfort and compliance. The use of rubber dam to isolate the tooth undergoing treatment, and to protect the patient from instruments and medicaments is mandatory.

Dental factors

Endodontic management should be considered within the overall context of occlusal development, with due consideration to occlusal guidance and space maintenance (See Chapter 11, Space maintenance). Under normal circumstances, the service life of a primary incisor is 5–8 years, and a primary cuspid or molar is 8–10 years. The early loss of a primary tooth may lead to localized space loss, delayed eruption and ectopic eruption of the permanent successor. Elective extraction may be considered within 3 years of anticipated exfoliation, because accelerated eruption of the permanent successor can be expected. Elective contralateral extraction may also be considered where appropriate to balance tooth loss.

Long-term success in endodontic therapy requires a coronal seal to prevent microleakage and the ingress of oral bacteria to the root canals. If the carious tooth is not restorable, it should be extracted. Pulpotomy and pulpectomy procedures require significant access cavity preparations, which have the potential to weaken the axial walls of the treated tooth. In general, full coverage restoration with a preformed metal crown or a composite resin crown is recommended.

Pulp capping

Indirect pulp capping

Sealing off the advancing carious lesion from the oral environment, produces a bacteriostatic response within the body of the lesion, and promotes pulpal healing with the formation of reactionary dentine. This is the basis for indirect pulp capping in both the primary and permanent dentition and is also known as caries control. Indirect pulp capping is also the basis for the atraumatic restorative technique (ART, see Chapter 5).

It is uncertain whether the carious lesion in dentine will become sterile and remineralize, or if it merely becomes quiescent with the potential to reactivate if there is leakage around the final restoration, hence there is debate over the necessity of re-entering the tooth to remove the residual caries once there is clinical and radiographic evidence of pulpal healing. Because of the known service life of the primary tooth, there is no indication for re-entering the primary tooth to remove residual caries when the clinical response is favourable.

Ozone and silver fluoride have both been proposed as adjunctive antimicrobial agents in conjunction with indirect pulp capping. At present there is a lack of evidence to support their superiority over sealing the lesion with standard restorative materials. Ozone may also promote remineralization by oxidization of the lactate–propionate buffering system (pH = 4) within the body of the carious lesion to bicarbonate and water. The depth of residual caries can be no greater than 2 mm when ozone is applied, as ozone will not penetrate more than 2 mm into carious dentine.

Large carious lesions and associated cavity preparations alter the mechanical properties of the treated tooth, reducing the rigidity of the cavity walls in normal function. This has the potential to increase the risk of microleakage. As indirect pulp capping relies on sealing off the residual caries from the oral environment, the residual tooth structure should be carefully evaluated. Areas of unsupported enamel should be removed. Weakened cavity walls, which are likely to flex in function thereby increasing the risk of microleakage, should be protected with either cusp capping or full coverage. This is of particular importance with approximal lesions where the buccal and lingual walls can be extensively undermined. Indirect pulp capping in lower first primary molars always requires a preformed metal crown.

Severely broken down first permanent molars can be effectively stabilized with preformed metal crowns to allow time for maturation of the pulp and dentine prior to definitive restoration. With growth, there is pulpal regression giving increased dentine thickness for crown preparation, and improved thickness of the radicular dentine giving better root strength. At the completion of dental growth, the restorative options for these teeth can be re-evaluated.

Indications
- Large carious lesion.
- Asymptomatic tooth or mild transient symptoms.
- Preoperative radiograph confirms the absence of radicular pathology.

Technique
- Pain control and isolation.
- Remove superficial caries.
- Remove all peripheral caries, leaving deep caries over pulp.
- Finalize cavity preparation.
- Restore tooth ensuring adequate coronal seal.

Direct pulp capping
Primary teeth
Small pulp exposures can be broadly classified as mechanical (iatrogenic) or carious. Direct pulp capping of carious pulp exposures in primary teeth has a poor prognosis, with failure occurring as a result of internal root resorption. The size of the pulp exposure does not affect prognosis. A pulpotomy should be undertaken in such cases. Uncontaminated mechanical pulp exposures are thought to have a more favourable response to direct pulp capping using hard-setting calcium hydroxide cements (Dycal, Life). There is inadequate evidence to support the use of other materials currently used, including antibiotic/corticosteroid (Ledermix), dentine-bonding resins, mineral trioxide aggregate (ProRoot MTA) in the primary dentition. Because of the difficulties

in determining the pulp status and the vastly superior prognosis of pulpotomy, direct pulp capping cannot be recommended in the primary dentition.

Immature permanent teeth
Direct pulp capping of pinpoint pulp exposures, either mechanical or carious, has a favourable prognosis in the immature permanent tooth. The use of calcium hydroxide and hard-setting calcium hydroxide cements (Dycal, Life), has been widely reported. There is limited evidence to support the use of other materials currently used including antibiotic/corticosteroid (Ledermix), dentine-bonding resins, and mineral trioxide aggregate (ProRoot MTA).

Pulpotomy

Primary teeth
Pulpotomy is the most widely used endodontic technique in the primary dentition. The suffix 'otomy' means 'to cut', so pulpotomy is 'to cut the pulp'. The aim of pulpotomy in the primary tooth is to amputate the inflamed coronal pulp and preserve the vitality of the radicular pulp, thereby facilitating the normal exfoliation of the primary tooth. A pulpotomy cannot be done if the pulp is necrotic.

The contemporary pulpotomy traces its origins to nineteenth-century techniques for the mummification of painful, inflamed or putrescent pulpal tissue. Over the twentieth century, the pulpotomy technique changed with fewer stages and reduced duration of application and concentration of medicament. Emphasis is now placed on the preservation of healthy radicular pulp rather than mummification.

Caries removal
The treated tooth must be rendered completely caries free before proceeding with the pulpotomy. The recommendation to remove caries from periphery to pulp not only prevents contamination of the pulpotomy site with carious debris but also reduces the risk of inadvertent pulp exposure. Access to the coronal pulp requires complete removal of the roof of the pulp chamber. Amputation of the coronal pulp requires a clean cut at the level of the pulpal floor. Residual tissue tags at the amputation site will create problems with haemostasis. High-speed rotary instrumentation with copious water spray irrigation creates the optimal cut. If the floor of the pulp chamber is perforated, the tooth must be extracted.

Haemostasis
Haemostasis at the pulpotomy site must be obtained before application of the therapeutic agent. This is achieved with continuous irrigation and gentle dabbing with cotton wool pellets and should occur within 5 minutes. If bleeding cannot be arrested, the pulpal inflammation is considered to have spread to the roots, and is associated with a poor prognosis. This is referred to as the 'bleeding sign'. Pulpectomy or extraction should be considered in these cases.

Pulp medicaments
The therapeutic medicament is applied to the pulpotomy site once haemostasis has been obtained. See the section 'Therapeutic agents used for pulpotomy in primary teeth' below.

Figure 6.6 Method of performing a pulpotomy. **A** Preoperative radiograph shows deep carious lesion. Clinical history revealed intermittent symptoms on eating with no history of spontaneous pain. **B** Carious lesion identified relative to dental anatomy. **C** Cavity preparation showing complete removal of peripheral caries. **D** After the tooth is rendered free of caries, the roof of the pulp chamber is removed completely, and the pulp is amputated to the level of the pulpal floor. Haemostasis must be achieved at this point before proceeding. **E** The therapeutic agent is applied to the pulpotomy site. **F** Base is applied to completely seal the pulpotomy site. **G** The tooth is built up with a core material. **H** The tooth is restored with a preformed metal crown.

⟶

The pulpotomy site is then covered with a therapeutic base. Traditionally this has been a zinc oxide-eugenol-based cement. However, eugenol in direct contact with pulp tissue causes chronic pulpitis. It is reasonable to substitute a eugenol-free cement as the therapeutic base. When MTA is used as the therapeutic agent, it will also act as the therapeutic base. Finally, a core material should be used to seal the tooth before the final restoration, ideally with a full coverage restoration.

Earlier texts have suggested that teeth, which are to have a preformed metal crown, should also have a routine electively pulpotomy, regardless of whether they have a carious pulp exposure. This position is no longer tenable given the predictable success of indirect pulp capping.

Indications for pulpotomy in primary teeth
- Carious pulp exposure.
- Tooth asymptomatic or mild transient pain.
- Preoperative radiograph confirms the absence of radicular pathology.
- Restorable tooth.

Technique (Figures 6.6, 6.7)
1. Pain control and rubber-dam isolation.
2. Complete removal of caries from peripheral to pulpal.
3. Removal of roof of pulp chamber.
4. Amputation of coronal pulp.
5. Arrest of bleeding at amputation site (see discussion of 'bleeding sign' above).
6. Application of therapeutic agent (see Therapeutic agents used for pulpotomy).
7. Place base directly on to pulp amputation site (IRM or Cavit).
8. Place core.
9. Restore tooth with adequate coronal seal. Full coverage with a preformed metal crown or composite crown) is preferred.
10. Regular radiographic assessment.

Therapeutic agents used for pulpotomy in primary teeth
A diverse range of chemicals have been used as pulpotomy agents. As most of these have not been subject to rigorous clinical trials, their use has been based on expert opinion and retrospective studies. In their review for the Cochrane Collaboration, Nadin et al (2003) concluded that based on the available randomized controlled trials (RCTs):

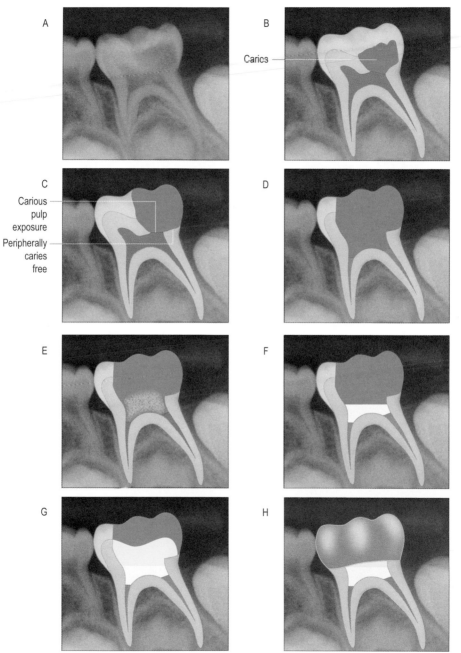

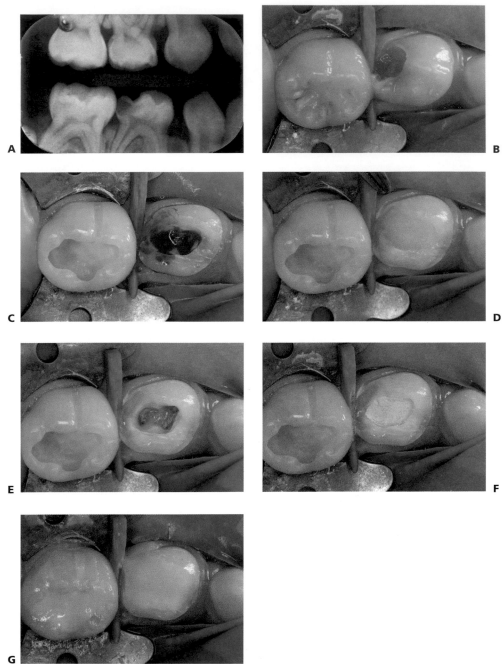

Figure 6.7 Clinical view of a pulpotomy procedure. **A** Bitewing radiographs show deep carious lesion in tooth 84. **B** Preoperative appearance of tooth with subgingival extension of caries. Preoperative wedging is used to protect gingival tissues, facilitate caries removal, and to prevent bleeding into cavity during preparation. **C** Removal of roof of pulp chamber and amputation of coronal pulp. **D** Application of cotton pledget moistened with formocresol to pulpotomy site. **E** Formocresol-treated pulpotomy site. **F** Cavit base completely sealing pulpotomy site. **G** Build-up of crown prior to restoration with a stainless steel crown. (Courtesy of Dr J Winters.)

There is no reliable evidence supporting the superiority of one type of treatment for pulpally involved primary molars. No conclusions can be made as to the optimum treatment or techniques for pulpally involved primary molar teeth due to the scarcity of reliable scientific research. High quality RCTs, with appropriate unit of randomisation and analysis are needed.

The available evidence suggests that formocresol, ferric sulphate, electrocautery and MTA have similar efficacy. Calcium hydroxide appears to have a consistently lower success rate in vital pulpotomy in deciduous teeth than these four agents. There are a number of other materials that are of historical significance, or have regional usage, and a number of experimental techniques including bone morphogenic protein and growth factors, which will not be discussed. All current therapeutic agents have toxic effects and must be correctly handled within their therapeutic range. Clinicians should carefully read the Materials Safety Data Sheet for these agents. Cases should be carefully selected within the guidelines recommended.

Formocresol
Formocresol has been used in dentistry for over 100 years, and for vital pulpotomy in deciduous teeth for over 80 years. Its efficacy has been extensively studied, with clinical success rates ranging from 70% to 100%, making it the standard against which newer techniques are compared. The formaldehyde component of formocresol is strongly bactericidal and reversibly inhibits many enzymes in the inflammatory process.

Originally, the aim of using formocresol was to completely mummify (fix) all residual pulpal tissue and necrotic material within the root canal. Current techniques however, aim to create a very superficial layer of fixation while preserving the vitality of the deeper radicular pulp. Contemporary pulpotomy is explicitly contraindicated in the presence of radicular pulpitis or pulp necrosis.

Formocresol is applied to the pulpotomy site on a cotton wool pledget. Any excess material should be blotted off the pledget prior to application. Traditionally, a 5-minute application time has been recommended; however, contact times of only a few seconds are probably equally effective. It is prudent to limit both dose and contact time. Formocresol should only be applied to the pulpotomy site after haemostasis has been obtained. It should never be applied to bleeding tissue.

In 2004, the International Agency for Research on Cancer (IARC) concluded that chronic exposure to high levels of formaldehyde causes nasopharyngeal cancer in humans. In assessing the potential risks of using formocresol clinically, however, it is important to consider the pharmacokinetics of formaldehyde. Formaldehyde is an important intermediate in normal cellular metabolism. It serves as a building block for the synthesis of purines, pyrimidines, many amino acids and lipids, and is a key molecule in one-carbon metabolism. Endogenous formaldehyde is present at low levels in body fluids, with a concentration of 2–3 mg/L in human blood. Application of formocresol results in systemic absorption of formaldehyde, however, the absorbed formaldehyde is rapidly metabolized to formate and carbon dioxide with a half-life of 1–2 minutes. The use of formocresol in dentistry falls within the current permitted exposure limits, and short-term exposure limits for formaldehyde. Formaldehyde does not bioaccumulate.

Ferric sulphate

Ferric sulphate is widely used in dentistry as a haemostatic agent (Astringident). It was initially used in pulpotomy as an aid to haemostasis prior to placement of calcium hydroxide. However, as an independent therapeutic agent, ferric sulphate pulpotomy has a success rate of 74–99%. Ferric sulphate is thought to react with the pulp tissue, forming a superficial protective layer of iron–protein complex. The predominant mode of failure is the result of internal resorption.

Ferric sulphate is burnished onto the pulp stumps (pulpotomy site) using a micro-brush for 15 seconds, then rinsed off with water and dried. Persistent bleeding after the application of ferric sulphate is an indication for pulpectomy or extraction.

According to criteria of Worksafe Australia, ferric sulphate is a hazardous, corrosive liquid, which has the potential to cause severe injury. Ferric sulphate decomposes to form sulphuric acid, which can cause superficial tissue burns if it is not confined to the pulpotomy site.

Electrosurgery

Electrosurgery uses radiofrequency energy to produce a controlled superficial tissue burn. It is both haemostatic and antibacterial. Excessive energy or contact time causes a deep tissue burn with necrosis of the radicular pulp and subsequent internal root resorption. Electrosurgical pulpotomy has a success rate of 70–94%.

The electrosurgery unit should be set to coagulate, with a low power setting. A small ball or round-ended tip is applied to the pulpotomy site and briefly activated. The site should immediately be flooded with water to remove excess heat. Each pulp stump is treated in turn. If necessary, electrocoagulation can be repeated to control persistent bleeding, until the total cumulative application time is 2 seconds. Persistent bleeding after this time is an indication for pulpectomy or extraction.

Electrosurgical equipment has the potential to interfere with pacemakers and implanted electronics. The patient must be correctly grounded with a dispersive plate to prevent earth leakage burns, which can occur in the extremities, a long way from the surgical site. Electrosurgical equipment should be set up, maintained and used according to the manufacturer's directions.

Mineral trioxide aggregate

MTA is a mixture of tricalcium silicate, bismuth oxide, dicalcium silicate, tricalcium aluminate and calcium sulphate. It is chemically similar to standard cement mix. MTA powder reacts water to form a paste, which is highly alkaline (pH = 13) during the setting phase, then sets to form an inert mass. Clinical success rates for MTA pulpotomy are similar to formocresol and ferric sulphate.

The MTA powder is mixed with water immediately prior to use. The resultant paste is applied to the pulpotomy site using a proprietary carrier or a plastic instrument and is left in situ to set. It is covered with a suitable base material prior to restoration of the tooth. The paste should only be applied after haemostasis has been obtained. Persistent bleeding from the pulpotomy site is an indication for pulpectomy or extraction.

Exposure to MTA dust can cause respiratory irritation, ocular damage and skin irritation. Dry powder contacting wet skin or exposure to moist or wet material may cause more severe skin effects including chemical burns due to its caustic nature while setting. Exposed persons may not feel discomfort until hours after the exposure and, in this case, significant injury may have already occurred. ProRoot MTA root canal repair material may contain trace amounts of free crystalline silica. Prolonged exposure to respirable free crystalline silica may aggravate other lung conditions. It also may cause delayed lung injury including silicosis, a disabling and potentially fatal lung disease, and/or other diseases. The IARC has determined that silica is a known human carcinogen.

Immature permanent tooth

The aim of pulpotomy in the immature permanent tooth is to amputate the inflamed coronal pulp and preserve the vitality of the remaining pulp to promote apexogenesis (see Chapter 5). Apexogenesis involves the continued normal development of the radicular pulp below the pulpotomy site, resulting in normal root length, thickness of radicular dentine and apical closure. Apexogenesis optimizes root anatomy and strength. The main risk of apexogenesis is the potential for dystrophic pulp calcification in the event that subsequent pulpectomy is required. The biomechanical properties of the root are more favourable after apexogenesis than after apexification, but apexification is the only option once pulp necrosis has occurred in the immature permanent tooth.

Unlike the primary dentition in which the pulpotomy is always at the level of the pulpal floor, a small carious exposure of the pulp horn of a permanent tooth can be managed by a superficial pulpotomy of only 1–2 mm. This is based on Cvek's pulpotomy. Where there is a large exposure, or multiple exposure sites, a deep pulpotomy is required to the opening of the root canals. The exposure site is continuously irrigated until haemostasis occurs prior to application of the therapeutic medicament. The therapeutic medicament can be calcium hydroxide powder or paste (Pulpdent, Ultracal) or MTA (ProRoot MTA). Antibiotic/corticosteroid (Ledermix) paste has also been used.

Clinical criteria

- Carious pulp exposure.
- Asymptomatic tooth – but may have mild episodic pain.
- Preoperative radiograph confirms immature roots with open apices.
- Absence of radicular pathology.
- Restorable tooth.

Technique

1. Pain control and rubber-dam isolation.
2. Complete removal of caries.
3. Removal of roof of pulp chamber.
4. Amputation of coronal pulp, either superficially, or deep to the opening of the root canal.

5. Arrest of bleeding at amputation site.
6. Application of therapeutic medicament (calcium hydroxide or MTA).
7. Place base directly over the therapeutic medicament (IRM or Cavit).
8. Restore tooth with adequate coronal seal.
9. Regular radiographic assessment.

Pulpectomy

Primary teeth

Pulpectomy is the complete removal of all pulpal tissue from the tooth. Pulpectomy can only be considered for primary teeth that have intact roots. Any evidence of root resorption is an indication for extraction. Severe infections including acute facial cellulitis associated with primary teeth do not respond well to pulpectomy. Extraction is usually recommended in these cases.

Although the root canal morphology of primary incisors is relatively simple, the root canal morphology of multi-rooted primary teeth is more complex than permanent teeth, with fins, ramifications and inter-canal communications. These anatomical factors inhibit complete chemo-mechanical debridement of the root canal space. The anatomical apex may be up to 3 mm from the radiographic apex, and frequently occurs on the lateral surface of the root, making it difficult to determine the true working length. Over-instrumentation of the primary tooth root canal has the potential to damage the underlying permanent tooth. Electronic measurement of the root canal can assist with the location of the anatomical apex of a primary tooth.

Obturation of the root canal space in a primary tooth must not interfere with normal exfoliation of the permanent successor. This requires a resorbable paste root filling. The exception to this would be where it is planned to retain a primary tooth that does not have a permanent successor. Suitable materials for obturation include unreinforced zinc oxide eugenol cement, calcium hydroxide paste (Pulpdent, Ultracal) and iodoform paste (Kri, Diapex).

Vital pulpectomy in primary incisors is more successful than ferric sulphate pulpotomy.

Indications for pulpectomy in primary teeth

- Pulp necrosis in any primary tooth, or carious exposure of vital primary incisor.
- Restorable tooth.
- Preoperative radiograph confirms intact non-resorbed root.
- Retention of tooth is required.

Technique

1. Pain control and rubber-dam isolation.
2. Complete removal of caries.
3. Chemo-mechanical cleaning and preparation of the root canal, taking care to force neither instruments nor debris beyond the anatomical apex. Copious irrigation with sodium hypochlorite.
4. Obturation with a resorbable paste (see above).

5. Restoration to ensure adequate coronal seal.
6. Regular radiographic assessment.

Immature permanent teeth (Figure 6.8)

Dental immaturity is defined by the lack of apical closure. Necrotic immature permanent molars have a poor long-term prognosis and, except in exceptional circumstances,
these teeth should be removed (see Chapter 11, Extraction of first permanent molars).
However, retention of such teeth may be important for alveolar development, behavioural reasons or may facilitate subsequent orthodontic treatment by holding space
until the optimal time for extraction.

By definition, these teeth have already lost significant amounts of tooth structure
due to caries. In addition, endodontic treatment would weaken an already compromised tooth, require apexification over many years (see Chapter 7) and involves
significant operative challenges (i.e. isolation, obturation, restoration).

Tables 6.1 and 6.2 summarize the treatment options for primary and immature
permanent teeth.

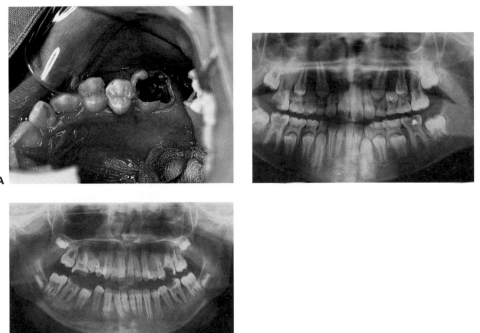

A

B

C

Figure 6.8 A, B The long-term prognosis and the ability to restore a tooth are the
overriding factors when assessing whether pulp therapy should be undertaken. In these cases,
it is often preferable to extract the first permanent molars and allow the second molars to
drift mesially. **C** In this case, the eruption of the second molars does not affect the decision to
remove the first molars due to the extensive carious breakdown in addition to the presence of
the third molars.

Table 6.1 Treatment options for primary teeth

Clinical event	Signs or symptoms	Pulpal status	Treatment choice
Caries without exposure	No spontaneous symptoms	Healthy or reversible pulpitis	Restore tooth
Caries with possible or near exposure	No spontaneous symptoms	Healthy or reversible pulpitis	Indirect pulp capping
Caries with possible or near exposure	Occasional pain on stimulation	Reversible pulpitis	Pulpotomy
Caries with possible or near exposure	Close to exfoliation		Consider elective extraction
Iatrogenic/non-carious exposure	No spontaneous symptoms	Healthy	Pulpotomy
Carious exposure	Minimal history of pain No mobility No radiographic evidence of pathology	Reversible pulpitis	Pulpotomy
Carious exposure	Spontaneous pain	Irreversible pulpitis	Pulpectomy Intermediate dressing Extraction
Carious exposure	Draining sinus Swelling Mobility Radiographic pathology (inter-radicular or periapical, root resorption)	Necrotic pulp	Pulpectomy with resorbable dressing or Extraction
Gross caries	Caries through bifurcation Extensive root resorption Tooth not restorable Furcation periapical pathology	Necrotic pulp	Extraction

Table 6.2 Treatment options for immature permanent teeth

Clinical event	Signs or symptoms	Pulpal status	Treatment choice
Caries without exposure	No spontaneous symptoms	Healthy or reversible pulpitis	Restore tooth
Caries with possible or near exposure	No spontaneous symptoms or Occasional pain on stimulation	Healthy or reversible pulpitis	Indirect pulp capping/caries control
Small pulp exposure	No spontaneous symptoms	Healthy	Direct pulp capping
Carious exposure	Minimal history of pain No mobility No radiographic evidence of pathology	Reversible pulpitis	Pulpotomy and apexogenesis
Carious exposure	Spontaneous pain	Irreversible pulpitis	Pulpectomy and apexification or Extraction
Carious exposure	Draining sinus Swelling Mobility Radiographic pathology	Necrotic pulp	Pulpectomy and apexification or Extraction
Gross caries	Tooth not restorable	Irreversible pulpitis or Necrotic pulp	Extraction

References and further reading

Casas MJ, Kenny DJ, Johnston DH et al 2004 Outcomes of vital primary incisor ferric sulfate pulpotomy and root canal therapy. Journal of the Canadian Dental Association 70:34–38

Huth KC, Paschos E, Hajek-Al-Khatar N et al 2005 Effectiveness of 4 pulpotomy techniques–randomized controlled trial. Journal of Dental Research 84:1144–1148

IARC Monographs 2006 Formaldehyde, 2-butoxyethanol and 1-tert-butoxypropan-2-ol. Lyons, IARC

Nadin G, Goel BR, Yeung CA et al 2003 Pulp treatment for extensive decay in primary teeth. Cochrane Database of Systematic Reviews 1: CD003220

Rodd HD, Waterhouse PJ, Fuks AB et al British Society of Paediatric Dentistry. Pulp therapy for primary molars. International Journal of Paediatric Dentistry 16(Suppl 1):15–23

7

Trauma management

Contributors
Angus Cameron, Richard Widmer, Paul Abbott, Andrew A C Heggie, Sarah Raphael

Introduction

The management of dentoalveolar trauma in children is distressing for both child and parent (Figure 7.1) and often difficult for the dentist. However, trauma is one of the most common presentations of young children to a paediatric dentist. The patient's emergency must be the dentist's routine. The child should be carefully assessed regarding treatment needs before commenting to parents because many cases are not as bad as they first appear. Initial reassurance to both parent and child is of great value. Trauma not only compromises a previously healthy dentition but may also leave a deficit that affects the self-esteem and quality of life and commits the patient to life-long dental maintenance.

Guidelines for management of dental injuries

The International Association of Dental Traumatology has published guidelines in 2007 with recommendations for the management of dental injuries based on a review of the literature and consensus opinions. These guidelines provide the most current views on care based on the published evidence and the opinions of professionals who practise in this field. As is stated in the guidelines, there is no guarantee of success and as further research is published, clearly the recommendations in these latest guidelines will be updated. The practitioner should be aware that clinical judgement is still required, depending on the presentation of each case.

Aetiology

Most injuries are caused by falls and play accidents. Luxation injuries to upper anterior teeth predominate in toddlers because of their frequent falls during play and attempts at walking. Injuries are generally more common in boys. Blunt trauma tends to cause greater damage to the soft tissues and supporting structures whereas high-velocity or sharp injuries cause luxations and fractures of the teeth.

Predisposing factors
- Class II division 1 malocclusion.
- Overjet 3–6 mm – double the frequency of trauma to incisor teeth compared with 0–3 mm overjet.

Figure 7.1 The presentation of a child with trauma is distressing for parent and child. The child in other instances may be oblivious to what has happened and is happily playing in the surgery.

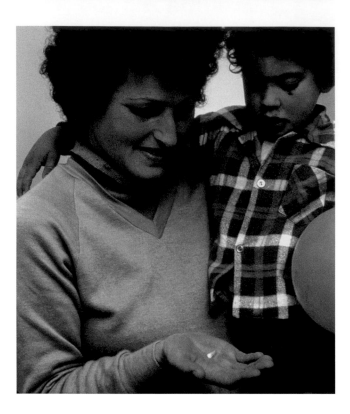

- Overjet >6 mm – threefold increase in the risk. The study in Table 7.1 by Hall (1994), from the Royal Children's Hospital in Melbourne, shows that falls and play accidents account for the majority of injuries. Importantly, although accounting for only 1% of all injuries, over 80% of child abuse occurs in the very young child.

Frequency
- 11–30% of children suffer trauma to primary dentition. This figure may represent up to 20% of all injuries in preschool children.
- 22% of children suffer trauma to permanent dentition by age 14 years.
- Male:female ratio is 2:1.
- Peak incidence is at 2–4 years and rises again at 8–10 years.
- Upper anterior teeth are most commonly involved.
- Usually single tooth, except in cases of motor vehicle accidents and sporting injuries.

Dog bites account for a significant number of injuries and every year several children are killed by dogs. It is common that the dog is known to the child and it cannot be stressed too highly that children must be supervised when around even the most timid of animals.

Table 7.1 Aetiology of maxillofacial injuries in children			
	% Injuries occurring at each age group		**% Total injuries**
	0–5 years	**5–10 years**	**10–15 years**	
Falls	50.1	32.8	17.1	43.2
Play accidents	39.5	43.5	17	17.7
Motor vehicle accidents	31.9	44.1	24	17.4
Sporting accidents	9	29.5	61.5	8.3
Dog bites	63.3	29.6	7.1	6.4
Fights and assaults	–	21.9	78.1	1.4
Child abuse	80	20	–	1
Others				4.6

Source: Hall (1994).

Child abuse

Child abuse is defined as those acts or omissions of care that deprive a child of the opportunity to fully develop his or her unique potential as a person either physically, socially or emotionally. There are four types of child abuse:

- Physical abuse.
- Sexual abuse.
- Emotional abuse.
- Neglect.

Dental neglect is the knowing failure of a parent or guardian to access treatment of orofacial conditions for a child. When left untreated such conditions may adversely affect a child's normal growth and development.

The true incidence of child abuse and neglect is unknown, and although there is increasing awareness and reporting, professionals are still reluctant to deal with it. The first step in preventing abuse is recognition and reporting. Dentists are in a strategic position to recognize and report mistreated children because they often see the child and parent/caretaker interacting during multiple visits and over a long period of time.

The orofacial region is commonly traumatized during episodes of child abuse (Figure 7.2). Injuries that do not match the given history, bruising of soft tissue not overlying bony prominences or injury that takes the shape of a recognizable object, and multiple injuries of different ages, may be the result of non-accidental trauma. Bite marks in children represent child abuse until proved otherwise. The characteristics and diagnostic findings of child abuse, and the protocol of reporting such cases, should be familiar to the dentist so that appropriate notification, treatment and prevention of further injury can be instituted.

Whenever injuries are inconsistent with the history, the patient must be investigated for abuse. There is a legal obligation in some countries or states to report the suspicion

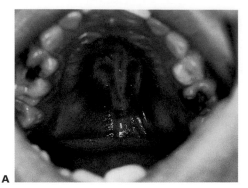

A

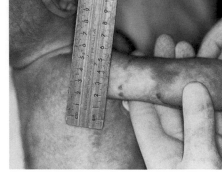

B

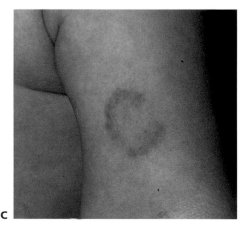

C

Figure 7.2 A Child abuse caused by sexual assault by a family member. Commonly the perpetrator is known to the child. **B, C** A 3-month-old infant and a 18-month-old infant who were bitten by older children. Good photographic records are required and the wounds should not be washed until specimens for DNA testing of saliva are taken. The child assault team will organize appropriate input from social workers, paediatricians and the police, if necessary. The dentist should also be aware of the legal requirements for recording of evidence (i.e. standardized photography with measuring scale).

of child abuse or sexual assault. In Australia, child abuse teams are available at all paediatric hospitals or through the departments of family and community services.

History

As dental injuries may become the subject of litigation or insurance claims, a thorough history and examination is mandatory. Where possible, injuries should be photographed. An accurate history gives important information regarding:
- Status of the dentition at presentation.
- Prognosis of injuries.
- Other injuries sustained.
- Medical complications.
- Possible litigation.

Questions to ask
- When did the trauma occur?
- How did the trauma occur?

- Were there any other injuries?
- What initial treatment was given?
- Have there been any other dental injuries in the past?
- Are current immunizations up to date?

Examination

Examination should be undertaken in a logical order. It is important to examine the whole body as the patient may present first to the dentist and other injuries may have occurred (Figure 7.3 and see Chapter 1).

Trauma examination and records
- Extra-oral wounds and palpation of the facial skeleton (Figure 7.4).
- Injuries to oral mucosa or gingivae.
- Palpation of alveolus.
- Displacement of teeth.
- Abnormalities in occlusion.
- Extent of tooth fractures, pulp exposure, colour changes.
- Mobility of teeth.
- Reaction to pulp sensibility tests and percussion.

Assessment of cranial nerves involved in facial trauma
I	Olfactory	Olfaction
II	Optic	Vision
III	Oculomotor	Movements of the globe
IV	Trochlear	Superior rectus
V	Trigeminal	Muscles of mastication
VI	Abducent	Lateral rectus

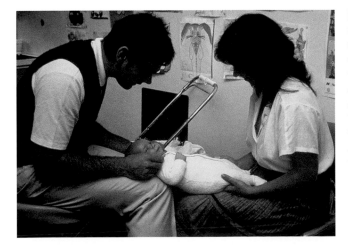

Figure 7.3 One of the most convenient ways to examine young children is with the child's head in the dentist's lap. The child can see the parent, who gently restrains the arms. This gives an excellent view of the upper teeth and jaws, where most trauma occurs.

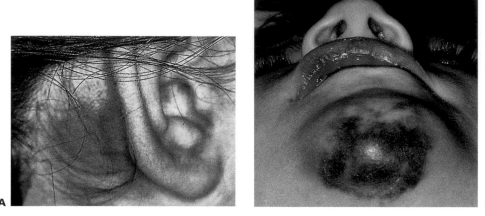

Figure 7.4 A The 'battle sign', or bruising of the mastoid region, is associated with a base-of-skull fracture. Examination must include all areas of the head and neck, which often requires parting the hair to detect lacerations and bruising. **B** Bruising is a collection of blood which will fall to the most dependent point. The chin-point ecchymosis shown here is often associated with gingival degloving, laceration and mandibular fracture.

VII	Facial	Muscles of facial expression
VIII	Vestibulocochlear	Hearing and balance
XII	Hypoglossal	Tongue function

Head injury

Closed head injury is the most common cause of childhood mortality in accidents. Between 25% and 50% of all accidents in children up to 14 years involve the head. If there is any suggestion that a head injury has been sustained, the child should be immediately medically assessed, preferably in a paediatric casualty department.

Signs of closed head injury

- Altered or loss of consciousness.
- Bleeding from the head or ears.
- Disorientation.
- Prolonged headache.
- Nausea, vomiting, amnesia.
- Altered vision or unilateral dilated pupil.
- Seizures or convulsions.
- Speech difficulties.

Dentoalveolar injuries take second place if there is central nervous system involvement. If there is any loss of consciousness, hourly neurological observations should be commenced (see Appendix S). The Glasgow Coma Scale is commonly used in accident and emergency departments to assess the severity of head injury and prognosis (see Appendix L).

Investigations

Radiographs
The request for radiographs is obviously made after a thorough investigation. There is great value in using extra-oral films in young children, e.g. panoramic radiographs. In the very upset or difficult child, it may be the only way that some clinical information can be gained in the acute phase of management.

When taking periapical films, several angulations should be taken for each traumatized tooth. This is especially important to determine the presence of root fractures and tooth luxations. As a baseline, all traumatized teeth should be radiographed to assess:

- Stage of root development.
- Injuries to root and supporting structures.

Guide to prescription of radiographs
Dentoalveolar injuries
- Anterior maxillary occlusal or anterior mandibular occlusal.
- Panoramic radiograph.
- True lateral maxilla for intrusive luxations of primary anterior teeth.

Condylar fracture (Figure 7.5)
- Panoramic radiograph, closed and open mouth.
- Cone-beam tomography or computed tomography (CT) scan
- Reverse Townes'.

Mandibular fracture
- Panoramic radiograph.
- True mandibular and anterior mandibular occlusal.
- Lateral oblique (this is rarely used today).

Maxillary fractures
- CT scan.

New imaging technologies have superseded older-style views such as the lateral oblique, the reverse Townes' and Waters' projection (occipitomental 30°). While such radiographs may be valuable in particular cases, contemporary practice demands the

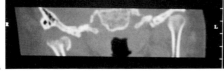
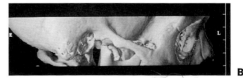

A   B

Figure 7.5 Use of computed tomographic reformatting to visualize fractures to the mandibular condyle. **A** Coronal section showing an intracapsular fracture with medical displacement of the condylar head due to the pull of medial pterygoid. **B** Three-dimensional reconstruction showing the degree of displacement of the condylar head following chin-point trauma.

use of CT or cone-beam tomography for an accurate assessment of middle third fractures in children.

Pulp assessment tests

Pulp assessment tests provide an essential baseline measure of pulpal status. It is common that the initial responses at presentation may be inaccurate; however, it is important that results are recorded for later comparison. Young children often find it difficult to discriminate between the touch of the tester and the actual stimulus itself, so the clinician must be aware of false results. In cases that are difficult to diagnose, isolation of individual teeth under rubber dam may be required.

Pulp sensibility testing

Pulp sensibility relates to the assessment of pulpal health. Previously termed 'vitality testing' this new terminology stresses the fact that neural and vascular components of the pulp tissue need individual consideration. A tooth may not respond to a thermal test but may have an intact blood supply. Such discrimination of the health of pulpal elements will be important in planning treatment.

Thermal sensitivity

Responses to cold stimuli give the most reliable and accurate records in children (even with immature teeth). The carbon dioxide pencil is regarded as being the most convenient, but is also the most expensive. Ethyl chloride spray, or ice may also be used. Cold thermal stimulation has the advantage that assessment of the pulp is possible under temporary crowns and splints.

Electrical stimulation

Electrical stimulation may give a graded response to stimuli. When using these instruments the rheostat should be slowly increased so that painful aversive stimulation of the tooth is avoided. The value of electrical stimulation is equivocal in the young child.

Percussion

There are two reasons to percuss teeth:

- Sensitivity in response to percussion gives information about the extent of damage to the apical tissues. Be aware that the percussion of luxated teeth will usually be painful.
- The sound in response to percussion is also an important indicator of the likelihood of ankylosis.

Transillumination (Figure 7.6)

This is an extremely useful, non-invasive technique to assess the presence of cracks and/or fractures, and subtle alterations in crown colour which may indicate a change in pulpal status.

Other considerations in trauma management

Having carefully assessed the patient, the only treatment necessary may be to reassure the child and parent and discuss possible sequelae such as pulp necrosis, resorption of intruded teeth, and facial swelling.

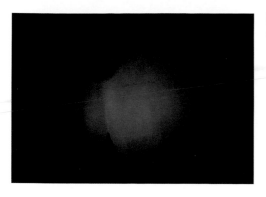

Figure 7.6 Transillumination to detect enamel infractions.

Fasting requirements

If the patient requires extensive work under general anaesthesia it is important to check fasting details. A child over 6 years of age must be fasted for at least 6 hours without solids or liquids. Children under the age of 6 years must be fasted for 6 hours without solids and 2 hours without liquids.

Immunizations

If a child has sustained an injury that involves contamination of the wound with soil, especially from a farm area, their tetanus immunization status must be determined. If the child has completed their normal immunization schedule, under normal circumstances boosters are not required (see vaccination schedules in Appendix F).

Maxillofacial injuries

Fractures of the facial bones are uncommon in children and account for less than 5% of all maxillofacial fractures. Consequently, few surgeons have extensive experience in this area and the management of these cases must embody an understanding of the implications of such injuries for the growing child (Figure 7.7).

Principles of management

Management of maxillofacial trauma is complicated in a child by the unerupted dentition, anxiety, growth considerations and the common association of closed head injuries that may delay definitive treatment. The use of internal fixation such as miniplates and screws must be undertaken with care due to the potential for damaging developing tooth buds. Intermaxillary fixation, occasionally in conjunction with transosseous wires is well tolerated in children. While arch bars may be used as dental fixation, silver cap splints may be still used effectively. With accurate reduction, fixation and immobilization, fractures unite within 3 weeks. Prophylactic antibiotic treatment and strict oral care must be maintained. Non-union or fibrous union is almost unknown.

Fractured mandible

Most mandibular fractures involve the parasymphyseal region (due to the position of the unerupted canine) and the condylar neck either in isolation or in combination.

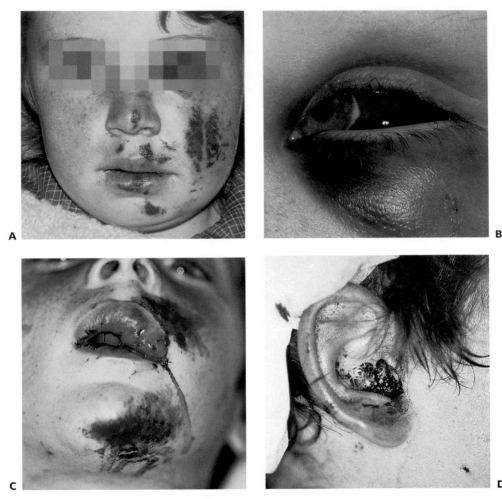

Figure 7.7 A, B This girl fell from a Tarzan rope onto her face. There is extensive ecchymosis and subconjunctival haemorrhage. While many of the signs of a zygomatic fracture are present, the immaturity of the frontozygomatic suture allowed for some displacement and there was no fracture evident. **C, D** Many children suffer chin-point trauma and it is important to check the mandibular condyles. This boy sustained a right subcondylar fracture. There was bleeding from the external meatus as the condyle had perforated the anterior wall of the meatus. Under no circumstances should the ear be suctioned because the ossicles may be removed if the tympanic membrane is ruptured.

Clinical signs
- Pain, swelling.
- Trismus.
- Occlusal discrepancies.
- Stepping of the lower border.
- Sublingual/buccal ecchymosis (Figure 7.8).

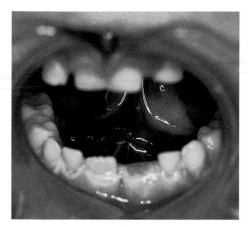

Figure 7.8 The sublingual haematoma is pathognomonic for a fractured mandible in the symphysis or in the canine region of the body.

- Chin asymmetry.
- Paraesthesia of the mental nerve distribution.

Management
- Reduction and fixation with arch bars and wire or elastic intermaxillary fixation.
- Splints may be attached with glass ionomer or black copper cement or retained with circum-mandibular wiring.

Condylar fractures
Fractures of the mandibular condyle are likely to be under-diagnosed in children and comprise up to two-thirds of all mandibular injuries. This injury usually results from trauma to the lower border of the chin. If a subcondylar fracture occurs, the condylar head is displaced anteromedially by the action of the lateral pterygoid muscle. Depending on the displacement of the fragments and the compensatory posturing of the mandible, there may be deviation of the chin to the affected side or there may be no occlusal disharmony. Bleeding from the external meatus may occur due to perforation of the anterior wall of the auditory canal by the condylar head (see Figure 7.7C, D). Bleeding or discharge from the ear should be investigated by an otolaryngologist but suctioning of the external meatus is contraindicated due to the potential for disturbance of the ossicular chain should there be a perforation of the tympanic membrane. Displacement of the condylar head into the middle cranial fossa has been reported but is a rare event.

Management
Treatment is almost always conservative with a short period of rest followed by active movement to prevent the temporomandibular joint ankylosis. Fractures involving telescoping of the condyle and distal fragment have been successfully treated with functional appliances for 2–3 weeks or longer, allowing better remodelling. Bilateral subcondylar fractures may result in significant displacement and an anterior open bite. A short period of intermaxillary fixation with posterior bite blocks to distract the fragments may be indicated. Where there has been gross displacement of the condylar head, or in severe cases of bilateral fracture, Botox (botulinum toxin) has been used

to paralyse the lateral pterygoid muscle, relieve the spasm in this muscle and minimize the fracture displacement.

As the condylar neck is relatively broader in the child with a greater volume of cancellous bone, fractures of the articular surface are more common than in the adult. In cases of intracapsular fracture (Figures 7.5, 7.9), follow-up over many years will enable detection of any growth disturbance. Should there be a limitation of opening or frank ankylosis, early intervention with a costochondral graft is recommended.

Maxillary fractures

Middle-third fractures are rare in children and usually present with other severe maxillofacial and head injures. Mid-facial fractures tend not to follow the typical 'Le Fort lines', as the craniofacial sutures are not closed and there is a tendency for greenstick fractures to occur.

Clinical signs

- Facial swelling and periorbital ecchymosis (Figure 7.10).
- Periorbital surgical emphysema.
- Subconjunctival haemorrhage, with no posterior limit.
- Diplopia with or without inferior ocular muscle entrapment.
- Orbital contour deformities.
- Midfacial mobility.
- Infraorbital paraesthesia (Figure 7.11).
- Cerebrospinal fluid rhinorrhoea and epistaxis.
- Occlusal discrepancies.
- Zygomatic stepping, orbital stepping or both.

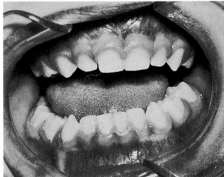 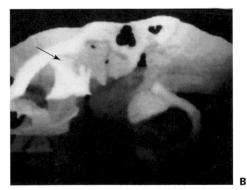

A   B

Figure 7.9 A, B Mandibular asymmetry caused by a dislocation of the left condyle after play equipment fell on this young girl. Imaging of these injuries can be difficult and in this case a CT scan was performed with three-dimensional reconstruction to detail the injury. The CT demonstrates the dislocation, with the condylar head (arrow) anterior to the articular eminence and lying under the zygomatic arch. As is common with these injuries in children, an intracapsular fracture-dislocation is present, which remodelled itself without treatment. Normal function was achieved within 6 months.

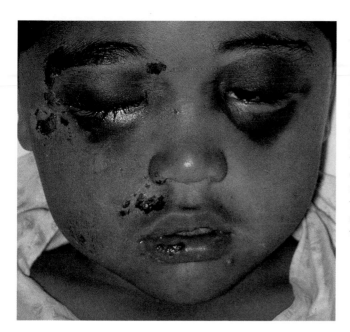

Figure 7.10 Middle-third fracture of the face in a child involved in a motor vehicle accident. Note the bilateral periorbital ecchymosis and swelling resulting in closure of the eyes. Despite the appearance, there was only minimal displacement of the maxilla, although external fixation was required to reduce the depressed nasal fracture.

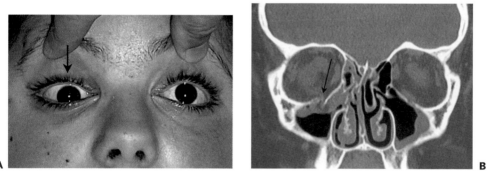

A   B

Figure 7.11 A Limitation of upward gaze associated with right orbital floor 'blow-out' fracture. **B** Coronal CT scan demonstrating 'trapdoor' orbital floor fracture with tissue entrapment.

Management

- Conservative management is usual unless there is displacement of the maxillary complex.
- Simple maxillary fractures are managed with cap splints or arch bars with inter-maxillary fixation.
- With marked displacement of the mid-facial complex, internal semi-rigid fixation or extra-oral fixation may be necessary.

Sequelae of fractures of the jaws in children

Closed head injury
Children who sustain middle-third injuries usually have concomitant head injuries. Head injuries occur in 25% of cases of facial trauma. These children spend extended periods in intensive care units, undergo personality changes, suffer post-traumatic amnesia and may have episodes of neuropathological chewing.

Tooth loss
Approximately 10% of children who sustain fractures of the jaws will also have loss of permanent teeth.

Developmental defects of enamel
In addition to the damage caused by displacement of primary teeth into the crypts of permanent successors (see 'Sequelae of trauma to primary teeth' later in the chapter), unerupted teeth in the line of jaw fractures may be also be damaged. Defects may include:
- Hypoplasia or hypomineralization of enamel.
- Dilaceration of crown and roots.
- Displacement of the developing tooth within the bone.
- Arrest of tooth development with pulp canal obliteration.

Intra-articular damage to the temporomandibular joint
There is always a risk of ankylosis of the temporomandibular joint after significant displacement of the condylar head, intracapsular fracture or a failure to achieve early mobilization of the joint. Treatment of the ankylosis involves condylectomy and joint reconstruction with a costochondral graft in later childhood.

Growth retardation
Maxillary (Figure 7.12) and mandibular growth retardation may occur following major trauma. Significant scarring of soft tissues and/or tissue loss may inhibit jaw growth. Mandibular asymmetry with antegonial notching may occur on the affected side after

Figure 7.12 Maxillary hypoplasia and growth retardation, in another patient with a middle-third fracture, 8 years after the trauma.

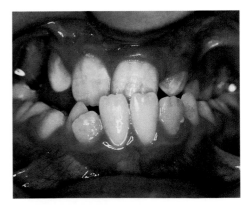

subcondylar fracture. The key to management is to correct asymmetries early to avoid secondary maxillary deformity.

Luxations in the primary dentition

General management considerations
There is general agreement that most injuries to the primary dentition can be managed conservatively and heal without sequelae

Immunization
If the child is not fully immunized then a tetanus booster is required: tetanus toxoid 0.5 mL by immediate intramuscular injection (see vaccination schedules, Appendix F).

Antibiotics
Unless there are significant soft-tissue or dentoalveolar injuries, antibiotics are not usually required. Antibiotics are prescribed empirically as a prophylaxis against infection, but are not a substitute for proper debridement of wounds. All drugs should be prescribed according to the child's weight (see Appendix M).

Luxations
Up to 2 years of age, the most common injuries to the primary teeth are luxations involving a displacement of the teeth in the alveolar bone.

Concussion and subluxation (Figure 7.13)
Concussion is an injury to the tooth and ligament without displacement or mobility of the tooth. Subluxation occurs when the tooth is mobile but is not displaced. Both involve minor damage to the periodontal ligament. All these teeth are tender to percussion, there is haemorrhage and oedema within the ligament, but gingival bleeding and mobility only occurs if the teeth have been subluxated.

Management
- Periapical radiographs as baseline.
- Soft diet for 1 week.
- Advice to the parents of possible sequelae, such as pulp necrosis.
- Individualized follow-up.

Intrusive luxation
Intrusive injuries (see Figure 7.11E, F) are the most common injuries to upper primary incisors. Newly erupted incisors often take the full force of any fall in a toddler. There is usually a palatal and superior displacement of the crown, which means that the apex of the tooth is forced away from the permanent follicle.

Management
- If the crown is visible and there is only minor alveolar damage – leave tooth to re-erupt.
- If the whole tooth is intruded – extract.

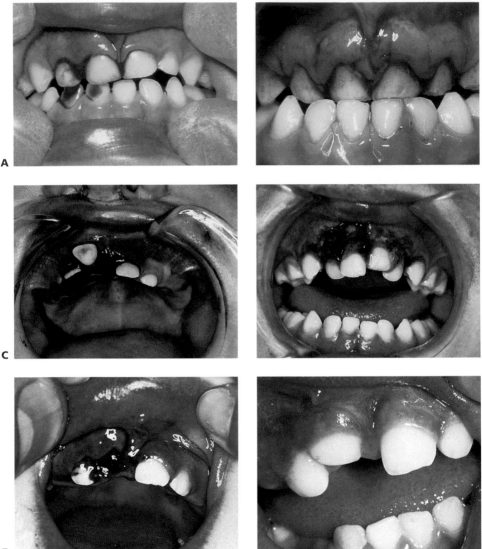

Figure 7.13 A Subluxation of the upper right incisors with minimal displacement. **B** Palatal luxation of the upper incisors resulting in an occlusal interference. These teeth should be repositioned digitally, only to relieve the interference. Further anterior movement may damage the permanent teeth. **C** Extrusive luxation of the upper right primary incisors. These should be removed. **D** Gross displacement of all upper anterior teeth with gingival degloving and loss of the labial plate. This child had the displaced teeth extracted, and debridement and suturing of the gingiva under general anaesthesia. **E** An intrusive luxation of the upper right central incisor in a 12-month-old child. Note the displacement of the gingiva, indicating that the tooth has not been avulsed. **F** The tooth partially re-erupted within a month.

Clinical Hint

Where the apex of the primary tooth has perforated the labial plate the tooth should be removed. The decision on whether to extract or to allow for re-eruption is very much a clinical one, and is based on the presentation of the injuries and the assessment of the child. More severe injuries, involving alveolar bone and gingiva, often necessitate extraction.

Extrusive and lateral luxation (Figures 7.13B–D, 7.14A, 7.15)

Treatment is dependent on the mobility and extent of displacement. If there is excessive mobility the tooth should be removed.

Avulsion (Figure 7.14)

- Avulsed primary teeth should not be replanted.
- Replacing an avulsed primary tooth may force the blood clot in the socket, or the root apex itself, into the developing permanent tooth. The other main reason is lack of patient cooperation. There are cases in which the parent or caregiver replants the tooth and it seems to be stable and viable; in these cases the tooth could be left in situ.
- Unless significant soft-tissue damage is present antibiotics are not required. Splinting of primary teeth may be difficult in young, traumatized children and if successfully placed, the splint must then also be removed later when the child is less compliant.

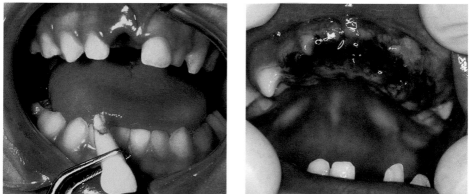

A   B

Figure 7.14 A There is almost no indication for the replantation of an avulsed primary tooth. There is more risk of damage to the permanent tooth than there is benefit gained by replacing the tooth. **B** A child involved in a motor vehicle accident resulting in six avulsed primary teeth. A chest radiograph was required to ensure that no teeth were swallowed or aspirated.

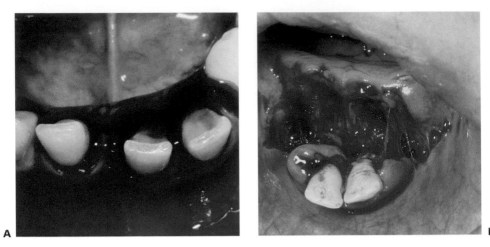

A   B

Figure 7.15 A Luxations in the mandible usually present with an anterior displacement of the incisors. This child presented 1 week after trauma with continued gingival oozing. He was subsequently diagnosed with Christmas disease (factor IX deficiency). **B** A dentoalveolar fracture in a 6-month-old infant. In these cases it is important to reposition the bone, with or without the teeth. A thick (2-0) nylon suture passed through both labial and lingual plates can be used to provide fixation for the fragment. Teeth usually survive this trauma and there are few untoward sequelae for the permanent teeth.

Fractures of primary incisors
Crown fractures not involving the pulp (Figure 7.16A)
Unlike the permanent dentition, primary teeth are more commonly displaced rather than fractured. Enamel and dentine may be smoothed with a disc and if possible cover the dentine with glass ionomer cement or composite resin. Paediatric strip crowns are often useful. A possible sequela is pulp necrosis and/or grey discoloration.

Complicated crown/root fractures (Figure 7.16C, D)
More commonly, fractures of primary teeth involve the pulp and extend below the gingival margin. Commonly, there are multiple fractures in individual teeth. In these cases it is not possible to adequately restore the tooth and so it should be removed. Often the fracture is not immediately evident, but the child may present several days after the trauma with a pulp polyp separating the fragments. Such a proliferative response is a protective mechanism and is not painful.

Management
- Most discomfort results from the movement of fractured pieces of enamel still held by the gingiva or periodontal ligament. In emergency management these loose tooth fragments should be removed.
- The remaining tooth can be extracted when convenient. This may necessitate the use of sedation or a short general anaesthetic.
- If a small piece of root remains in the socket after a fracture it may be safely left in situ where it will be resorbed as the permanent tooth erupts. It is important to keep parents adequately informed in these situations.

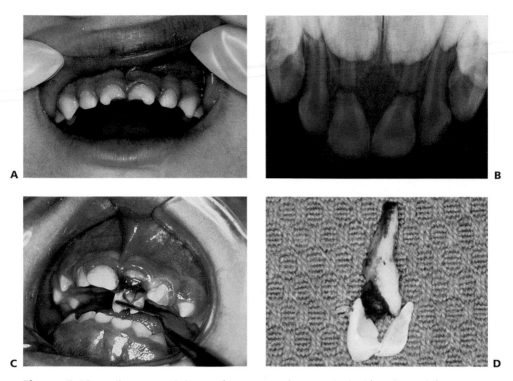

Figure 7.16 A Minor enamel/dentine fractures can be smoothed with a disc or left untreated. **B** Root fractures, again, require no treatment unless the coronal fragments are excessively mobile. The apical portions remain vital and resorb normally. **C** A complex crown/root fracture involving the upper left primary central incisor. These teeth are not restorable and need to be extracted. The extent of the subgingival fracture can be seen in **D**. The pulpal polyp that forms usually causes no discomfort.

Root fractures (Figure 7.16B)

As mentioned above, when children fracture primary incisors, there is usually a complex crown/root fracture that extends below the gingival margin and extraction is indicated. Isolated root fractures are uncommon. No treatment is usually necessary for primary incisors. If, at regular review, the pulp shows signs of necrosis, with excessive mobility or sinus formation, the coronal portion should be removed. Apical root fragments are always removed by resorption as the permanent tooth erupts.

Dentoalveolar fracture (Figure 7.15B)

This is more common in the mandible with the anterior teeth displaced anteriorly with the labial plate. It is often desirable to reposition the teeth with the bone to maintain the alveolar contour. This can be achieved with a thick nylon suture (2-0) passed through the labial and lingual plates of the bone. Teeth that are excessively mobile should be carefully dissected out of the sockets preserving the labial plate, which is then repositioned and sutured.

Sequelae of trauma to primary teeth (Figures 7.17, 7.18)

It is important to discuss with parents the sequelae of luxated or avulsed primary incisors. Although it may be difficult to accurately predict the prognosis for permanent teeth, parents appreciate having an idea of possible outcomes. In cases that have been followed, up to 25% of children are left with some developmental disturbance of the permanent tooth.

Damage to the permanent dentition occurs more often with intrusive luxation and avulsion in very young children. It is important to warn parents of possible problems with permanent teeth and also to reassure them that, with modern restorative materials, minor defects are easily repaired. Sequelae in the permanent dentition depend on:

- Direction and displacement of the primary root apex (Figure 7.17).
- Degree of alveolar damage.
- Stage of formation of the permanent tooth.

Possible damage to primary and permanent teeth

- Necrosis of the pulp of the primary tooth with grey discoloration and possible abscess formation.
- Internal resorption of the primary tooth.
- Ankylosis of the primary tooth. Commonly, intruded primary teeth will fail to fully erupt but will exfoliate normally. In rare cases, extraction may be required just prior eruption of the permanent incisor.
- Hypoplasia (Figure 7.18E) or hypomineralization (Figure 7.18B) of succedaneous teeth.
- Dilaceration of the crown, or root, varies by developmental stage (Figure 7.18C, D).
- Resorption of the permanent tooth germ.

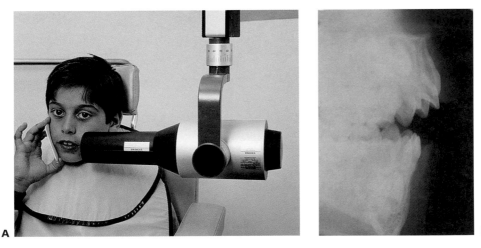

A B

Figure 7.17 A Technique of taking a true lateral maxillary radiograph. This film gives a good localization of the position of the primary root apex in relation to the central incisors. **B** The root apex is clearly visible, just underneath the anterior nasal spine, having perforated the labial plate. In this situation, damage to the unerupted permanent tooth is less likely.

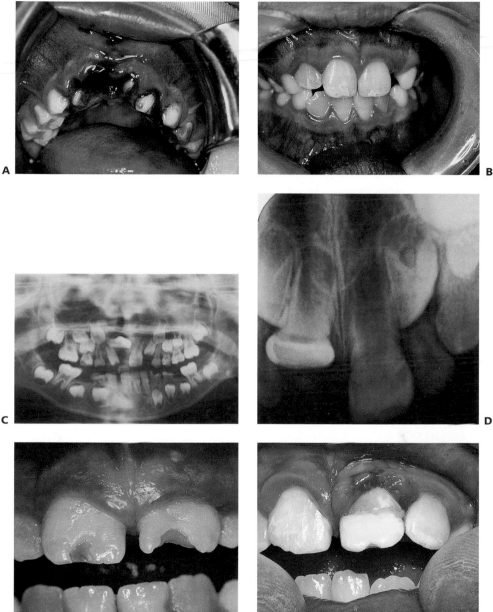

Figure 7.18 A It is often difficult to predict sequelae. For example, this case of severe intrusion, and alveolar disruption, has caused little damage other than mild hypocalcification of the permanent incisors (**B**). **C** Displacement and dilaceration of the upper-right permanent central incisor, following avulsion of the primary precursor tooth, at 18 months of age. **D** Severe dilaceration of the crown of the upper left central incisor. **E** Hypoplasia of the permanent central incisors resulting from trauma in the primary dentition. **F** Restoration of dilacerated teeth is extremely difficult, especially when the defect involves the gingival margin.

Treatment options
- If the primary tooth is discoloured, but asymptomatic, no treatment is usually indicated, however, masking a discoloured tooth with composite resin may be an option if aesthetics are of concern. If an abscess is present, pulpectomy or extraction is indicated.
- Hypoplasia and hypomineralization of the permanent teeth can be restored with composite resin.
- Dilaceration of the crown or root of the permanent tooth often necessitates surgical exposure and bonding of chains or brackets for orthodontic extrusion (see Chapter 11 for details of surgical procedure). Severe cases may be untreatable and such teeth may need to be removed.

Crown and root fractures of permanent incisors

Crown infractions
An incomplete fracture (or crack) of the enamel without loss of tooth structure. Fractures do not cross the dentinoenamel junction and usually require transillumination or indirect light to be viewed (see Figure 7.6).

Management
- Pulp sensibility test.
- Periapical radiographs.

Review
- Pulp sensibility testing after 3 and 12 months.
- Radiographs after 12 months.

Uncomplicated enamel and enamel/dentine fractures
Uncomplicated fractures are confined to enamel or enamel and dentine but do not involve the pulp. The most common presentation is an oblique fracture of the mesial or distal corner of an incisor.

Management
- Baseline periapical radiographs and pulp sensibility tests. Several angulations may be required to exclude other injuries.
- Enamel-only fractures – smooth over sharp edges with a disc or restore with composite resin if required.
- Enamel and dentine fractures – cover dentine with glass ionomer cement and then restore the crown with composite resin either immediately or at review.

Review
- Pulp sensibility testing after 6–8 weeks and then at 12 months.
- Radiographs at each review.

Clinical Hint

It is extremely important to cover the exposed dentine of permanent incisors as soon as possible. This is to prevent direct irritation of the pulp via the dentinal tubules. Parents have often saved the fractured piece of permanent incisor that can sometimes be used to restore the tooth by being bonded back onto the tooth with composite resin (Figure 7.19).

In the very immature tooth, where there is a questionable pulp exposure, an elective Cvek pulpotomy (see below) may be indicated. This will ensure normal development of the apex and prevent the need for any possible open apex endodontic procedure (apexification).

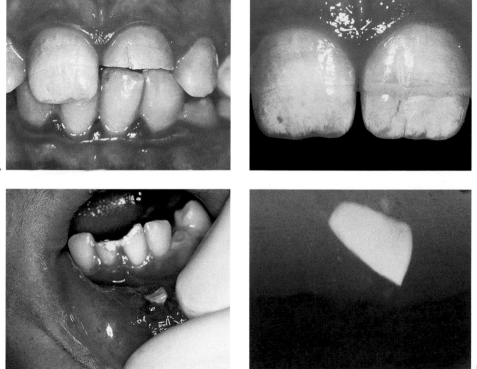

A   B

C   D

Figure 7.19 Cementation of a fractured enamel fragment. **A** A chamfer or bevel is placed around the fragment and remaining crown and the dentine covered with glass ionomer cement. **B** Composite resin is then used to bind the fragment to the crown. It is often impossible to re-create the subtle hypocalcific flecks in a crown with composite resin alone; the replacement of the fractured piece is a good alternative technique if the fragment can be found. **C** Always look for fragments of tooth in the soft tissues. It is essential that they are removed at the time of the trauma as they are extremely difficult to find once the tissues have healed. **D** Radiographs are useful in localizing tooth fragments within the lip.

Figure 7.20 Assessment of any pulp exposure is essential, especially in cases where the tooth is immature. Immediate coverage and dressing will help to prevent pulp necrosis and the need for an open apex endodontic procedure.

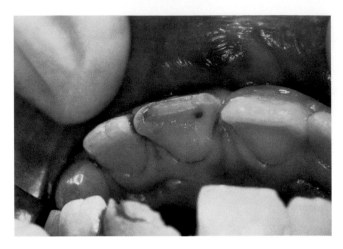

Prognosis
Pulp necrosis after extensive proximal fracture:
- No protective coverage of dentine: 54%.
- With dentine coverage: 8%.

Complicated crown fractures (Figure 7.20)
- Fractures involving enamel, dentine and exposure of the pulp.
- Involves laceration and exposure of the pulp to the oral environment.
- Healing does not occur spontaneously and untreated exposures will result in pulp necrosis.

The time elapsed since the injury and the stage of root development will influence treatment. If the tooth is treated within hours of the exposure conservative management is appropriate. After several days, microabscesses occur within the pulp, and more radical pulp amputation is required.

Management
- Periapical radiographs at different angulations.
- Aim is to preserve vital, non-inflamed pulp tissue, biologically walled off by a hard-tissue barrier (Cvek 1978).

In almost all situations, if vital pulp tissue can be covered with a calcium hydroxide dressing, it is possible to form a dentine bridge over the defect. It is undoubtedly preferable to preserve tooth vitality rather than start root canal treatment.

Incomplete root apex with vital pulp
Cvek pulpotomy (apexogenesis) (Figure 7.21)
The Cvek pulpotomy procedure involves the removal of contaminated pulp tissue with a clean round high-speed diamond bur, using saline or water irrigation. A non-setting calcium hydroxide is placed directly onto uncontaminated vital tissue (see step 4 below). The steps are as follows:
1. Local anaesthesia.
2. The use of rubber dam is mandatory.

3. The pulp is washed with saline until the haemorrhage stops. Any clot should then be gently rinsed away.
4. Non-setting calcium hydroxide is placed over the pulp remnant and this is then covered with a setting calcium hydroxide. It is essential that the calcium hydroxide is placed over vital tissue, it must not be placed over a blood clot.
5. Glass ionomer cement base is placed over the dressings and the tooth is restored with composite resin.

This technique does not need to be limited to the coronal pulp. A 'partial pulpotomy' may be performed at any level of the root canal as there are great benefits in preserving the vitality of traumatized incisors.

Review

- 6–8 weeks and then at 12 months with pulp sensibility tests.
- Radiographs at review to check for hard-tissue barrier formation and continued root development (Figure 7.22).

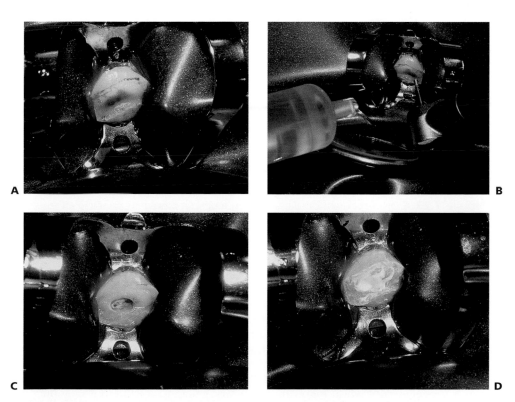

Figure 7.21 Cvek pulpotomy. **A** Traumatic exposure of an upper central incisor. **B** Obtaining access to the pulp chamber with a high-speed diamond bur with copious saline irrigation. **C** Removal of 2 mm of pulpal tissue to a level of vital uncontaminated tissue. **D** Placement of non-setting calcium hydroxide dressing over the vital pulp tissue.

Figure 7.22 A Pulp exposure in an immature central incisor. **B** A Cvek pulpotomy (apexogenesis) has allowed normal root development with a dentine barrier in the crown. This significantly strengthens the root, especially at the cementoenamel junction.

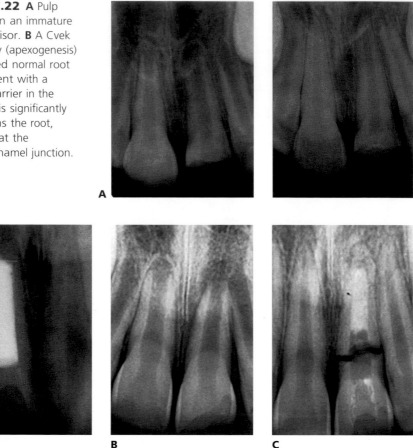

A   B

A   B   C

Figure 7.23 A Open apex root canal treatment is a difficult procedure, requiring an apexification procedure. **B, C** The long-term prognosis of these teeth is poor with over 75% sustaining root fractures within 5 years because of inherent weakness in the cervical region.

Prognosis
- Success rates 80–96%.

Incomplete root apex with necrotic pulp (Figure 7.23)

If the pulp of a tooth with a complicated crown fracture is necrotic then extirpation and root canal treatment is required. Although there is no difference in prognosis of the root filling in immature teeth, compared with mature teeth, long-term survival of any tooth with an open apex is reduced. This is caused by the thin cervical dentine and a shortened root which make the tooth susceptible to fracture not only during endodontic procedures but also during function. Endodontic treatment in immature anterior teeth is difficult because of the inability to create an apical seat, the thin dentinal walls, and the difficulty in obturating the canal by the traditional method of lateral condensation. Fifty per cent of teeth will suffer root fracture within 5 years.

Management
Aim to create an apical hard-tissue barrier (apexification) against which the root canal filling can be placed, by using calcium hydroxide treatment.

Technique (apexification)
1. Local anaesthesia.
2. Create access cavity under rubber dam.
3. Extirpate the necrotic pulp tissue.
4. Mechanically prepare the canal 1 mm short of the radiographic apex.
5. The canal should be carefully instrumented to completely remove necrotic debris, but preserve as much tooth structure as possible. The apical root, being very thin, is weak and may fracture if undue pressure is exerted.
6. Irrigate thoroughly with 1% sodium hypochlorite to dissolve pulp tissue remnants and to disinfect the canal system.
7. Ledermix paste should be placed as the initial dressing followed by calcium hydroxide.
8. Re-dress with non-setting calcium hydroxide paste after 1–2 weeks, with a paste filler.
9. Compress the calcium hydroxide with a cottonwool pellet to ensure good condensation in the canal and to allow contact with apical tissues.
10. Place glass ionomer cement or zinc oxide eugenol (an intermediate restorative material (IRM)) temporary dressing.

Review
Review the child 3–6 monthly. The formation of a calcific bridge may take up to 18 months. Once the bridge has formed the canal may be obturated. The calcium hydroxide should be changed every 2–3 months. This fresh dressing ensures an adequate concentration of calcium hydroxide and reduces the chances of infection.

Obturation is performed with gutta-percha using either a warm vertical condensation technique, or lateral condensation. An impression of the apical seat may be made with softened gutta-percha which is then cemented into the canal with an endodontic sealer. Whichever technique is used, it should be stressed that gentle pressure must be applied to avoid root splitting or pushing the calcified barrier through the apex (Figure 7.23A). Thermoplasticized gutta-percha delivery systems are often invaluable in these cases.

In immature teeth there is occasionally development of a small root apex, although the pulp otherwise appears necrotic. This appears to be caused by surviving remnants of Hertwig's epithelial root sheath.

Mature root apex
If the pulp of a permanent anterior tooth is exposed by trauma, and the period of exposure is short, it need not be removed, regardless of the apical development. The Cvek (partial) pulpotomy can be used to attempt to preserve the vitality of the pulp. If there are restorative considerations (i.e. the need for a post) it may be better to perform a complete extirpation and root canal treatment immediately.

Root fractures

- A fracture involving enamel, dentine and the cementum may or may not involve the pulp. Pulp necrosis occurs in 25% of cases and is related to the degree of displacement of the fragments. Progressive inflammatory or replacement root resorption is rare.
- To check for horizontal root fractures, alter the vertical angulation of periapical radiographs. When looking for vertical root fractures, change the horizontal angulation.
- Sometimes, a horizontal root fracture is not initially evident. This is because the fracture site opens up under the influence of an inflammatory exudate several days after the injury. Thus, for all traumatized teeth it is important to take a subsequent radiograph within 2 weeks (Figure 7.24).

Frequency
- Primary dentition: 0.5–7%.
- Permanent dentition: 2–4%.

Healing of root fractures
- Hard-tissue union with calcified tissue (osseo-dentine).
- Interposition of bone.
- Interposition of fibrous connective tissue.
- Granulation tissue indicating coronal pulp necrosis.

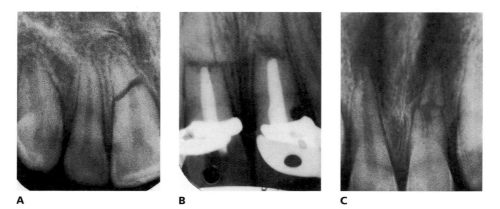

A   **B**   **C**

Figure 7.24 **A** High apical fractures often require no treatment. In most cases the apical fragment is not necrotic. **B** When the coronal fragments are necrotic, root canal treatment should only be performed up to the fracture line. Long-term calcium hydroxide treatment is required because the 'apex' at the fracture site will be wide open. In this case, bone is interposed between the two fragments. **C** Not all coronal fragments become necrotic. Healing of an apical third root fracture. The apical fragment is vital and there has been pulp canal obliteration in the coronal two thirds. In this case, there is probably bone interposed between the two fragments.

Management
- Radiographs – several vertical and/or horizontal angulations of periapical radiographs are usually required to adequately determine the extent of the fracture.
- Repositioning of coronal fragment.
- Rigid splinting with composite resin and wire or orthodontic appliances for at least 4 months if coronal fragment is mobile.
- High apical root fractures often require no treatment.

Review
- Review at 4 weeks, 8 weeks with pulp sensibility testing.
- Remove splint at 4 months.
- Review at 6 months, 12 months and 5 years.
- Radiographs at recall appointment.

Pulp necrosis of coronal fragment
It is uncommon for the apical fragment to develop pulp necrosis. If pulp necrosis of the coronal fragment occurs, there will be radiographic signs of bone loss at the level of the fracture. Other symptoms, such as pain, excessive mobility or gingival swelling and sinus formation, may also be present.
- Extirpate the pulp from coronal fragment to 1 mm below the fracture line. Never advance an instrument through the fracture site.
- Place non-setting calcium hydroxide paste to induce hard-tissue barrier formation at the fracture site (Figure 7.24B). This may take up to 18 months.
- Obturate with gutta-percha once the barrier has formed.

Pulp necrosis of both apical and coronal fragments
When the apical fragment shows signs of necrosis the prognosis is poor. Extirpation and obturation of the coronal fragment should be performed followed by periapical surgery to remove the apical fragment. There have been reports of intra-radicular splinting and endodontic implants, but both have a very poor long-term prognosis.

Crown/root fractures

The coronal fragments should always be removed to fully assess the extent of the fracture (Figure 7.25).

Uncomplicated crown/root fracture
Where the fracture extends just below the gingival margin, cover the dentine with a glass ionomer initially and then restore the tooth with composite resin or a crown.

Complicated crown/root fracture (pulp exposure)
If the fracture extends below the crestal bone and the root development is complete remove the coronal fragments to assess the extent of the fracture and extirpate the pulp. Calcium hydroxide or Ledermix paste may be placed as the initial endodontic dressing.

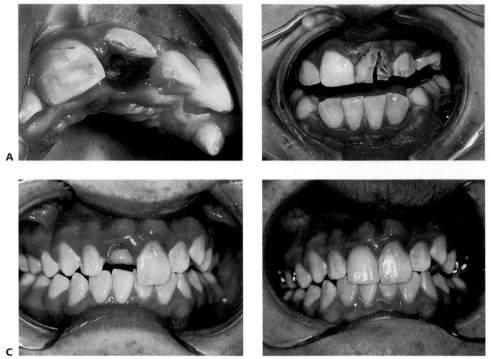

Figure 7.25 A The coronal fragment of a crown/root fracture should always be removed to investigate the extent of the fracture. In this case it is just above the alveolar crest on the palate, about 4 mm below the gingival margin. Treatment will involve periodontal-flap surgery and placement of a crown with an extended shoulder. Alternatively, orthodontic extrusion may be required. **B** Vertical fractures are virtually untreatable. They may be held together with an orthodontic band or composite resin, but their prognosis is very poor. Retention in the short term may be valuable to preserve bone while planning for possible orthodontics, or implants, when growth has finished. **C** A crown/root fracture in an immature tooth with a poor prognosis. **D** A removable appliance was constructed with the pontic covering the retained root. Retention of the root will maintain alveolar bone prior to the consideration of long-term restorative needs.

If the crown/root fracture does not extend below the crestal bone, and the root development is complete, a Cvek pulpotomy may be performed. This type of fracture may be restorable with composite resin whereas the more deeply extending fracture may need a cast restoration or necessitate surgical treatment.

The prognosis for a tooth with a complicated crown/root fracture is poor.

Options for management
- Gingivectomy to expose fracture margin. If the fracture is minimal, and just below the gingival margin, then restoration of the root surface may be performed with glass ionomer cement and a crown build-up in composite resin.
- Cast crown with extended shoulder with or without periodontal flap procedure.

- Orthodontic extrusion of the root to expose the fracture margin.
- Extraction.
- Root burial.

Orthodontic extrusion

This may be a viable option in management provided there is adequate root length to support a crown. A gingivoplasty will almost always be required to reposition the gingival margin after the completion of retention. Fixed appliances are placed to extrude the root so that the margin is exposed. Retention may be difficult and a pericision is advisable. Because of the narrower emergence profile of the root compared with the crown of a normal tooth, a satisfactory aesthetic result may be difficult to achieve.

Root burial or decoronation (Figure 7.26)

In cases of subalveolar root fracture, root burial (decoronation) may be an alternative to extraction to preserve alveolar bone. The root is buried below the alveolar crest and a coronally repositioned flap raised to cover the defect with periosteum. In this way, it is possible for bone to grow over the root surface (Figure 7.26E). The root may be vital or obturated with gutta-percha. This technique in valuable in the preservation of labiopalatal width, that may be essential if an osseointegrated implant is required later. It may negate the need for ridge augmentation.

Crown/root fractures in immature teeth

When complex crown/root fractures occur in teeth with incomplete apical formation, consideration should be given to maintaining the pulp vitality, where possible, to allow continuation of root development. However, if the pulp has undergone necrosis and infection, then endodontic treatment including apexification will be necessary. It is worth noting, however, that complicated crown/root fractures tend to occur in mature teeth where consideration of apical development is unnecessary. As a general comment, if the complex fracture extends below the crestal bone then the prognosis is poor.

Luxations in the permanent dentition

Concussion and subluxation

These teeth are treated symptomatically. Concussed teeth will have a marked response to percussion, but the tooth will be firm in the socket. A subluxated tooth will exhibit increased mobility but will not have been displaced and there are no radiographic abnormalities. They are tender to percussion and mobility is usually increased.

Management

- Relieve from occlusion, splinting is not usually required.
- Soft diet for 2 weeks.

Review

- Pulp sensibility testing at 1, 3 and 12 months.
- Radiographs at each review.
- It is important to follow up these teeth for at least 12 months clinically, checking pulpal status, colour, mobility and radiographically assessing changes in the size of the pulp chamber and in root development.

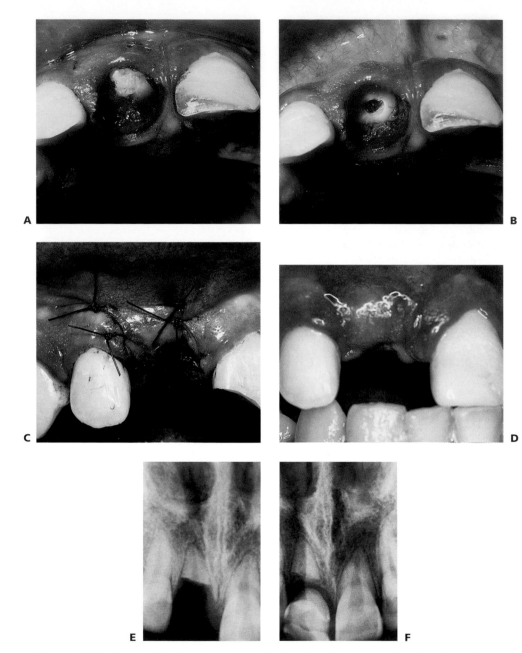

Figure 7.26 Root burial of a tooth fractured below the alveolar crest. Root burial may be an alternative to extraction in these cases. **A** This root has been traumatized with the fracture extending from the gingival margin on the labial to a level below the alveolar crest on the palatal. **B** The root is sectioned 1–2 mm below the crestal bone, and **C** covered with a coronally repositioned mucoperiosteal flap. **D** Healing after 2 weeks. **E, F** Bone growth has been stimulated over the root. This preserves the alveolar height for later prosthodontic work. The original crown has been contoured and attached to adjacent teeth with composite resin.

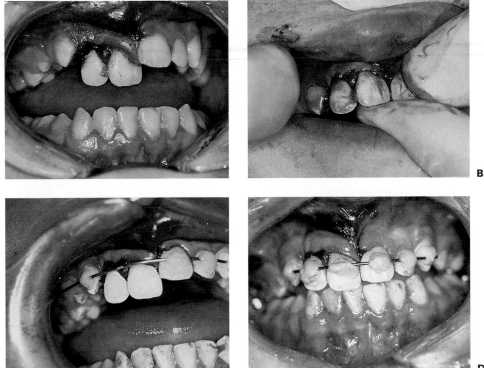

Figure 7.27 A Lateral luxation (palatal) with a dentoalveolar component involving the upper right central and lateral incisors. **B** The block of teeth and bone is manually replaced with finger pressure. **C, D** A rigid composite resin and wire splint is placed. When placing a splint, attach and stabilize uninvolved teeth before splinting the displaced segment.

Prognosis
- Pulp necrosis in 3–6%.

Lateral and extrusive luxation
Teeth may be luxated in any direction and, depending on the extent of luxation, the teeth may need repositioning and splinting. This can be achieved with digital pressure or with forceps. If the latter are used, care must be taken to avoid damage to the root surface and the tooth should be held by the crown only. The teeth will be visibly displaced, potentially mobile with radiographic changes in the periodontal ligament. Pulp sensibility tests may give negative results initially.

Management
1. Repositioning with local anaesthesia. Early repositioning is important (Figure 7.27A, B) as it is often extremely difficult to mobilize the tooth if the patient presents after 24 hours.
2. Suture gingival lacerations.

3. Flexible splinting with composite resin, and wire (Figure 7.24C, D) or orthodontic appliances, for 2 weeks for extrusive luxation, and 4 weeks for lateral luxation because of concomitant alveolar bone fracture.
4. Antibiotics, tetanus prophylaxis, and 0.2% chlorhexidine gluconate mouthrinse if required.

Lateral luxations always have a component of dentoalveolar fracture and it is important to mould the bone back into the correct position. Those fragments of bone attached to periosteum should be retained.

Review
- Review every 2 weeks while the splint is in place, then 1, 3, 6 and 12 monthly up to 5 years.
- Pulp sensibility testing.
- Radiographs at each visit.

Prognosis
- Dependent on the degree of displacement and apical development, with excellent healing in immature teeth.
- Pulp necrosis occurs in 15–85% of cases and is more prevalent in teeth with closed apices.
- Pulp canal obliteration often occurs in teeth with immature apices.
- Resorption is rare.
- Transient apical breakdown (2–12%) is an expansion of the apical periodontal ligament space. There is no indication for starting root canal treatment, unless there are other indicators of infection of the pulp canal.

Intrusion
Intrusion (caused by the compression of the root into alveolar bone) is one of the worst injuries that can occur. There is extensive damage to the supporting structures and the neurovascular bundle. There is much discussion about whether intrusively luxated teeth should be repositioned or allowed to re-erupt on their own. Treatment may well depend on the state of apical development and, as a general rule, the partial disimpaction and flexible splinting of severely intruded teeth with incomplete root formation is preferred.

Management
Current opinion suggests that early repositioning of intruded permanent teeth is essential. The aims of disimpaction are to avoid ankylosis, minimize pressure necrosis of the periodontal ligament and allow access to the palatal surface of the tooth to extirpate the pulp within 21 days.

Repositioning
Teeth with incomplete root formation
- If the crown remains visible and there is a very wide immature apex (>2 mm) the tooth may be allowed to re-erupt spontaneously.
- If there is no improvement in position then rapid orthodontic repositioning.
- (Gentle) surgical repositioning may be required to mobilize the tooth.

Teeth with complete root formation

- Immediate repositioning is preferred for mature teeth.
- Fixed orthodontic appliances can be used to apply traction to the intruded tooth over a 2-week period (Figure 7.28)

OR

- Gently reposition the tooth with fingers or with forceps applied only to the crown. Avoid rotating the tooth in the socket.
- Extrusion should be rapid so that the palatal surface is exposed and an access cavity can be made.

Endodontics

- Extirpation of the pulp is essential in almost all cases. Ledermix paste should be placed as the initial dressing for up to 3 months, followed by calcium hydroxide for 3 months before obturation.
- If the apex is immature, then a further period of calcium-hydroxide therapy will be required for apexification before root-canal obturation.
- The only exceptions are partially intruded extremely immature teeth which are being left to re-erupt (with regular monitoring).

Review

- It is essential that these teeth are regularly followed up. Progressive inflammatory resorption occurs very rapidly and an immature tooth may be lost within a number of weeks.
- Review every 2 weeks during mobilization phase, then at 6–8 weeks, 6 months, 12 months and yearly for 5 years.

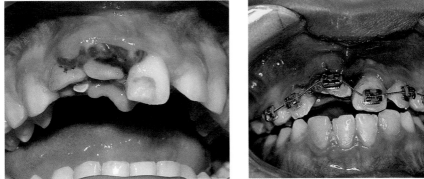

A   B

Figure 7.28 A Intrusion of the upper right permanent incisors and canine. This child was involved in a motor vehicle accident and unfortunately no dental treatment was available. At presentation, 2 months later, the intruded teeth had become ankylosed and could not be moved orthodontically. They subsequently underwent replacement resorption and a denture was constructed. Early mobilization is essential to prevent ankylosis and allow access to the palatal surface to perform pulp extirpation. **B** An example of orthodontic appliances being used to extrude a partially intruded tooth. If the crown is completely intruded, a flap should be raised and the tooth mobilized surgically.

Prognosis
- Mature teeth undergo pulp necrosis in almost all cases (96%), and there is a high prevalence of root resorption and ankylosis.
- Immature teeth that re-erupt show pulp necrosis in 60% of cases and ankylosis in up to 50% of cases.
- Teeth treated early have a much better prognosis.

Dentoalveolar fractures
With luxation of teeth, the alveolar plate can be fractured or deformed. Use firm finger pressure on the buccal and lingual plates to reposition. It should be remembered that alveolar fractures can occur without significant dental involvement. These alveolar fractures should be splinted for 4 weeks in children (or 6–8 weeks in adults). Luxated or avulsed teeth usually result in alveolar bone fracture and/or displacement. Firm pressure is needed to realign bony fragments. Splinting may be rigid or semi-rigid and is dependent on the degree of injury and the numbers of teeth involved.

Pulp vitality
Current pulp sensibility tests only test the ability of the pulpal nerves to respond to the stimulus; they do not provide any information about the presence or absence of blood supply or the histological status of the pulp. When determining the status of the pulp in luxated permanent teeth beware of false test results. Negative results may arise because of damage of sensory nerves of the pulp, even though the tooth's vascularity is maintained. It may take up to 1 year (or never) to get a positive response from such a pulp. Thus, one must be careful to judge the patient's signs and symptoms before commencing endodontics. Regular radiographs are required to assess root development and growth, evidence of external or internal root resorption, and changes in the shape of the pulp chamber. Clinically, changes in colour, excess mobility, tenderness to percussion and sinus formation are important diagnostic signs.

Radiographs
It is important to remember that when teeth have been luxated they may have had a crown or root fracture. The crown fractures are usually obvious but root fractures may be hidden or not yet apparent. Therefore, radiographs are always essential.

Avulsion of permanent teeth

If a permanent incisor is avulsed, the chance of successful retention is enhanced by minimizing the extra-oral time. Even if the tooth has been out of the mouth for an extended period, it is usually still better to replant the tooth, with the knowledge that success might be unlikely. In the mixed dentition this is important, as replantation of even questionable teeth will allow normal establishment of the arch and occlusion. Furthermore, orthodontic treatment planning is simpler if the tooth remains in the socket. These teeth are usually lost by replacement resorption, which has the benefit of preserving the alveolar bone height, making prosthodontic replacement much simpler.

First aid advice

Always check the patient's clothing for avulsed teeth that are thought to be lost. It is important that parents, caregivers and teachers have access to appropriate advice on the management of avulsed teeth. Timing is essential and this information can be given over the telephone:

- Keep the child calm.
- Do not allow the child to eat or drink. If sedation or anaesthesia is required in extensive injuries then the child may need to be fasted.
- Locate the tooth and hold by the crown only.
- Replant the tooth immediately if clean. If the tooth is dirty, it should be washed briefly under cold water (10 seconds only) or with milk if available.
- Hold the tooth in place by biting gently on a handkerchief or clean cloth, or use some aluminium foil or similar and seek urgent dental treatment.
- If unable to replant, store the tooth in isotonic media to prevent dehydration and death of the periodontal ligament cells. Use:
  - preferably milk or
  - saline (i.e. contact lens solution) or hold in the mouth adjacent the molars
  - wrap in plastic cling wrap
  - **do not use water** as this will result in hypotonic lysis of ligament cells.
- Seek urgent dental treatment.

Time is essential! The long-term prognosis of the tooth is severely reduced after 10 minutes. Do not waste time searching for an ideal storage medium, replant the tooth!

Management in the dental surgery

The following are guidelines for replanting avulsed permanent teeth (after Flores et al (IADT) 2007a,b).

Tooth replanted prior to arrival

Debride the mouth but do not extract the tooth.

Tooth maintained in storage solution with extra-oral time less than 60 minutes

1. Gently debride the root surface under copious saline, milk or tissue-culture media (Hanks balanced salt solution) irrigation. When holding teeth always do so by the crown in a wet gauze square (teeth can be very slippery, see Figure 7.29A).
2. Give local anaesthesia and gently debride the tooth socket with saline, taking care not to curette the bone or remaining ligament (Figure 7.29B).
3. Replant the tooth gently under finger pressure. The tooth usually 'clicks' back into the correct position if there has not been too much bony damage (Figure 7.29C).

Tooth is dry or extra-oral time is greater than 60 minutes

1. Remove any necrotic periodontal ligament with a wet gauze.
2. Extirpate the pulp prior to replantation.
3. Give local anaesthesia and gently debride the tooth socket with saline, taking care not to curette the bone or remaining ligament.
4. Replant the tooth gently under finger pressure.

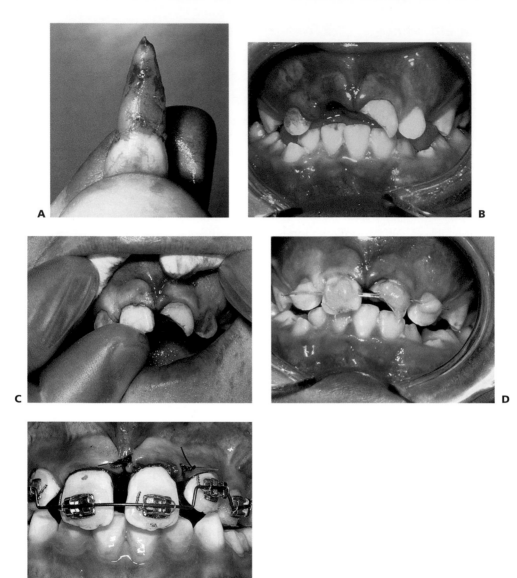

Figure 7.29 Management of avulsion. **A** Always hold the tooth by the crown and gently debride the root surface with saline. **B** The socket should be irrigated and clear of debris. **C** Replant with firm pressure. The tooth will usually click back into position. **D** Splint with a flexible splint, such as composite and nylon fishing line, to allow some physiological movement. **E** Orthodontic appliances are extremely useful when splinting traumatized teeth. The wire should be passive and allow physiological movement. Placement of a wire through orthodontic brackets allows the splint to be removed and the mobility of the tooth assessed.

Management following replantation

1. Splint for 14 days (Figure 7.29D).
2. Reposition any degloved gingival tissues and suture if required.
3. Prescribe high-dose, broad-spectrum antibiotics and check current immunization status.
4. Account for any lost teeth. A chest radiograph may be required.
5. Normal diet and strict oral hygiene including chlorhexidine gluconate 0.2% mouthwash.

Splinting of avulsed teeth

- Composite resin and nylon fibre (0.6 mm diameter) such as fishing line (20 kg breaking strain)

or

- Orthodontic brackets with archwire (0.014"). Orthodontic appliances are particularly useful as the time taken to apply the brackets is half that to set composite resin.

Splints should be flexible to allow normal physiological movement of the tooth. This helps to reduce the development of ankylosis; however, if there is a bone or root fracture present, then a rigid splint must be used so that there is no movement of the teeth and bony segments.

Splints should generally stay in place for 14 days if there are no complicating factors such as alveolar or root fractures. Avulsed teeth with immature apices that are dry may require splinting up to 4 weeks. The occlusion may need to be relieved when the degree of overbite or luxation is such that the tooth will receive unwanted masticatory force. This can be achieved by minimal removal of enamel, or construction of an upper removable appliance, or placement of composite resin on the molars to open the bite. However, some physiological movement is necessary.

Replanting of dry teeth

As a general rule, all teeth should be replanted whether wet or dry. Although the prognosis of the tooth may be poor, it is usually preferable to have the tooth present for 5 years during growth than not at all. Always keep options open for future treatment.

1. Gently remove the dead periodontal ligament with wet gauze.
2. Do not scale or root plane the cementum at all.
3. Create access cavity and extirpate the pulp.
4. Rinse the tooth in 2% sodium fluoride (pH 5.5) for 20 minutes. The aim is to incorporate fluoride into the dentine and cementum that may reduce ankylosis.
5. Place Ledermix paste in the root canal.
6. Replant and splint for 14 days.
7. Replace the Ledermix with calcium hydroxide after 3 months and complete the root canal filling after 6–12 months if there is no sign of inflammatory resorption.

Endodontics

Immature root apex

If the tooth has been avulsed, replanted within a short period and the apex is **extremely** immature (>2 mm) and the child is <8 years, endodontic treatment is only needed if the symptoms and clinical signs indicate that the pulp space has become infected.

If the canal becomes infected, Ledermix is placed initially for 3 months and then calcium hydroxide treatment commenced to induce apexification. The calcium hydroxide should be non-setting and placed so as to fill the radicular pulp space, and sealed with Cavit or glass ionomer cement. This is changed 3-monthly until an apical barrier is formed and obturation is possible. The rate of survival of immature teeth is only 30% even if replanted early.

Mature root apex
In all other situations, in which the apex of the avulsed tooth is less than 2 mm open or closed, endodontics should be commenced within 2 weeks. Initial dressings should be Ledermix paste for 3 months followed by calcium hydroxide. The root canal filling should be completed after 6–12 months.

Generally, it is best to always replant teeth even if they have a poor prognosis. With appropriate treatment, these teeth will be lost by progressive replacement resorption, the positive benefit being that alveolar height is maintained. The only exceptions are those cases with very immature roots where ankylosis will prevent alveolar bone growth and may complicate future orthodontic and prosthodontic management.

Complications in endodontic management of avulsed teeth

External inflammatory root resorption (Figure 7.30A)
- The progressive loss of tooth structure by an inflammatory process caused by the presence of infected and necrotic debris in the root canal.
- This resorption can be prevented or managed with appropriate treatment.
  Factors in prevention and management include:
- **Prophylactic antibiotics**: high-dose, broad-spectrum antibiotics (amoxicillin) should be given as soon as possible after avulsion and continued for 2 weeks. The benefits of tetracyclines are controversial and these should be avoided in children where staining of other teeth may occur.
- **Pulp extirpation**: This should be completed as soon as possible after the replantation. It may be done at the time of trauma, but not outside the mouth. It must be done within 10 days.

Avoid medicaments that may cause inflammation, such as calcium hydroxide, in the first 3 months after trauma. Ledermix paste is an ideal first-dressing medicament as it has been shown to prevent inflammatory root resorption and inhibit the action of clastic cells.

Management
If inflammatory resorption is detected the canal must be thoroughly re-instrumented and dressed with Ledermix paste for 3 months, but changing the dressing every 6 weeks. Calcium hydroxide can then be placed for a further 3 months after which time, if there is no progression of the resorption, the canal can be filled.

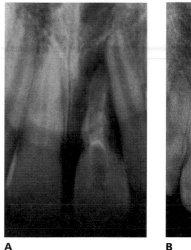
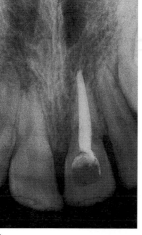
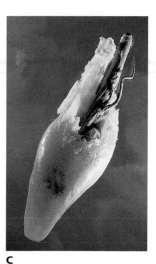

A   **B**   **C**

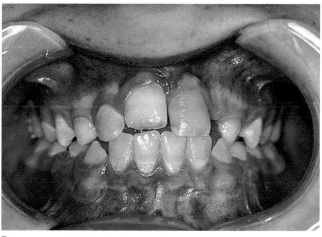

D

Figure 7.30 A Inflammatory root resorption resulting from a failure to adequately instrument and medicate the root canal. **B** The root is being replaced by bone around the gutta-percha root filling. Note the slight infraocclusion of this tooth. **C** Replacement resorption of an avulsed central incisor. Note the ankylosed bone on the labial aspect of the root. **D** Ankylosis and subsequent infraocclusion is a significant problem when permanent teeth are traumatized before the cessation of growth. There is retardation of alveolar growth and the tooth is ultimately lost.

External replacement root resorption (Figure 7.30B–D)

This is the progressive resorption of tooth structure, and replacement with bone, as part of continual bone remodelling. It results from cemental damage greater than 2 mm or from replantation of dry teeth. It cannot be treated, so the aim must be to prevent replacement resorption and subsequent ankylosis. Factors in prevention and management include:

- **Extra-oral time**: prognosis decreases dramatically after 15 minutes if tooth is dry. Fifty per cent of periodontal ligament cells are dead after 30 minutes. All are dead after 60 minutes.
- **Storage media**
  - Milk is the best medium and may keep cells viable for up to 6 hours. It has the advantage that it is pasteurized, with few bacteria, is readily available and is cold. There appears to be no difference between low-fat and skimmed milk, but yoghurt and sour milk should be avoided.
  - Saliva is suitable for up to 2 hours.
  - Saline and plastic cling wrap will maintain cells for 1 hour.
  - Water is hypotonic and causes cell lysis.
  - Tissue culture media such as Hank's balanced-salt solution or RPMI (1640 (Roswell Park Memorial Institute tissue culture medium) is also appropriate, if available, and may give up to 24 hours' cell survival.
- **Mechanical damage**: ankylosis will result if >2 mm of cementum has been removed or damaged.
- Risk increases with increased handling during transport and replantation.
- **Splinting**: flexible splinting allows physiological movement and results in less ankylosis and replacement resorption.

Management
- No treatment is possible.

Future options for management of resorption
Emdogain
The use of enamel matrix protein derivatives has been proposed in the management of avulsed teeth. Emdogain is a commercially available porcine enamel matrix derivative which has been successfully used to treat periodontal defects. The enamel matrix derivative composed of amelogenins has a key role in both enamel formation and the development of acellular cementum. Amelogenins are secreted from Hertwig's epithelial root sheath cells initiating the formation of cementum which provides the foundation for periodontal ligament attachment to the tooth. Emdogain has been shown to be successful in the treatment of buccal dehiscence lesions in monkeys and periodontal defects in humans. As a result of this early success, there was hope that the product would reduce ankylosis in avulsed teeth. However, recent research has tempered the initial enthusiasm and questioned its clinical benefit (Schjøtt & Andreasen 2005).

Alendronate
This is another topical agent that may show promise. It is a third generation bisphosphonate which exhibits osteoclastic inhibitory activity.

Both these products may allow regeneration of the periodontal ligament and inhibit or prevent replacement resorption that is the major cause of tooth loss after avulsion.

Questions concerning the management of avulsed teeth
- Despite a plethora of literature supporting the different procedures for managing avulsed teeth, the clinical reality remains that teeth that have been out of the mouth for more than 30 minutes have a poor prognosis.

- There is good evidence to support the use of specialized storage media, however, they are rarely available at the scene of an accident. Anecdotally, many dental injuries occur on weekends during sport. It is interesting to calculate the average time taken to get a traumatized child to a dentist on a Saturday afternoon.
- There is a social cost following trauma including absence from school (for the child) and work (for the parent) in attending multiple appointments, and self-esteem. There are also financial considerations of complex restorative and endodontic treatment for teeth that often have a very poor outcome.

Parents and children should be given a clear indication about the probably outcome of treatment. Heroic work is often performed with all good intentions when the prognosis is questionable (Barrett & Kenny 1997). In some cases it will be preferable to retain hopeless teeth where replacement resorption will preserve bone. In other cases, the retardation of alveolar bone growth accompanying ankylosis in a growing child may necessitate early removal. Consider the following questions:

- What is the long-term prognosis of the tooth?
- Are there orthodontic considerations such as the implications of ankylosis or space loss?
- Is the tooth important in the development of the occlusion?

Always keep your options open.

Autotransplantation (Figure 7.31)

Autotransplantation has been successfully used in the management of tooth loss following trauma. It may be used in management of complicated crown/root fractures, replacement of the missing anterior teeth, and after avulsion injuries.

Good case selection is essential.

Indications
- Traumatized anterior tooth with poor long-term prognosis.
- Cases with Class I or Class II malocclusion with moderate to severe crowding involving extraction of premolars. Autotransplantation must be considered as part of an overall treatment plan for the patient and other alternatives such as orthodontic space closure, fixed and removable prosthodontics and osseo-integrated implant placement must be considered.

Success rates
- 94% success rate for open apex.
- 84% success rate for closed apex.

Procedure for autotransplantation
1. Selection of donor tooth (Table 7.2).
2. Analysis of recipient site:
   - size and shape of recipient area
   - need for socket expansion or instrumentation

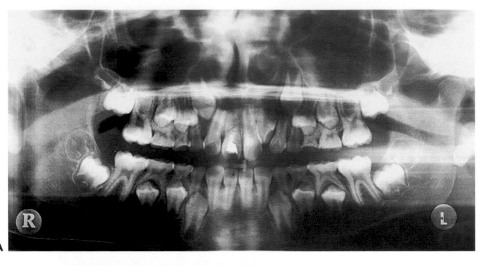

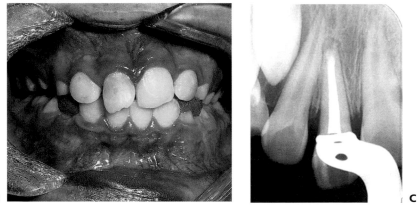

Figure 7.31 Autotransplantation. **A** The upper right central incisor in this boy was avulsed and undergoing resorption. A supplemental lateral incisor was present lying palatal to the upper left central incisor. This tooth was autotransplanted into the socket of the traumatized central. **B** Healing after 2 months. **C** Completion of root canal therapy at 6 months post op showing good bone and periodontal healing.

- stage of root development
- optimal time for transplantation when root is ½ to ¾ formed.
3. Surgical procedure:
   - remove the traumatized incisor
   - prepare the socket – the socket can be enlarged if required and then irrigated with saline. Any necrotic or foreign debris such as gutta-percha, intracanal medicaments, or granulation tissue must be removed
   - extract the donor tooth (usually premolar)

Table 7.2 Selection of donor tooth for autotransplantation

Donor tooth	Recipient site
Third molars	First molars
Lower first premolar	Upper central incisor
Lower second premolar	Upper lateral incisor
Supernumerary/supplemental teeth	Upper incisors
Lower incisors	Upper lateral incisor
Upper premolars	Depends on root shape

- make an incision into the periodontal ligament through the gingival margin. a collar of attached gingiva may be included with the graft
- gently extract the tooth, avoiding damage to the root surface
- position donor tooth into recipient site. This usually involves rotation of a pre-molar tooth about 45°
- splint with a flexible splint
- follow-up as per protocols for avulsed teeth.

The need for endodontic treatment will depend on the degree of root development (see Table 7.3).

Reasons for failure
- Inflammatory or replacement ankylosis:
  - closed apex – 20% root resorption
  - open apex – 3% root resorption.
- Pulp necrosis.
- Infraocclusion.
- Incomplete root formation.
- No primary healing.

Details of healing and prognosis are shown in Table 7.3.

Bleaching of non-vital incisors

One consequence of loss or trauma is tooth discoloration. Bleaching is a common procedure following root canal treatment. The integrity of the root canal seal is paramount and, above all, bleaching should not be carried out below the cementoenamel junction because of the risk of initiating cervical resorption.

Method
1. Bleaching must be carried out under rubber dam.
2. Ensure adequate root canal obturation and remove gutta-percha to a level 3 mm below the cementoenamel junction.

Table 7.3 Healing and prognosis after autotransplantation of premolars

Root development	Root resorption		Pulp revascularization	Root formation
	Inflammatory resorption	**Replacement resorption**		
Stage 1 Initial root formation				77% normal root length
Stage 2 ¼ root formation	3%	6%	100% pulp revascularization	66% arrested root formation
Stage 3 ½ root formation				88% normal root length
Stage 4 ¾ root formation			87% pulp revascularization	Up to 98% normal root length
Stage 5 Root formation complete with apical foramen wide open	9%	18%	No revascularization	Up to 98% normal root length
Stage 6 Root formation complete with apical foramen half closed				
Stage 7 Root formation complete with apical foramen closed	25%	38%	0% pulp revascularization	Complete root development

After: Andreasen et al (1990).

3. Place a zinc phosphate or Cavit base just above the cementoenamel junction.
4. Ensure that the access cavity is clean and free of all debris.
5. Acid etch the access cavity to open dentinal tubules and place a cotton pellet soaked in 30% hydrogen peroxide into the access cavity for 3 minutes.
6. Remove the cotton pellet and place a mixture of sodium perborate and hydrogen peroxide into the cavity and seal with a cotton pellet and temporary sealer such as Cavit. The perborate powder and peroxide is mixed to form a thick paste that can be packed into the chamber. This should remain in the tooth for 1 week, after

which the success of the procedure is evaluated. This may be repeated several times if required.

7. The pulp chamber is then filled with a glass ionomer base and the access cavity restored with composite resin.

Soft-tissue injuries

Alveolar mucosa and skin

Bruising (Figure 7.32)

The simplest and most common type of soft-tissue injury is bruising. This will often be present without any dental involvement. Treatment is symptomatic. However, be careful to check in the depths of the labial and buccal sulci for any deep soft-tissue wounds or degloving-type injuries.

Lacerations (Figures 7.33, 7.34)

- Often a full-thickness laceration of the lower lip can be undetected because of the natural contours of the soft tissues or the tentative examination of an upset child. If there has been dental injury, always look for tooth remnants in the lips.
- Careful suturing of skin wounds will be needed to avoid scarring and should be performed only by those who are competent to do so. Skin wounds must be closed within the first 24 hours and preferably within 6 hours.
- Any debris, such as gravel and dirt, must be removed by scrubbing with a brush wetted with an antiseptic surgical preparation such as 2.5% povidone iodine or 0.5% chlorhexidine acetate.
- Skin edges are ideally excised with a scalpel to remove necrotic tags and irregular margins.

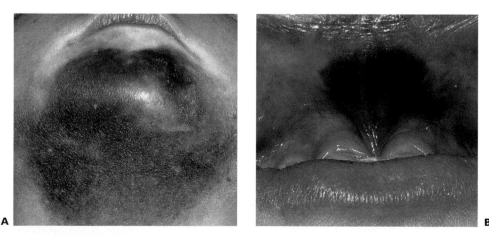

A   B

Figure 7.32 **A** Bruising of the chin is usually associated with severe degloving (see Figure 7.35B). **B** Bruising of the labial frenum may occur from a blow across the face; child abuse should always be suspected.

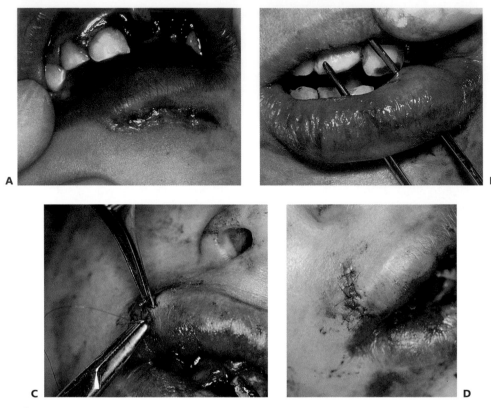

Figure 7.33 A When upper teeth are intruded, the lip is often bitten and a through-and-through laceration should be identified. **B** These lacerations must be closed in three layers: the muscle, mucosa and skin. Always check lip lacerations for the presence of any tooth fragments if there are fractured teeth. **C, D** When closing lacerations that cross the lip margin it is essential to reposition the vermillion border first. The remainder of the defect can be closed with interrupted nylon 6-0 sutures.

- Muscle closure and deep suturing is achieved with a fine resorbable material such as polyglactin or polyglycolic acid.
- Final skin closure is with 6-0 monofilament nylon on a cutting needle.

Attached gingival tissues
Degloving (Figure 7.35)
One of the most common injuries is degloving. A full-thickness mucoperiosteal flap is stripped off the bone, the separation line usually being the mucogingival junction (Figure 7.35A). These injuries tend to occur after blunt trauma and a common presentation is a large collection of blood in the submental region (Figure 7.32A). The flap is tightly sutured and a pressure dressing placed if the lower arch is involved. This prevents the pooling of blood and prevents swelling in the submental region, which may embarrass the airway.

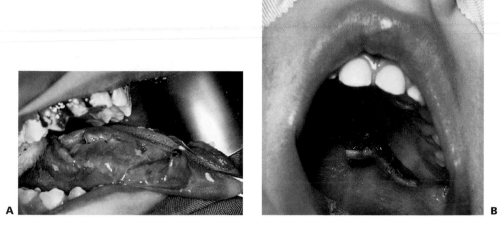

Figure 7.34 A Lacerations may be caused by self-mutilation. This child has a peripheral sensory neuropathy (congenital indifference to pain). Attempts to make splints that would stop her behaviour failed and, after much agonizing, a full clearance was performed. **B** A severe laceration of the palate caused by this child falling with a straw in her mouth. In many cases, small lacerations will granulate and heal without intervention, however, large ones require suturing.

Interdental suturing of displaced gingival tissue is very important, especially where palatal tissue is involved. The close re-adaptation of tissues to the tooth surface will help preserve alveolar bone especially interdentally. Suturing will also help keep the tooth in position.

Suturing (see Table 7.4)
Suturing of torn or lacerated gingival tissues should be considered using a fine suture such as 5-0 resorbable suture (Dexon or Vicryl). Polyglactin or polyglycolic acid sutures have good traction strength for at least 3 weeks and have less tissue reaction than catgut. As a braided material they are not as clean as monofilament sutures, but they are resorbable. Where strength is required, and removal of the sutures is not an issue, monofilament nylon is an excellent material.

Suturing may prevent a periodontal defect from lack of keratinized tissue, or at least reduce the extent of periodontal work subsequently required. Suturing may reduce the sequestration of displaced bony fragments and may prevent bacterial contamination of the gingival sulcus. Furthermore, there is much less pain from the wound if exposed bony defects are well covered with periosteum and gingival tissues.

Prevention

Education of parents and caregivers
- Seat belts and child restraints.
- Helmets for bike riding.

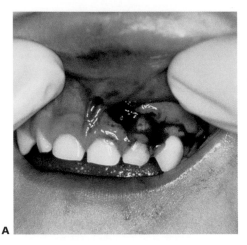

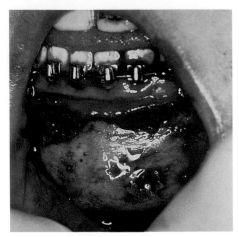

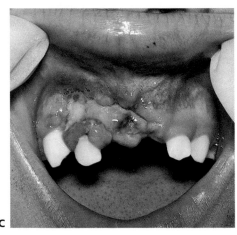

Figure 7.35 A Gingival degloving in a young child. Small tears such as this can be repositioned without suturing and will granulate well. **B** Severe degloving of the mandible separating at the mucogingival junction from molar to molar and to the level of the hyoid. The mental nerve on the left was severed. **C** Inadequate repositioning of degloving injury has resulted in delayed healing and soft tissue loss. It is essential that these injuries should be treated early.

- Mouthguards.
- Supervision of pets, especially dogs.

While seat belts and child restraints are covered by legislation, and more recently helmets for bike riders became mandatory in Australia, the failure of parents to observe these regulations often results in unnecessary childhood craniofacial trauma. It has been the authors' experience that there is often little trauma seen from sports, as most children are wearing mouthguards; nevertheless, there is a disproportionate amount of trauma seen from leisure activities such as skateboarding, swimming and other 'non-contact' sports.

Educating parents, caregivers and teachers about primary care for dental trauma is essential. The correct protocols for dealing with avulsed teeth should be available to all schools.

Table 7.4 Some indications for the selection of suture materials in paediatric dentistry

Suture	Indications	Size	Needle	Absorption	Tissue reaction	Notes
Surgical gut	Extraction suture	3-0	Cutting	Completely digested by 70 days. Effective strength for 2–3 days in the oral cavity	Moderate	Used for tissue closure where strength is required for 1–2 days
Chromic catgut	General closure	4-0	Taper	Completely digested by 110 days, but in the oral cavity it has effective strength for up to 5 days	Moderate but less than plain gut	Excellent for oral tissue closure when longer life is required compared with plain gut
Polyglycolic acid	Alveolar mucosa	4-0 5-0	Taper	Completely absorbed by hydrolysis after 90 days. Faster absorption when exposed to the oral environment. Good strength for a least 2 weeks.	Mild	Polyglycolic acid has great advantages for use in the oral cavity in children. It has good strength over 7 days and is resorbable. It is often retained for longer periods, however, and has a tendency to accumulate plaque due to its braided nature Taper needles are useful where tissues are friable
Polyglactin	Attached gingiva	3-0 4-0	Cutting			
	Large flaps where strength is required but a resorbable suture is desirable	3-0	Cutt ng			
Monofilament Nylon	Large flaps where strength is required (i.e. palate)	3-0 4-0	Cutting	Essentially a non-resorbable material, but degrades at 15–20% per year	Extremely low	Excellent tissue reaction and strength Monofilament material is extremely clean and allows good would healing but needs to be removed
	Skin	6-0	Cutting			Skin closure must be performed with 6-0. Sutures should be removed before 7 days
Surgical silk	General closure of most oral tissues where a non–resorbable suture is required	3-0 4-0	Cutting	Is completely degraded by 2 years	Moderate	Traditional suture material, used where strength was required Its use has diminished with the availability of materials such as polyglycolic acid Is a braided material and therefore not as clean as monofilament

References and further reading

Assessment

Gassner R, Tuli T, Hächl O et al 2004 Craniomaxillofacial trauma in children: a review of 3,385 cases with 6,060 injuries in 10 years. Journal of Oral and Maxillofacial Surgery 62:399–407

Hall R 1994 Pediatric orofacial medicine and pathology. Chapman and Hall Medical, London

Kopel HM, Johnson R 1985 Examination and neurological assessment of children with orofacial trauma. Endodontics and Dental Traumatology 18:252–268

Schatz JP, Joho JP 1994 A retrospective study of dento-alveolar injuries. Endodontics and Dental Traumatology 10:11–14

Stockwell AJ 1988 Incidence of dental trauma in the Western Australian School Dental Service. Community Dentistry and Oral Epidemiology 16:294–298

Facial fractures

Ferreira P, Marques M, Pinho C et al 2004 Midfacial fractures in children and adolescents: a review of 492 cases. British Journal of Oral and Maxillofacial Surgery 42:501–505

Posnick JC, Wells M, Pron GE 1993 Pediatric facial fractures: evolving patterns of treatment. Journal of Oral and Maxillofacial Surgery 51:836–844

Schweinfurth JM, Koltai PJ 1998 Pediatric mandibular fractures. Facial and Plastic Surgery 14:31–44

Zachariades N, Mezitis M, Mourouzis C et al 2006 Fractures of the mandibular condyle: a review of 466 cases. Literature review, reflections on treatment and proposals. Journal of Craniomaxillofacial Surgery 34:421–432

Zimmermann CE, Troulis MJ, Kaban LB 2006 Pediatric facial fractures: recent advances in prevention, diagnosis and management. International Journal of Oral and Maxillofacial Surgery 35:2–13

Child abuse

American Academy of Pediatrics Committee on Child Abuse and Neglect; American Academy of Pediatric Dentistry; American Academy of Pediatric Dentistry Council on Clinical Affairs 2005–2006 2005 Guideline on oral and dental aspects of child abuse and neglect. Paediatric Dentistry 7(Reference Manual):64–67

Cairns AM, Mok JY, Welbury RR 2005 Injuries to the head, face, mouth and neck in physically abused children in a community setting. International Journal of Paediatric Dentistry 5:310–318

Primary trauma

Brin I, Ben-Bassar Y, Zilberman Y et al 1988 Effect of trauma to the primary incisors on the alignment of their permanent successors in Israelis. Community Dentistry and Oral Epidemiology 16:104–108

Christophersen P, Freund M, Harild L 2005 Avulsion of primary teeth and sequelae on the permanent successors. Dental Traumatology 21:320–323

Sennhenn-Kirchner S, Jacobs HG 2006 Traumatic injuries to the primary dentition and effects on the permanent successors – a clinical follow-up study. Dental Traumatology 2:237–241

Spinas E, Melis A, Savasta A 2006 Therapeutic approach to intrusive luxation injuries in primary dentition. A clinical follow-up study. European Journal of Paediatric Dentistry 7:179–186

Permanent trauma

Andreasen JO, Andreasen FM, Bakland LK et al 2003 Traumatic dental injuries: a manual, 2nd edn. Munksgaard, Copenhagen

Andreasen FM, Andreasen JO 1985 Diagnosis of luxation injuries: the importance of standardized clinical, radiographic and photographic techniques in clinical investigations. Endodontics and Dental Traumatology 1:160–169

Andreasen JO, Borum MK et al 1995 Replantation of 400 avulsed permanent incisors:1–4. Endodontics and Dental Traumatology 11:51–89

Andersson L, Bodin I, Sorensen S 1988 Progression of root resorption following replantation of human teeth after extended extra-oral storage. Endodontics and Dental Traumatology 5:38–47

Cvek MJ 1978 A clinical report on partial pulpotomy and capping with calcium hydroxide in permanent incisors with complicated crown fracture. Journal of Endodontics 4:232–237

Rowe NL, Williams JW 1985 Maxillofacial injuries. Volumes I and II. Churchill Livingstone, Edinburgh

Options for management

Andreasen FM, Andreasen JO, Bayer T 1989 Prognosis of root-fractured permanent incisors – prediction of healing modalities. Endodontics and Dental Traumatology 5:11–22

Andreasen JO, Paulson HU, Yu Z et al 1990 A long-term study of 370 autotransplanted premolars. Part II: tooth survival and pulp healing subsequent to transplantation. European Journal of Orthodontics 12:14–24

Barrett EJ, Kenny DJ 1997 Survival of avulsed permanent maxillary incisors in children following delayed replantation. Endodontics and Dental Traumatology 13:269–275

Barrett EJ, Kenny DJ, Tenenbaum HC et al 2005 Replantation of permanent incisors in children using Emdogain. Dental Traumatology 21:269–275

Campbell KM, Casas MJ, Kenny DJ 2007 Development of ankylosis in permanent incisors following delayed replantation and severe intrusion. Dental Traumatology 23:162–166

Chaushu S, Becker A, Zalkind M 2001 Prosthetic considerations in the restoration of orthodontically treated maxillary lateral incisors to replace missing central incisors: a clinical report. Journal of Prosthetic Dentistry 85:335–341

Cohenca N, Stabholz A 2007 Decoronation – a conservative method to treat ankylosed teeth for preservation of alveolar ridge prior to permanent prosthetic reconstruction: literature review and case presentation. Dental Traumatology 23:87–94

Filippi A, Pohl Y, Von Arx T 2001 Treatment of replacement resorption with Emdogain – preliminary results after 10 months. Dental Traumatology 17:134–138

Flores MT, Andersson L, Andreasen JO et al 2007a International Association of Dental Traumatology. Guidelines for the management of traumatic dental injuries. I. Fractures and luxations of permanent teeth. Dental Traumatology 23:66–71

Flores MT, Andersson L, Andreasen JO et al 2007b International Association of Dental Traumatology. Guidelines for the management of traumatic dental injuries

Kenny DJ, Barrett EJ, Casas MJ 2003 Avulsions and intrusions: the controversial displacement injuries. Journal of the Canadian Dental Association 69:308–313

Humphrey JM, Kenny DJ, Barrett EJ 2003 Clinical outcomes for permanent incisor luxations in a pediatric population. I. Intrusions. Dental Traumatology 19:266–273

Lee R, Barrett EJ, Kenny DJ 2003 Clinical outcomes for permanent incisor luxations in a pediatric population. II. Extrusions. Dental Traumatology 19:274–279

Nguyen PM, Kenny DJ, Barrett EJ 2004 Socio-economic burden of permanent incisor replantation on children and parents. Dental Traumatology 20:123–133

Nikoui M, Kenny DJ, Barrett EJ 2003 Clinical outcomes for permanent incisor luxations in a pediatric population. III. Lateral luxations. Dental Traumatology 19:280–285

Paulsen HU 2001 Autotransplantation of teeth in orthodontic treatment. American Journal of Orthodontics and Dentofacial Orthopedics 119:336–337

Schjøtt M, Andreasen JO 2005 Emdogain does not prevent progressive root resorption after replantation of avulsed teeth: a clinical study. Dental Traumatology 21:46–50

Self-mutilation

Altom RL, Di Angelis AJ 1989 Multiple autoextractions: oral self mutilation reviewed. Oral Surgery Oral Medicine Oral Pathology 67:271–274

8 Paediatric oral medicine and pathology

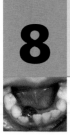

Contributors

Michael J Aldred, Angus Cameron

Introduction

Although some disorders are confined to the mouth, oral lesions may be a sign of a systemic medical disorder. Although much oral pathology in children is benign, it is essential to identify or eliminate more serious illnesses. The presentation of pathology in children is often different from adult pathology and the subtleties of these differences are often important in diagnosis. In addition, many lesions change in form or extent with growth of the body. As a diagnostic aid, conditions have been grouped according to presentation.

Orofacial infections

Differential diagnosis
- Bacterial infections:
  - odontogenic
  - scarlet fever
  - tuberculosis
  - atypical mycobacterial infection
  - actinomycosis
  - syphilis
  - impetigo
  - osteomyelitis.
- Viral infections:
  - primary herpetic gingivostomatitis
  - herpes labialis
  - herpangina
  - hand, foot and mouth disease
  - infectious mononucleosis
  - varicella.
- Fungal infections:
  - candidosis.

Odontogenic infections
The basic signs and symptoms of oral infection should be familiar to all clinicians.

Acute infection usually presents as an emergency:
- A sick, upset child.
- Raised temperature.
- Red, swollen face.
- Anxious and distressed parents.

Chronic infection typically presents as an asymptomatic or indolent process:
- A sinus may be present (usually labial or buccal).
- Mobile tooth.
- Halitosis.
- Discoloured tooth.

Presentation
- Children tend to present with facial cellulitis rather than an abscess with a large collection of pus. The child is usually febrile. Pain is common, although if the infection has perforated the cortical plate the child may not be in pain. The mainstay of treatment is removal of the cause of the infection. Too often, antibiotics are prescribed without consideration of extraction of the tooth or extirpation of the pulp.
- Maxillary canine fossa infections are predominately Gram positive or facultative anaerobic infections (Figure 8.1A). They may be misdiagnosed as a periorbital cellulitis (which is typically caused by *Haemophilus influenzae* or *Staphylococcus aureus* from haematogenous spread). Posterior spread may lead to cavernous sinus thrombosis and a brain abscess.
- Mandibular infections which spread may compromise the airway and there is the possibility of mediastinal involvement.
- Young patients may be dehydrated at presentation. It is important to ask about their fluid intake and ascertain whether the child has urinated during the previous 12 hours (see Appendix B, Fluid and electrolyte balance).

Management
The treatment of infection follows two basic tenets:
- Removal of the cause.
- Local drainage and debridement.

Criteria for hospital admission
- Significant infection present or spiking temperatures >39°C.
- Floor of mouth swelling.
- Dehydration.

Use of antibiotics
- Antibiotics should not be considered automatically as a first line of treatment unless there is systemic involvement. In a child, a temperature of 39°C or higher can be considered a significant rise (normal ~37°C).
- If a child has a systemic infection resulting from a local focus of dental infection (i.e. a sick child with a high temperature, an obvious spreading infection of the face and regional lymphadenopathy) antibiotics should be administered (see Appendix M).

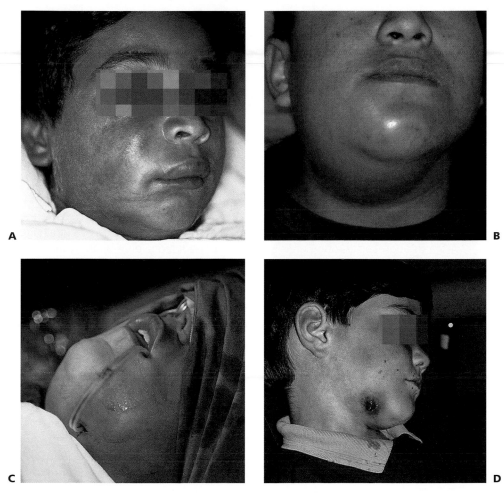

Figure 8.1 Severe facial swellings associated with odontogenic infections. **A** The left eye was almost closed from the spreading infection. **B** This child required extra-oral drainage of the facial swelling, which was caused by involvement of the floor of mouth, as well as the submandibular and sublingual spaces. He required hospitalization and was placed on high-dose intravenous penicillin supplemented with metronidazole. **C** Extra-oral drainage in place. **D** Draining sinus from inappropriately managed abscess in relation to a mandibular right first permanent molar. Although this child was placed on repeated courses of antibiotics, no attempt was made to remove the cause of the infection, namely, a carious tooth.

- Immunosuppressed patients or those with cardiac disease should receive antibiotics if infection is suspected.

General considerations
- Extraction of involved teeth

or

- Root canal treatment for permanent teeth if it is considered important to save particular teeth (see Chapter 6).
- Oral antibiotics if systemic involvement.

Amoxicillin is usually the drug of first choice. This has the advantage that it is given only three times a day, achieves higher blood levels and is a more effective antibiotic than, for example, phenoxymethylpenicillin. Often the extraction of the abscessed tooth alone will bring about resolution without antibiotic treatment.

Severe infections
- Hospital admission.
- Extraction of involved teeth. It is impossible to drain a significant infection solely through the root canals of a primary tooth.
- Drainage of any pus present. If the diagnosis or the correct management of an infection in the mandible has been delayed and the swelling has crossed the midline, or if there is swelling of the floor of the mouth, then extra-oral drainage with a through-and-through drain should be considered (Figure 8.1B, C). If a flap is raised, any granulation tissue should be removed and the area well irrigated. Flaps should be apposed but not tightly sutured. Soft flexible drains such as Penrose drains are better tolerated in children than are corrugated drains.
- Swabs for culture and sensitivity. It is important to take specimens for culture, even though empirical antibiotic treatment needs to be commenced immediately. Should the infection not respond to the initial antibiotic treatment, the results of the culture and sensitivity tests can be used to determine subsequent management.
- Intravenous antibiotics. Benzylpenicillin is the drug of first choice (up to 200 mg/kg/day).
- First-generation cephalosporins may be used as an alternative however, if the child is allergic to penicillin, there is cross-allergenicity and in these cases it would be prudent to avoid cephalosporins. In these cases, clindamycin would be a better choice.
- In severe infections, particularly deep-seated infections and those involving bone, metronidazole can be added. The flora of most odontogenic infections is of a mixed type and anaerobic organisms are thought to have a significant role in their pathogenesis.
- For any antibiotics administered, adequate doses must be used – treat serious infections in the head and neck seriously!
- Maintenance fluids, adding 10–12% for every degree over 37.5°C until the child is drinking of their own accord.
- 0.2% chlorhexidine gluconate rinses.
- Adequate pain control with paracetamol suspension (orally), 15 mg/kg, 4-hourly, or by suppository (rectally).
- If the eye is closed because of collateral oedema, it may be appropriate to apply 0.5% chloramphenicol eye drops or 1% ointment to prevent conjunctivitis.

Osteomyelitis
Rarely, odontogenic infection may lead to osteomyelitis, most commonly involving the mandible. Radiographically, the bone has a 'moth-eaten' appearance. Curettage of

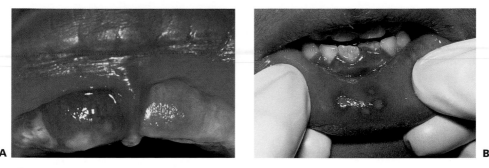

A   B

Figure 8.2 Different presentations of primary herpetic gingivostomatitis. **A** Infection with primary herpes often occurs at the time of eruption of primary teeth. **B** Common presentation with multiple small ulcers on the lower lip, and gingival swelling and inflammation.

the area is required to remove bony sequestra, and antibiotics are given for at least 6 weeks, depending on the results of microbiological culture and sensitivity test results. A variant of osteomyelitis has been reported in children and adolescents, termed juvenile mandibular chronic osteomyelitis. In this condition there is often no obvious odontogenic source of infection; there is limited response to a number of different treatment modalities.

Primary herpetic gingivostomatitis (Figure 8.2)
This is the most common cause of severe oral ulceration in children. It is caused by herpes simplex type 1 virus. Occasional cases of type 2 (the usual cause of genital herpes) infection have been reported, mainly in cases of sexual abuse. The clinical effects of the two different strains of herpes simplex virus are, however, clinically identical in the orofacial region. Although the majority of the population has been infected with the virus by adulthood, less than 1% manifest an acute primary infection. This usually occurs after 6 months of age, often coincident with the eruption of the primary incisors. The peak incidence is between 12 and 18 months of age. Incubation time is 3–5 days with a prodromal 48-hour history of irritability, pyrexia and malaise. The child is often unwell, has difficulty in eating and drinking and typically drools. Stomatitis is present, with the gingival tissues becoming red and oedematous. Intra-epithelial vesicles appear and rapidly break down to form painful ulcers. Vesicles may form on any part of the oral mucosa, including the skin around the lips. Solitary ulcers are usually small (3 mm) and painful with an erythematous margin, but larger ulcers with irregular margins often result from the coalescence of individual lesions. The disease is self-limiting and the ulcers heal spontaneously without scarring within 10–14 days.

Diagnosis
- History and clinical features.
- Exfoliative cytology showing the presence of multinucleated giant cells and viral inclusion bodies can be used for rapid diagnosis if laboratory support is at hand.
- Viral antigen can be detected by polymerase chain reaction (PCR) amplification. This can sometimes be useful in early confirmation of the diagnosis.

- Viral culture. Viral culture can take days or weeks to yield a result.
- Viral antibody detection in blood samples during the acute and convalescent phases. A rise in antibody titre can only provide late confirmation of the diagnosis.

Management
- Symptomatic care.
- Encourage oral fluids.
- If oral fluids cannot be taken then hospital admission is mandatory and intravenous fluids must be commenced.
- Analgesics – paracetamol, 15 mg/kg, 4-hourly.
- Mouthwashes for older children – chlorhexidine gluconate, 0.2%, 10 mL 4-hourly. In children over 10 years of age, tetracycline or minocycline mouthwashes may be beneficial, but must be avoided in younger children to prevent possible tooth discoloration.
- In young children with severe ulceration, chlorhexidine can be swabbed over the affected areas with cotton wool swabs. Much of the pain from oral ulceration is probably as a consequence of secondary bacterial infection. Chlorhexidine 0.2% mouthwash has been shown to be beneficial in the management of oral ulceration. A mouthwash containing chlorhexidine 0.12% and benzydamine hydrochloride (Difflam C) may offer some advantages over chlorhexidine alone.
- Topical anaesthetics: lidocaine viscous 2% or lidocaine (Xylocaine) spray. *Note:* topical anaesthetics are often advocated; however, the effect of a numb mouth in a young child is often more distressing than the pain from the illness and can lead to ulceration from the decrease in sensation and subsequent trauma. In addition, it is often difficult to initiate swallowing with a soft palate that has been anaesthetized.
- Antiviral chemotherapy. Aciclovir oral suspension or intravenously for immunosuppressed patients. This treatment is only worthwhile in the vesicular phase of the infection, i.e. within the first 72 hours. *Note:* the use of antiviral medications is contentious and usually reserved for children who are immunocompromised. There is some evidence to suggest, however, that the administration of aciclovir in the first 72 hours of the infection may be beneficial.
- Adequate pain control is also required with regular administration of paracetamol.
- Antibiotics are unhelpful.
- Severely affected young children often present dehydrated, being unable to eat or drink. Hospital admission is required for these cases with maintenance intravenous fluids.

Clinical Hint

An obviously ill child with puffy erythematous gingivae is most likely to have primary herpetic gingivostomatitis.

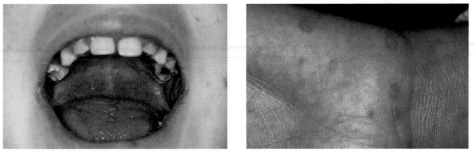

Figure 8.3 Infections caused by Coxsackie group A viruses. **A** Herpangina with characteristic palatal and pharyngeal ulceration and inflammation. **B** Cutaneous lesions in hand, foot and mouth disease.

Herpangina and hand, foot and mouth disease

These infections are caused by the Coxsackie group A viruses. As with primary herpes, both of the above conditions have a prodromal phase of low-grade fever and malaise that may last for several days before the appearance of the vesicles. In herpangina (Figure 8.3), a cluster of four to five vesicles are usually found on the palate, pillars of the fauces and pharynx, whereas in hand, foot and mouth disease up to 10 vesicles occur at these sites and elsewhere in the mouth, in addition to the hands and feet (Figure 8.3B). The skin lesions appear on the palmar surfaces of the hands and plantar surface of the feet and are surrounded by an erythematous margin. The severity of both diseases is usually milder than primary herpes and healing occurs within 10 days. Both diseases occur in epidemics, mainly affecting children.

Diagnosis
- Clinical appearance and history.
- Known epidemic.
- Viral culture from swab.

Management
- Symptomatic care, as for other viral infections.

Infectious mononucleosis (Figure 8.4A)
- This infection is caused by Epstein–Barr virus (EBV) and mainly affects older adolescents and young adults. The disease is highly infective and is characterized by malaise, fever and acute pharyngitis. In young children, ulcers and petechiae are often found in the posterior pharynx and soft palate. The disease is self-limiting.

Diagnosis
- History and clinical features.
- Paul–Bunnell agglutination test and atypical monocytes on blood film.

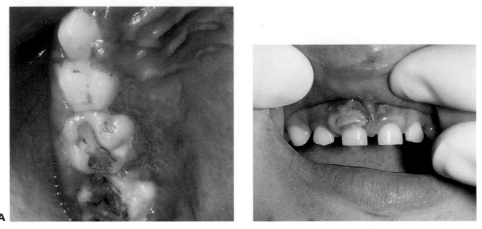

A   B

Figure 8.4 **A** Gingival ulceration and stomatitis during an acute episode of infectious mononucleosis. **B** Gingival ulceration in chickenpox infection. Note skin lesions at the angle of the mouth.

Varicella (Figure 8.4B)

This is a highly contagious virus causing chickenpox in younger subjects and shingles in older individuals. There is a prodromal phase of malaise and fever for 24 hours followed by macular eruptions and vesicles. In chickenpox, oral lesions occur in around 50% of cases but only a small number of vesicles occur in the mouth. These lesions may be found anywhere in the mouth in addition to other mucosal sites such as conjunctivae, nose or anus. Healing of oral lesions is uneventful.

Diagnosis

- Clinical appearance and history.

Candidosis

Acute pseudomembranous candidosis

The most common presentation of candidal infection in infants is thrush. White plaques are present, which on removal reveal an erythematous, sometimes haemorrhagic, base. In older children, thrush occurs when children are immunocompromised such as in acquired immune deficiency syndrome (AIDS) or in diabetes, or when prescribed antibiotics, steroids, or during chemotherapy and radiotherapy for malignancies.

> **Clinical Hint**
>
> White lesions which can be rubbed off are typical of thrush.

Median rhomboid glossitis

This characteristic uncommon lesion is a candidosis (rather than a developmental anomaly as was thought for many years), occurring on the dorsal surface of the tongue anterior to the circumvallate papillae, often in response to the use of antibiotics.

Diagnosis
Fifty per cent of children will have *Candida albicans* as a normal commensal, and culture is of little benefit. Smears or scrapings for exfoliative cytology reveal hyphae when disease is present, but the clinical picture may be diagnostic.

Management
- Antifungal medication for 2–4 weeks. Most antifungal treatment is unsuccessful because of poor compliance or instruction by the clinician.
- Amphotericin B lozenges or nystatin drops.
- Fluconazole orally (100 mg daily for 14 days) for cases of mucocutaneous candidosis in which the organism does not respond to topical treatment as described above.

Ulcerative and vesiculobullous lesions

Differential diagnosis
- Traumatic:
  - post-mandibular block anaesthesia
  - Riga–Fedé ulceration.
- Infective (see above):
  - primary herpetic gingivostomatitis
  - herpangina
  - hand, foot and mouth disease
  - infectious mononucleosis
  - varicella.
- Others:
  - recurrent aphthous ulceration
  - erythema multiforme
  - Stevens–Johnson syndrome
  - Behçet's syndrome
  - epidermolysis bullosa
  - lupus erythematosus
  - neutropenic ulceration
  - orofacial granulomatosis/Crohn disease
  - pemphigus
  - drug-induced (chemotherapy) lesions
  - lichen planus.

Lip ulceration after mandibular block anaesthesia
This is one of the most common causes of traumatic ulceration. Parents should be warned and children reminded not to bite their lips after mandibular block anaesthesia (Figure 8.5A).

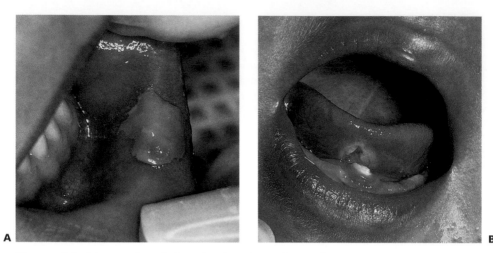

Figure 8.5 A Traumatic oral ulceration from biting the lip after a mandibular block injection. **B** Riga–Fedé ulcer on the ventral surface of the tongue arising from rubbing on the solitary mandibular incisor.

Riga–Fedé ulceration

This is ulceration of the ventral surface of the tongue caused by trauma from continual protrusive and retrusive movements over the lower incisors (Figure 8.5B). Once a common finding in cases of whooping cough, it now is seen almost exclusively in children with cerebral palsy.

Management

Smoothen sharp incisal edges or place domes of composite resin over the teeth. Rarely, in severe cases, extraction of the teeth might be considered.

Recurrent aphthous ulceration (Figure 8.6)

Recurrent aphthous ulceration (RAU) has been estimated to affect up to 20% of the population. Three types are identified:

- Minor aphthae.
- Major aphthae (Figure 8.6B).
- Herpetiform ulceration.

Minor aphthae account for the majority of cases, with crops of two to five shallow ulcers measuring up to 5 mm and occurring on non-keratinized mucosa. There is a typical central yellow slough with an erythematous border. Ulcers heal within 10–14 days without scarring. The cause of RAU is contentious. There is some evidence for a genetic basis for the disorder, with an increased incidence of ulceration in children whose both parents have RAU. Some studies have suggested that RAU is associated with nutritional deficiency states and so haematological investigation can be helpful. In major aphthae the keratinized mucosa may also be involved, the ulcers may be larger, last longer and heal with scarring.

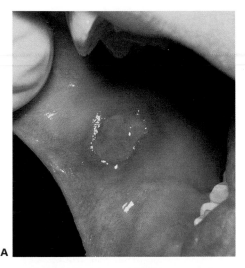

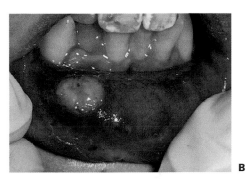

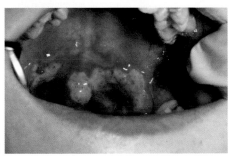

Figure 8.6 A Minor recurrent aphthae in an adolescent girl. These lesions were extremely painful. Haematological investigations revealed a low folate level, which when corrected eliminated further ulceration. **B, C** Major recurrent aphthous ulceration is a debilitating condition and heals with scarring. This girl's ulcers were managed with systemic steroids.

Diagnosis
- Clinical appearance and history.
- Blood tests for full blood, iron studies (including serum ferritin), serum vitamin B$_{12}$ levels and red cell folate in particular (if anaemia or latent anaemia suspected).

Management
- Symptomatic care with mouthrinses:
    - chlorhexidine gluconate 0.2%, 10 mL three times daily
    - minocycline mouthwash, 50 mg in 10 mL water three times daily for 4 days for children over 8 years of age
    - benzydamine hydrochloride 1.2% and chlorhexidine mouthwash (Difflam C).
- Topical steroids:
    - triamcinolone in Orabase (though this may be difficult to apply in children)
    - beclometasone dipropionate or fluticasone propionate asthma inhalers sprayed onto the ulcers
    - betamethasone (Diprosone OV) ointment.

- Systemic corticosteroids only in most severe cases of major aphthous ulceration.
- Herpetiform ulceration seems to respond best to minocycline mouthwashes.

Biopsy should only be considered if there is any doubt about the clinical diagnosis. Haematological investigations should be carried out to exclude anaemia or haematinic deficiency states (when appropriate, replacement can improve the ulceration or bring about resolution). As with all oral ulceration, symptomatic care with appropriate analgesics and antiseptic mouthwashes is appropriate. In those cases of severe recurrent oral ulceration, systemic corticosteroids may be used, although their use is best avoided in children. Minocycline mouthwashes should not be used in children under the age of 8 years to avoid tooth discoloration. Major aphthae tend to occur in older children.

> ### Clinical Hint
>
> Minor aphthae occur in recurrent crops of two to five ulcers, sparing the palate and dorsum of the tongue.

Behçet's syndrome

This condition is characterized by recurrent aphthous ulceration together with genital and ocular lesions, although the skin and other systems can also be involved. Lesions may affect other parts of the body. Behçet's syndrome can be subdivided into four main types:

- Mucocutaneous form – classical form with involvement of oral and genital mucosa and conjunctiva.
- Arthritic form with arthritis in association with mucocutaneous lesions.
- Neurological form with central nervous system involvement.
- Ocular form with uveitis with signs in addition to oral and genital lesions.

Diagnosis
- Clinical presentation.

Management
As for recurrent aphthous ulceration, but systemic treatment (corticosteroids) is usually required.

Erythema multiforme, Stevens–Johnson syndrome and toxic epidermal necrolysis

Three conditions exist that present with similar clinical signs and histological appearances. Like many conditions, varied nomenclature and misdiagnosis have clouded and confused the diagnosis/es). There is now a view that that these are distinct pathological entities and, perhaps importantly, might be initiated by quite distinct aetiological agents. The alternative view is that these disorders represent different presentations of the same basic disorder, distinguished by the severity and extent of the lesions.

Erythema multiforme (von Hebra) (Figure 8.7A–D)

The original description of erythema multiforme was that of a self-limiting but often recurrent and seasonal skin disease with mucosal involvement limited to the oral cavity. The lips are typically ulcerated with blood-staining and crusting. The characteristic macules ('target lesions') occur on the limbs but with less involvement of the trunk or head and neck. These lesions are concentric with an erythematous halo and a central blister. Although the lesions are extremely painful, the course of the illness is benign and healing and uneventful.

Stevens–Johnson syndrome (Figure 8.7E,F)

The condition presents with acute febrile illness, generalized exanthema, lesions involving the oral cavity and a severe purulent conjunctivitis. The skin lesions are more extensive than those of erythema multiforme. Stevens–Johnson syndrome is characterized by vesiculobullous eruptions over the body, in particular the trunk and severe involvement of multiple mucous membranes including the vulva, penis and conjunctiva. The course of the condition is longer and scarring may occur. Some authors have used the term erythema multiforme major for Stevens–Johnson syndrome, defining the condition as a severe form of erythema multiforme, but this is disputed by others. Although Stevens–Johnson syndrome patients are acutely ill, death is rare.

Toxic epidermal necrolysis

Similar to the clinical presentation of Stevens–Johnson syndrome, toxic epidermal necrolysis (TEN) or Lyell's syndrome is a severe, sometimes fatal, bullous drug-induced eruption where sheets of skin are lost. It resembles third degree burns or staphylococcal scalded skin syndrome. Oral involvement is similar to Stevens–Johnson syndrome. TEN may be misdiagnosed as a severe form of Stevens–Johnson syndrome (given the controversy over nomenclature), but the use of steroids is contraindicated, given an increase in mortality with their use in this disease.

Aetiology

Erythema multiforme is often initiated by herpes simplex reactivation. There is some evidence that Stevens–Johnson syndrome is initiated by a *Mycoplasma pneumoniae* infection or drug reaction. TEN is drug-induced.

Clinical presentation

A summary of the three conditions is shown in Table 8.1. There is an acute onset of fever, cough, sore throat and malaise, followed by the appearance of the lesions on the body and oral cavity ranging from 2 days to 2 weeks after the onset of symptoms. These break down quickly in the mouth to form ulcers. The most striking feature is the degree of oral mucosal involvement that may lead in all three cases to a pan-stomatitis and sloughing of whole oral mucosa. There is extensive ulceration and crusting around the lips, oral haemorrhage and necrosis of skin and mucosa leading to secondary infection. There may be difficulty in eating and drinking which complicates the clinical course, and there is usually extreme discomfort from both the skin and oral lesions that may necessitate narcotic analgesics.

Management

If there is a known precipitating factor such as herpes simplex infection then antivirals such as topical aciclovir can be used as a form of prophylaxis. Management is generally

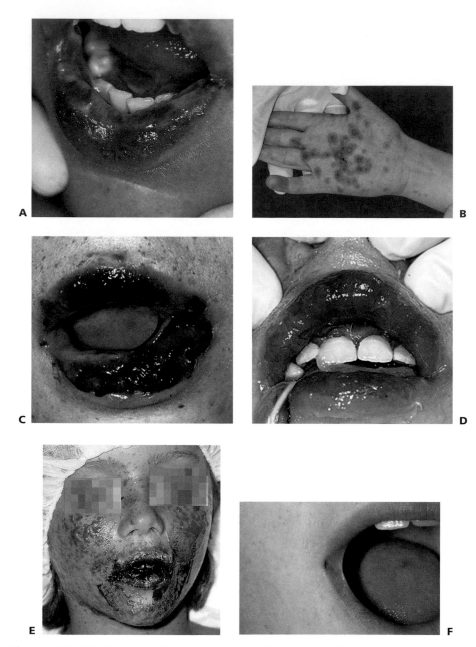

Figure 8.7 A Erythema multiforme presenting with pan-stomatitis and severe dehydration. Treatment included rehydration and symptomatic care of the ulceration. **B** Typical target lesions seen in erythema multiforme. **C** Ulceration of the lips may be severe, and resulted in the lips becoming fused together by the slough and crusting in this case. **D** The mouth was debrided under general anaesthesia. **E** Stevens–Johnson syndrome with severe mucocutaneous involvement. This child required admission to the intensive care unit for 3 days. **F** Stricture of the lateral commissure of the lips due to scarring following an episode of Stevens–Johnson syndrome.

Table 8.1 Differential diagnosis of erythema multiforme (EM), Stevens–Johnson syndrome and toxic epidermal necrolysis

Signs	Erythema multiforme (EM minor)	Stevens–Johnson syndrome (EM major)	Toxic epidermal necrolysis (Lyell's syndrome)
Aetiology	HSV re-activation in some cases	HSV re-activation? *Mycoplasma*? Drug-related	Drug-related – trimethoprim and sulfamethoxazole (Bactrim), carbamazepine lamotrigine
Recurrence	75% have multiple recurrences – two to three per year	Usually single but may recur	May recur in response to initiating agent
Target lesions	Yes Typical concentric target lesions on extremities	No or atypical Vesiculobullous eruptions on trunk, head and neck	Skin involvement is so severe that no separate lesions are ever seen
Skin	Raised papules acrally distributed	Multiple tissue involvement usually severe	Severe skin involvement, similar to burns Confluent sloughing of the skin
Mucosa	Crusting and bleeding of lips	Crusting and bleeding of lips Severe multiple mucosal involvement Oral, ocular and genital	Severe multiple mucosal involvement
Course	Within 2 weeks	>2 weeks Oral lesions may take months	Healing phase will take many months
Management	Short course of high dose systemic steroids Fluid maintenance	Fluid maintenance Debridement of oral lesions Narcotic analgesics/ sedation? Antibiotics for *M. pneumoniae*? Short course of high dose systemic steroids	Similar to burns management Resuscitation and fluid maintenance Narcotic analgesics Intubation and intensive care unit admission
Sequelae	Healing without scarring	May be scarring and oral stricture	Blindness may occur and there is a high mortality
Histopathology	Similar in all three conditions: subepidermal vesicles and bullae		

HSV, herpes simplex virus.

symptomatic and supportive. A major problem during the course of the illness is fluid balance and pain, much of which arises from secondary infection of the oral lesions. Debridement of the oral cavity with 0.2% chlorhexidine gluconate or benzydamine hydrochloride and chlorhexidine (Difflam C) is effective in removing much of the necrotic debris from the mouth. Extensive areas of ulceration tend to be less responsive to chlorhexidine and a minocycline mouthwash may prove more effective. The role of systemic steroids is controversial but they may be necessary in severe cases requiring hospital admission.

Management also includes:

- Adequate fluid replacement and total parenteral nutrition if required.
- Pain control which may necessitate the use of narcotics and sedation.

> **Clinical Hint**
>
> Crusted, blood-stained lips are typical of erythema multiforme.

Pemphigus

Pemphigus is an important vesiculo-bullous disease mainly affecting adults; however, children can be also affected. The lesions are intra-epithelial and rapidly break down so that affected individuals are often unaware of blistering, complaining instead of ulceration, mainly affecting the buccal mucosa, palate and lips.

Diagnosis

There may be positive Nikolsky's sign (separation of the superficial epithelial layers from the basal layer produced by rubbing or gentle pressure) and cytological examination can reveal the presence of Tzanck's cells. Direct immunofluorescence using frozen sections from an oral biopsy will reveal intracellular immunoglobulin (IgG) deposits in the epithelium, which are diagnostic for this disease. Indirect immunofluorescence on blood samples is sometimes used to monitor patients.

Management

- Systemic corticosteroid therapy.
- Antiseptic or minocycline mouthwashes and analgesia as necessary.

Epidermolysis bullosa

Epidermolysis bullosa is a term used to describe several hereditary vesiculo-bullous disorders of the skin and mucosa. The most recent classification is based on four different types:

- Intra-epithelial, non-scarring form transmitted as an autosomal dominant or X-linked trait.
- Junctional form with hemi-desmosome defect and severe scarring, transmitted as an autosomal recessive trait.
- Dermal form with scarring and skin atrophy, transmitted as an autosomal dominant trait.
- Acquired form (epidermolysis bullosa acquisita).

Blisters may form from birth or appear in the first few weeks of life depending on the form of the disease. Corneal ulceration may also be present and pitting enamel hypoplasia has been reported, mainly in the junctional forms of the disease.

Management

Management is often extremely difficult because of the fragility of the skin and oral mucosa. Intensive preventive dental care is essential to prevent dental caries, combined with treatment of early decay. Supportive care is required with the use of chlorhexidine gluconate mouthwashes and possibly topical anaesthetics such as lidocaine (Xylocaine viscous). Fortunately, children may receive dental treatment under general anaesthesia without laryngeal complications. Because of oral stricture, however, access into the mouth is often difficult and in the older patients surgical release of the commissure may be necessary. It is important to cover instruments with copious lubricant, and the use of rubber dam is essential.

Systemic lupus erythematosus

Systemic lupus erythematosus is a chronic inflammatory multisystem disease occurring predominantly in young women. The hallmark of systemic lupus erythematosus is the presence of antinuclear antibodies which form circulating immune complexes with DNA. Oral ulceration often occurs in systemic lupus erythematosus and treatment of the condition usually involves systemic steroids.

Orofacial granulomatosis and Crohn disease (Figure 8.8)

Although not primarily an ulcerative condition, oral ulceration may be the presenting sign in orofacial granulomatosis. Orofacial granulomatosis may be confined to the

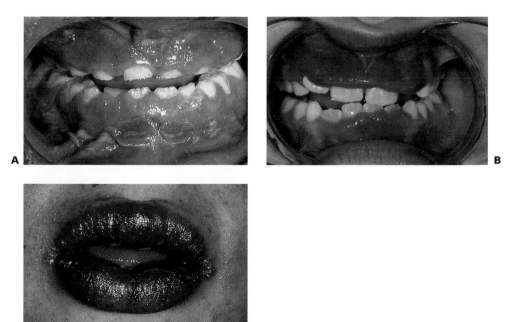

Figure 8.8 Presentations of orofacial granulomatosis/Crohn disease. **A** The intra-oral appearance is pathognomonic with swelling of the gingivae, a cobblestone appearance of the buccal mucosa and ulceration of the labial and buccal sulci. **B** A different presentation with bright red swollen gingivae. **C** The patient initially presented with a painless swelling of the lips and had evidence of malabsorption, perianal fissuring and bowel problems, and was diagnosed with Crohn disease. Management was with systemic corticosteroids.

orofacial region or be a manifestation of Crohn disease, an inflammatory condition of the gastrointestinal tract, or of sarcoidosis.

Presentation

- Diffuse swelling of the lips and cheeks, often initially recurrent and then becoming persistent.
- Diffusely swollen gingivae (Figure 8.8B).
- Linear ulceration or fissuring of the buccal and labial sulcus. A characteristic 'cobblestone' appearance of the buccal mucosa (Figure 8.8A).
- Polypoid tags of vestibular and retromolar mucosa.
- Children may also present with diarrhoea, failure to thrive, weakness, fatigue, anorexia and perianal fissuring or skin tags as manifestation of Crohn disease.
- Oral changes have been found in between 10% and 25% of patients with Crohn disease and, importantly, their appearance may precede other systemic symptoms.

Diagnosis

- Biopsy of oral lesions.
- Blood tests including:
  - full blood count, differential white cell count (to exclude leukaemia), erythrocyte sedimentation rate (ESR) and C-reactive protein
  - serum angiotensin-converting enzyme (ACE) level to identify or exclude sarcoidosis.
- Barium studies, endoscopy and biopsy of bowel if Crohn disease is suspected.

Management

- Some cases of orofacial granulomatosis have been shown to be a response to topical medicaments or dietary components. An exclusion diet can be considered to identify food intolerance.

Crohn disease

- Prednisolone. Steroids are usually commenced at a high dosage (2–3 mg/kg daily for 6–8 weeks) to gain control of the disease and is then reduced.
- Sulfasalazine.
- Dietary management for malabsorption.
- Metronidazole for perianal disease.

More recently methotrexate, budesonide and infliximab (a monoclonal antibody which neutralizes tumour necrosis factor (TNF) α) have also been used in the management of Crohn disease. Research continues into the use of paratuberculosis therapy (rifabutin, clarithromycin and clofazimine) and of thalidomide for refractory adult cases.

Melkersson–Rosenthal syndrome

Melkersson–Rosenthal syndrome is regarded by some as a form of orofacial granulomatosis.

Presentation
- Recurrent/persistent orofacial swelling lasting from 1 hour to several months.
- Facial nerve paralysis.
- Fissured (plicated) tongue.

Melkersson–Rosenthal syndrome is a diagnosis sometimes made without this triad – there is controversy regarding its existence or place within the disorders characterized by orofacial granulomata.

Pigmented, vascular and red lesions

If a lesion is red or bluish in colour there should be the suspicion of a vascular lesion. These lesions will blanch on pressure with a glass slide (or end of a test tube if access is difficult) as the blood is removed from the vessels. Melanotic lesions are rare in children (other than racial pigmentation). A characteristic melanin-pigmented oral lesion in young children is the melanotic neuroectodermal tumour of infancy.

Differential diagnosis
- Racial pigmentation (Figure 8.9).
- Vascular lesions:
  - haemangioma
  - other vascular malformations
  - haematoma
  - petechiae and purpura
  - hereditary haemorrhagic telangiectasia
  - Sturge–Weber syndrome.
- Pigmented lesions (containing melanin):
  - melanotic neuroectodermal tumour of infancy
  - Peutz–Jeghers syndrome
  - Addison's disease.

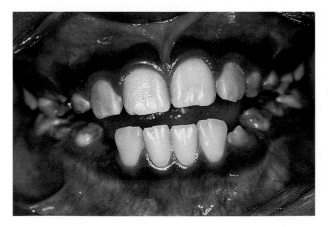

Figure 8.9 Racial pigmentation of the attached gingiva. This should not be confused with heavy metal toxicity which is limited to the marginal gingivae.

- Other red/blue/purple lesions:
  - giant cell epulis/peripheral giant cell granuloma
  - eruption cyst
  - Langerhans' cell histiocytosis
  - geographic tongue
  - median rhomboid glossitis
  - hereditary mucoepithelial dysplasia
  - cyanosis
  - heavy metal toxicity.

Lesions of vascular origin

Haemangioma (Figure 8.10A, B)

Haemangiomas are endothelial hamartomas. Typically present at birth, they may grow with the infant but then may regress with time to disappear by adolescence. As such, they require no treatment other than observation, excepting cosmetic concerns.

Other vascular malformations

Arteriovenous malformations include birthmarks, blood vessel and lymphatic anomalies. These may be life-threatening conditions which can occasionally present with

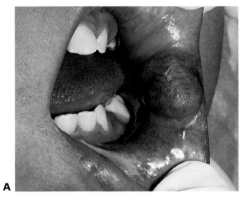

A

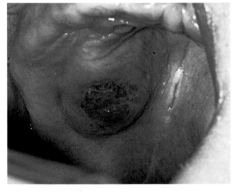

B

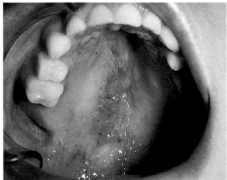

C

Figure 8.10 A, B Two presentations of haemangioma in infants. **C** Lymphangioma in the palate.

profound haemorrhage. Arteriovenous malformations have been classified by Kaban and Mulliken (1986) according to their flow characteristics. They are either:

- Low-flow lesions – capillary, venous, lymphatic or combined port-wine stains, Sturge–Weber syndrome

or

- High-flow lesions – arterial with arteriovenous fistulae (Figure 8.11). Present with mobile and sometimes painful teeth, a bruit and palpable pulses, bleeding from gingivae and bony involvement.
- Combined lesions – extensive combined venous and arteriovenous malformations.

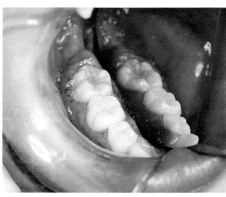

A

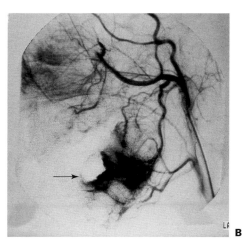

B

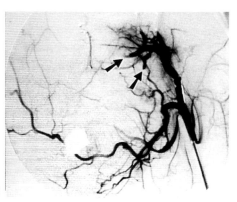

C

Figure 8.11 A high-flow arteriovenous malformation in the mandible. This child presented with an unusual erythematous enlargement of the gingivae around the mandibular right first permanent molar in addition to mobile teeth (**A**). During the biopsy 350 mL (20% of total volume) of blood was lost after extraction of the second primary molar. The haemorrhage was controlled with an iodoform pack (arrowed) (**B**). **B** Subsequently, an angiogram was ordered. The extent of the lesion posterior to the pack is seen. **C** The lesion was managed by embolizing the inferior alveolar and maxillary arteries (arrow), and the mandible was resected later.

Diagnosis

- Presentation may be subtle, such as prolonged bleeding from the gingivae after tooth brushing, or alternatively a torrential single episode haemorrhage.
- Vascular lesions are often warm to touch (though this can be difficult to determine if wearing latex gloves).
- Radiographically, there may be enlargement of the periodontal ligament space and a diffuse abnormal trabeculation of the bone.
- A bruit or pulse may be felt over high-flow lesions.
- Teeth may be hypermobile and may have pulsatile movements.
- Facial asymmetry may be present as lesions expand.
- Digital subtraction angiography (Figure 8.11B) is required for definitive diagnosis of feeder vessels and the distribution of the lesion.
- Magnetic resonance angiography can be used to aid diagnosis; however, digital subtraction angiography has the advantage that embolization can be performed at the same time.

Management

- Low-flow lesions can be removed by careful surgery with identification and ligation of feeder vessels. Larger lesions can be managed with cryotherapy, laser ablation or injection of sclerosing solutions.
- High-flow lesions require selective embolization of vessels, but these will generally recur after embolization due to revascularization from contralateral supply and recanalization of the embolized artery. Repeat embolization and resection of the entire lesion is often necessary involving jaw reconstruction.
- If a tooth is accidentally removed and a torrential haemorrhage results, some clinicians suggest that the extracted tooth should be immediately replaced and additional measures used to control haemorrhage.

> **Clinical Hint**
>
> Vascular lesions blanch on pressure.

Lymphangioma (Figure 8.10C)

- Diagnosis of developmental lymph vessel abnormalities must exclude vascular involvement. Surgical excision is only necessary if of functional or aesthetic concern.
- **Cystic hygroma** is a term used to describe a large lymphangioma involving the tongue, floor of mouth and neck. Expansion of the lesion may cause respiratory obstruction and treatment usually involves multiple resections over time, management with laser ablation, or cryosurgery.

Petechiae and purpura

Petechiae are small pinpoint submucosal or subcutaneous haemorrhages. Purpura or ecchymoses present as larger collections of blood. These lesions are usually present in

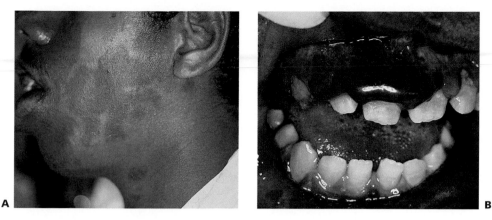

A   B

Figure 8.12 A, B Sturge–Weber syndrome showing the extent of the capillary vascular malformation in the face which is contiguous with the intra-oral involvement.

patients with severe bleeding disorders or coagulopathies, leukaemia and other conditions such infective endocarditis. Initially bright red in colour, they will change to a bluish-brown hue with time as the extravasated blood is metabolized.

Hereditary haemorrhagic telangiectasia (Rendu–Osler–Weber disease)

An autosomal dominant disorder presenting as a developmental anomaly of capillaries. Lesions may be small flat or raised haemorrhagic nodules or spider naevi. Bleeding as a result of involvement of the gastrointestinal tract and respiratory tract can lead to chronic anaemia.

Sturge–Weber syndrome (Figure 8.12)

This syndrome typically presents with:
- Encephalotrigeminal angiomatoses.
- Epilepsy.
- Intellectual disability.
- Calcification of the falx cerebri.
- Vascular lesions involve the leptomeninges and peripheral lesions appear along the distribution of the fifth nerve.

Extraction of teeth within regions of the affected jaws should be performed with caution and only after thorough investigation of the extent of the anomaly although it has been reported that they are usually uncomplicated (see Other vascular malformations above).

Maffucci's syndrome

Presents with multiple haemangiomas and enchondromas of the small bones in the hands and feet. Only a small number of cases will manifest with oral lesions, mainly haemangiomas.

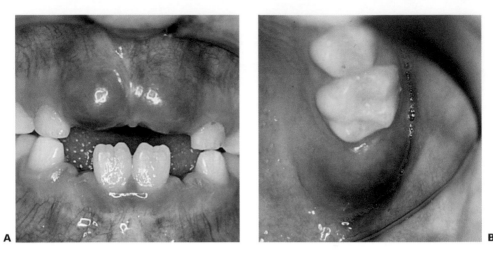

Figure 8.13 Eruption cysts may be associated with any tooth. **A** Two eruption cysts associated with the maxillary central incisors. **B** Eruption cyst of the maxillary first permanent molar.

Melanin-containing lesions
Peutz–Jeghers syndrome
An autosomal dominant disorder, manifesting as multiple small, pigmented lesions on oral mucosa and circumoral skin appearing almost like dark freckles. There is an important association with intestinal polyposis coli which requires gastrointestinal investigation.

Red lesions
Eruption cyst or haematoma
Follicular enlargement appearing just prior to eruption of teeth. These lesions tend to be blue-black as they may contain blood. They usually require no treatment unless infected. The parents and child should be reassured and the follicle allowed to rupture spontaneously or it may be surgically opened if infected (Figure 8.13).

Hereditary mucoepithelial dysplasia
A rare disorder where there is a reduced number of desmosomes attaching the epithelial cells to each other. Lens cataracts, corneal lesions leading to blindness, skin keratosis and alopecia are associated with a fiery red mucosa involving both keratinized and non-keratinized mucosa. Diagnosis is confirmed by gingival and/or mucosal biopsy. Transmission electron microscopy is necessary to demonstrate reduced number of desmosomes and amorphous intracellular inclusions. The oral lesions are usually asymptomatic. Loss of sight is progressive due to corneal vascularization. Corneal grafts are unsuccessful as they too undergo vascularization.

Geographic tongue (Figure 8.14A)
This condition is also termed glossitis migrans, benign migratory glossitis, erythema migrans or wandering rash of the tongue. It presents as areas of depapillation and

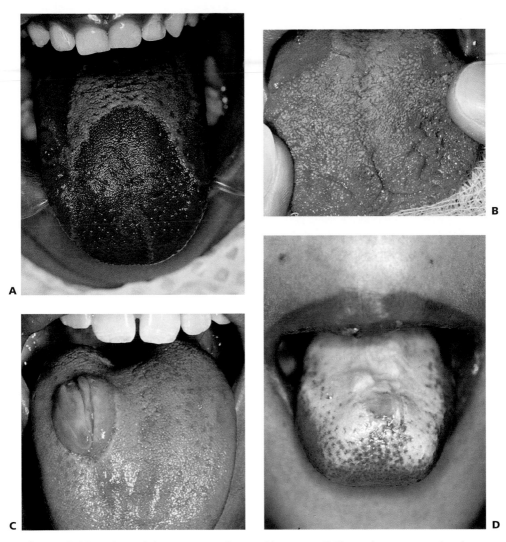

Figure 8.14 Lesions of the tongue. **A** Geographic tongue. **B** Fissured tongue associated with mild geographic tongue. **C** A large swelling (an ulcerated fibroepithelial hyperplasia) on the dorsal surface of the tongue with a central area of ulceration caused by a palatal expansion appliance (quad helix). **D** Acute pseudomembranous candidosis or thrush with typical white plaques on the dorsum of the tongue in an immunocompromised child.

erythema with a heaped keratinized margin on the lateral margins and dorsal surface of the tongue. The lesions appear as map-like areas (hence the 'geographic') and may change in their distribution over a period of time (hence the 'migratory'). The areas affected may return to normal and new lesions appear at different sites on the tongue. Sometimes symptomatic, topical corticosteroids may be beneficial for those children in pain.

Fissured tongue (Figure 8.14B)

Also termed plicated tongue, scrotal tongue, fissured tongue or lingua secta. The tongue in these patients is fissured, the fissures being perpendicular to the lateral border. Although this is usually considered a variation of normal, it is a commonly found condition in children with Down's syndrome. Some patients with a fissured tongue will also have geographic tongue. Fissuring of the tongue is also a feature of Melkersson–Rosenthal syndrome.

Epulides and exophytic lesions

Differential diagnosis

- Inflammatory hyperplasias:
  - fibrous epulis/pyogenic granuloma
  - giant cell epulis/peripheral giant cell granuloma.
- Congenital epulis of the newborn.
- Squamous papilloma/viral warts.
- Condyloma acuminatum.
- Eruption cyst/haematoma.
- Melanotic neuro-ectodermal tumour of infancy.
- Tuberous sclerosis.
- Mucocoele.
- Lymphangioma.

Fibrous epulis (Figure 8.15A)

One of the most common epulides that is seen in children resulting from an exuberant fibro-epithelial reaction to plaque. Commonly arising from the interdental papillae, they range in colour from pink to red to yellow. Those appearing yellow are ulcerated. The term pyogenic granuloma is used by some to describe such lesions which are extremely vascular.

Management

Oral hygiene and surgical excision. Lesions may recur, particularly if good oral hygiene is not maintained.

Clinical Hint

Fibrous epulides involve the marginal gingivae.

Giant cell epulis/peripheral giant cell granuloma (Figure 8.15B)

These lesions usually occur in the region of the primary dentition. The colour of these lesions tends to be dark purple. Bone loss of the alveolar crest can sometimes be observed as 'radiographic cupping'. It is important to ensure that there is no intra-osseous component radiographically as in this case the diagnosis would be a central

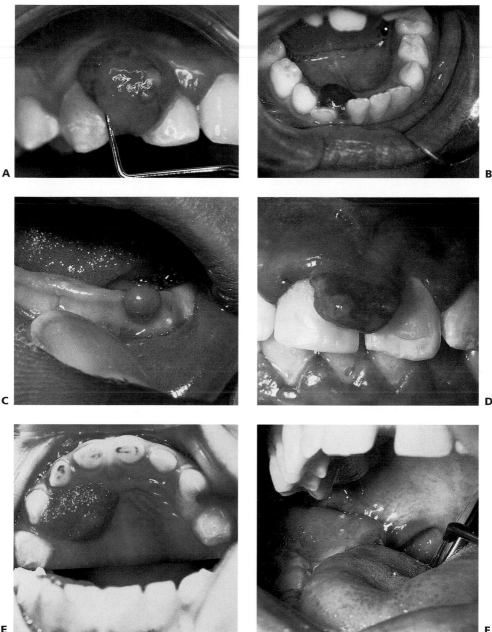

Figure 8.15 Gingival swellings. **A** Fibrous epulis. **B** Peripheral giant cell granuloma/giant cell epulis. **C** Congenital epulis. **D** Epulis associated with angiomata in a child with tuberous sclerosis. **E** A papilloma in the palate of a young child. In this case the lesion was associated with viral warts on the extremities, hence this is assumed to be a viral papilloma. **F** A large gingival swelling in the retromolar triangle proved to be a metastatic fibrosarcoma. The primary lesion was in the posterior abdomen and secondary lesions had invaded the pelvis, lungs and mandible.

giant cell granuloma. As with all giant cell lesions of the jaws, hyperparathyroidism should be considered in the differential diagnosis.

Management
- Surgical excision.
- Haematological investigations for calcium, phosphate, alkaline phosphatase and parathyroid hormone.
- Lesions may regrow if not totally excised.

Squamous papilloma (Figure 8.15E)
A squamous papilloma is a benign neoplasm, presenting as a cauliflower-like growth on the mucosa. The colour of the lesion depends on the degree of keratinization. The lesion is clinically indistinguishable from a viral wart.

Management
Surgical excision including the stalk and a border of normal tissue.

Viral warts
A viral infection by the human papilloma virus. Lesions may be single or multiple and it is important to consider the presence of warts on other areas of the body, especially on the hands and fingers.

Management
Surgical excision. If multiple lesions are present extra-orally, dermatological management may also be required.

Congenital epulis (Figure 8.15C)
The congenital epulis is a rare benign lesion of unknown origin found only in neonates. Lesions are equally distributed between maxillary and mandibular arches and may in multiple in about 10% of reported cases; they are 10 times more common in girls than in boys. It arises from the gingival crest but is thought not to be odontogenic in origin. The swelling is characterized by a proliferation of mesenchymal cells with a granular cytoplasm and is usually pedunculated. There is controversy over the histogenesis of this lesion. The congenital epulis is histologically indistinguishable from the extra-gingival granular cell tumour, which is usually seen on the tongue. Immunohistochemically, the congenital epulis is S100 negative whereas the granular cell tumour is positive for both CD68 and S100. It has been suggested that the congenital epulis is a non-neoplastic, perhaps reactive lesion arising from primitive gingival perivascular mesenchymal cells with the potential for smooth muscle cytodifferentiation.

Alternative terminology
Congenital granular cell tumour, Neumann tumour, granular cell epulis, gingival granular cell tumour.

Management
Lesions often regress with time, although large lesions which interfere with feeding may require surgical excision. Large lesions are sometimes present at birth and may be life-threatening because of respiratory obstruction. The eruption of the primary

dentition is unaffected by either surgical or conservative management and recurrence is uncommon.

Tuberous sclerosis (Figure 8.15D)

Tuberous sclerosis is an autosomal dominant disorder characterized by seizures, mental retardation and adenoma sebaceum of the skin. Epulides or generalized nodular gingival enlargement may be present. Some of these may result from vascular malformations and may bleed profusely when excised. Hypoplasia of the enamel is often observed as surface pitting; this can be demonstrated particularly effectively by the use of disclosing solutions.

Gingival enlargements (overgrowth)

Differential diagnosis
- Drug-induced hyperplasia:
  - phenytoin
  - ciclosporin A
  - nifedipine
  - verapamil.
- Syndromes with gingival enlargement as a presenting feature:
  - hereditary gingival fibromatosis
  - other syndromes.

Phenytoin enlargement (Figure 8.16A, B)

Not all patients taking phenytoin have gingival enlargement. Principally there is enlargement of the interdental papilla. There may be delayed eruption of teeth because of the bulk of fibrous tissue present and ectopic eruption. Overgrowth has been suggested to result from decreased collagen degradation and phagocytosis, as well as increased collagen synthesis. Withdrawal of the drug will bring about resolution in all but severe cases. Oral hygiene is most important in controlling overgrowth.

Management
- Maintenance of oral hygiene.
- Use of chlorhexidine 0.2% mouthwashes.
- Gingivectomy may be required to allow eruption of teeth or for aesthetics.

Ciclosporin A-associated enlargement (Figure 8.16C, D)

A significant number of children now undergo kidney, liver, heart or combined heart/lung transplantation. The mainstay of immunosuppressive anti-rejection chemotherapy is ciclosporin A. Gingival overgrowth occurs in between 30% and 70% of patients and is not strictly dose-related but may be more severe if the drug is administered at an early age. Individual patients appear to have a threshold below which gingival overgrowth will not occur.

Nifedipine and verapamil enlargement

Both these drugs are calcium-channel blockers, used to control coronary insufficiency and hypertension in adults; their main use in children is to control ciclosporin-induced

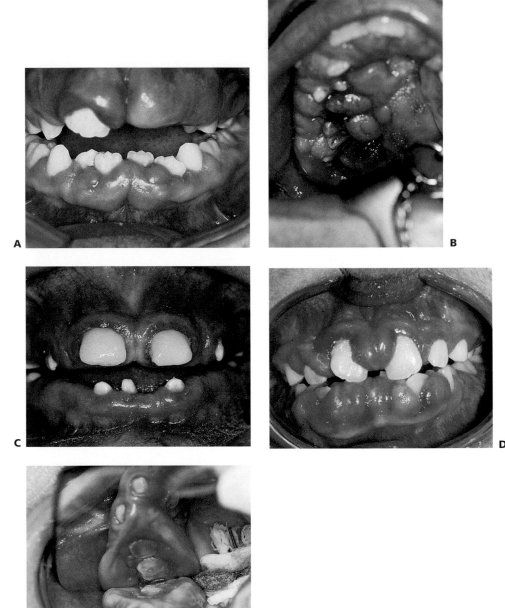

Figure 8.16 A Phenytoin-associated gingival enlargement. This initially involves the interdental papillae and then adjacent tissues. **B** The enlargement can become so extensive as to cover the whole palate. An acute periodontal abscess was associated with this case. **C** Ciclosporin A-associated gingival enlargement in a child following end-stage renal failure and kidney transplantation. The enamel is malformed due to the effects of the renal disease. **D** Ciclosporin A-associated gingival enlargement in a child following heart transplantation. **E** Hereditary gingival fibromatosis.

hypertension after transplantation. An increase in the extra-cellular compartment volume is responsible for enlargement that occurs in addition to the enlargement caused by ciclosporin A, which is invariably used in these patients.

Management
- As with phenytoin hyperplasia, maintenance of oral hygiene is mandatory.
- Gingivectomy if required.
- In children with severe enlargement, a full mouth procedure may be required. In these cases periodontal flap procedures are preferable as primary closure can be achieved.

Hereditary gingival fibromatosis (Figure 8.16E)
Gingival enlargement may be a feature of several syndromes, some of which include learning disabilities. These syndromes may occur sporadically or as an autosomal dominant or an autosomal recessive trait.

Management
Gingivectomy or periodontal flap procedures as required to allow tooth eruption and maintain aesthetics. Histopathological examination of the excised tissue may assist in diagnosis of some of the rarer causes of syndromic gingival enlargement (e.g. juvenile hyaline fibromatosis).

Premature exfoliation of primary teeth

Premature loss of primary teeth is a significant diagnostic event. Most conditions which present with early loss are serious and a child presenting with unexplained tooth loss warrants immediate investigation. Teeth may be lost because of metabolic disturbances, severe periodontal disease, connective tissue disorders, neoplasia, loss of alveolar bone support or self-inflicted trauma.

Differential diagnosis
- Neutropenias:
  - cyclic neutropenia
  - congenital agranulocytosis.
- Qualitative neutrophil defects:
  - prepubertal periodontitis
  - juvenile periodontitis
  - leucocyte adhesion defect
  - Papillon–Lefèvre syndrome
  - Chèdiak–Higashi disease
  - acatalasia.
- Metabolic disorders:
  - hypophosphatasia.
- Connective tissue disorders:
  - Ehlers–Danlos syndrome (Types IV and VIII)
  - erythromelalgia

- acrodynia
- scurvy.
- Neoplasia:
  - Langerhans' cell histiocytosis
  - acute myeloid leukaemia.
- Hypophosphatasia.
- Self-injury:
  - hereditary sensory neuropathies
  - Lesch–Nyhan syndrome
  - psychotic disorders.

Periodontal disease in children (Figure 8.17D)

Although gingivitis is not uncommon in children, periodontitis with alveolar bone loss is usually a manifestation of a serious underlying immunological deficiency. Two forms of periodontal disease in children, prepubertal periodontitis and juvenile periodontitis, are associated with characteristic bacterial flora including *Actinobacillus actinomycetemcomitans*, *Prevotella intermedia*, *Eikenella corrodens* and *Capnocytophaga sputigena*. The presence of these bacteria is thought to be related to decreased host resistance, specifically neutropenia or neutrophil function defects. Although B-cell defects show few oral changes, altered T-cell function will manifest with severe gingivitis, periodontitis and candidosis.

Neutropenias and qualitative neutrophil defects
Neutropenia
- Peripheral blood levels <1500/mL.
- Acute forms usually fatal.
- Chronic forms have indolent progression.
- Cyclic (see below) characterized by recurrent episodes.
- Intermittent as part of Shwachman's syndrome.

Cyclic neutropenia (Figure 8.17A, B)

In this condition there is an episodic decrease in the number of neutrophils every 3–4 weeks. Peripheral neutrophil counts usually drop to zero and during this time the child is extremely susceptible to infection. Recurrent oral ulceration often occurs when cell counts are low. Gingival and periodontal involvement occurs with the appearance of teeth and is progressive.

Management
- Early preventive involvement.
- Dental care through all stages of cycle.
- Chlorhexidine 0.2% mouthwashes or gel.
- Elective extraction of primary teeth may be considered in severe cases.
- In some familial cases the condition appears to totally regress during adolescence.

Leucocyte adhesion defect (Figure 8.17C, D)

A rare autosomal recessive condition associated with a reduced level of adhesion molecules on peripheral leucocytes resulting in severely reduced resistance to infection.

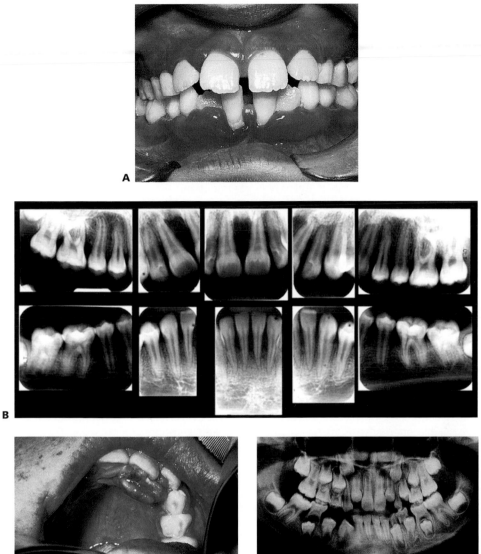

Figure 8.17 **A** Gross gingival inflammation in an adolescent with cyclic neutropenia. This girl lost most of her primary teeth by the age of 7 years. **B** Periapical radiographic survey showing the extent of bone loss and angular defects in another child with cyclic neutropenia. **C** Severe unexplained palatal ulceration in a child with a leucocyte adhesion defect. The maxillary left incisor exfoliated a short time later. **D** Prepubertal periodontitis, also associated with a leucocyte adhesion defect. It is important to assess normal eruption patterns and to be suspicious of loss of teeth in the absence of caries or other pathology.

The CD11/CD18 molecules are necessary for effective phagocytosis. Children present with delayed wound healing, persistent severe oral ulceration, cellulitis without pus formation, severe gingival inflammation, periodontitis and premature loss of primary teeth. Also present is a persistently high leucocytosis and reactive marrow, without evidence of leukaemia. One important indicator of this condition is late separation of the umbilical cord after birth.

Diagnosis

Diagnosis is confirmed by examining leucocytes for surface expression of CD11/CD18 markers using immunofluorescence techniques and cytofluorographic analysis.

Management

- Most children succumb to overwhelming infection.
- Granulocyte transfusion and bone marrow transplantation may be effective in some cases.

Papillon–Lefèvre syndrome (Figure 8.18)

An autosomal recessive condition manifesting as hyperkeratosis of the palms and feet and progressive exfoliation of all teeth from periodontal disease. *A. actinomycetem-comitans* has been implicated in the periodontal disease which is associated with a qualitative neutrophil defect and mutations in the lysosomal protease cathepsin C gene on 11q14-21. Primary teeth commence shedding from the time of eruption, with no evidence of root resorption. All primary teeth are usually lost before the permanent teeth erupt, when they in turn are exfoliated.

Diagnosis

- The oral changes and skin lesions are pathognomonic for this condition.
- Selective anaerobic culturing for *A. actinomycetemcomitans* is difficult, and a more reliable alternative is to use an enzyme-linked immunosorbent assay (ELISA) to detect IgG antibodies against this organism.

Management

No treatment is particularly successful. Extraction of any remaining primary teeth before eruption of the permanent teeth has been advocated. Intensive periodontal therapy with metronidazole and chlorhexidine to eliminate or reduce *A. actinomy-cetemcomitans* may be successful in delaying the inevitable exfoliation of teeth, although the basic neutrophil function defect remains. Treatment of other family members has also been recommended, including pets (especially dogs) if they are found to harbour the bacteria. Several papers have reported the use of vitamin-A derivatives in management that may improve the prognosis. All patients require planned full clearances and dentures to avoid pain and disfigurement. It is important to consider proceeding with extractions in the permanent dentition to minimize excessive bone loss.

Chèdiak–Higashi disease

This is a rare autosomal recessive disorder affecting lysosomal storage and causing a qualitative neutrophil defect. There is defective neutrophil chemotaxis and abnormal degranulation that results in poor intracellular killing. There is also reported to be

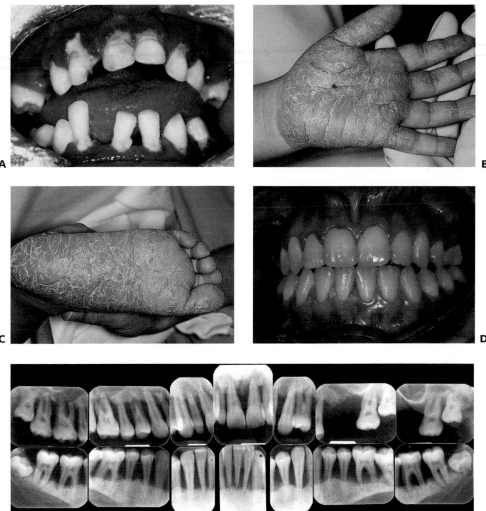

Figure 8.18 Papillon–Lèfevre syndrome. **A** The initial presentation of the child with severe periodontal disease-associated tooth mobility. Many of these teeth exfoliated within 6 months. **B, C** The characteristic appearance of the hands and feet in the same child. **D, E** The permanent dentition in a boy of 17 years, following long-term antibiotic treatment that has failed to improve the prognosis of the dentition.

abnormal B-cell and T-cell function and thrombocytopenia. Most children die by 10 years of age because of overwhelming sepsis. Teeth are shed because of severe periodontal disease with rapid alveolar bone loss.

HIV-associated periodontal disease in children

There are few cases documenting periodontal disease in young children. In adolescents there are reports of acute necrotizing ulcerative gingivitis (ANUG) and a characteristic linear marginal gingival erythema. Excellent oral hygiene and plaque control are essential combined with supportive therapy including chlorhexidine and metronidazole as required.

Langerhans' cell histiocytosis (disseminated) (Figure 8.19)

This condition was previously termed histiocytosis X and included the conditions eosinophilic granuloma, Hand–Schüller-Christian disease and Letterer–Siwe disease. The abnormality in common is a proliferation of Langerhans' cells. Oral lesions characteristically occur in all four quadrants and characteristically affect the tissues overlying or supporting the primary molar teeth. The lesions typically extend forward to the canines, but rarely involve the incisors.

Presentation
- Malaise, irritability.
- Anogenital and postauricular rash.
- Diabetes insipidus.
- Premature exposure by alveolar resorption and subsequent loss of primary teeth, especially molars.

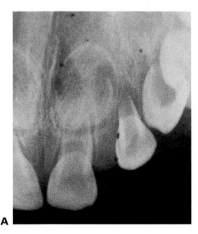

A

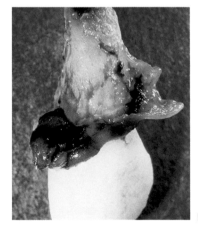

B

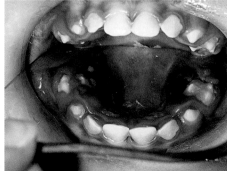

C

Figure 8.19 A Necrotic central incisor presenting with long-standing palatal ulceration. This child had Langerhans' cell histiocytosis, the lesion is shown in **B**. **C** Characteristic appearance of disseminated Langerhans' cell histiocytosis with lesions in all four quadrants.

- Radiographically, teeth appear to be 'floating in air'.
- Typically, all four quadrants are involved.

Diagnosis
- Biopsy of oral or skin lesions – cells positive for S100.
- Transmission electron microscopy of Langerhans' cells shows characteristic Birbeck's bodies.

Management
- Excision and curettage of oral lesions and extraction of involved teeth is required to control oral lesions.
- Multiagent chemotherapy is required for disseminated disease and is most effective if commenced early.

Hypophosphatasia (Figure 8.20)
A decrease in serum alkaline phosphatase and an increase in the urinary excretion of phosphoenolamine (PEA) are pathognomonic for hypophosphatasia. The more usual form is transmitted as an autosomal dominant trait, whereas the autosomal recessive form is invariably lethal. Loss of at least some of the incisor teeth usually occurs before 18 months. Several authors have identified groups of children who manifest only dental changes, namely the early loss of teeth without any rachitic bone changes – the term odontohypophosphatasia has been suggested for these patients but this is inappropriate as the presentation of loss of teeth alone is only one end of the spectrum in the variable expression of this disease. In these children there are less severe changes and we have observed that the permanent dentition is unaffected.

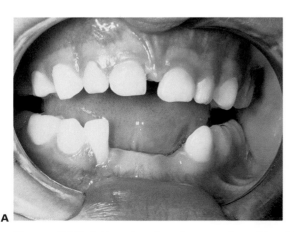
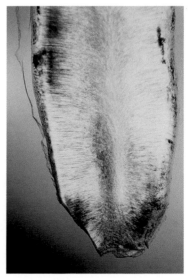

A **B**

Figure 8.20 A Hypophosphatasia presenting with exfoliation of the maxillary and mandibular anterior teeth around 2 years of age. There is minimal gingival inflammation and hard-tissue sections (**B**) show absent cementum.

Diagnosis

- Serum alkaline phosphatase level less than 90 U/L. The normal range is 80–350 U/L, however, growing children often have levels well in excess of these values (>400 U/L).
- Urinary PEA and serum pyridoxal-5-phosphate (vitamin B_6) tests are required to confirm the diagnosis. A skeletal survey of the long bones is necessary as rachitic changes may be present in severe cases.
- Sections of the exfoliated teeth show abnormal or absent cementum.

Self-mutilation (Figure 8.21)

A number of conditions exist which present with self-mutilation:

- Hereditary sensory neuropathies (congenital insensitivity to pain syndrome).
- Lesch–Nyhan syndrome (hypoxanthine guanine phosphoribosyltransferase deficiency).

Hereditary neuropathies are rare inherited disorders affecting the number and distribution of small myelinated and unmyelinated nerve fibres. Most categories in classification systems arose from the varied clinical presentations – terms used have included congenital indifference or insensitivity to pain, dysautonomia, sensory anaesthesia, painless whitlows of the fingers and recurrent plantar ulcers with osteomyelitis.

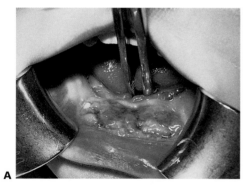

A

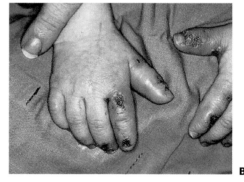

B

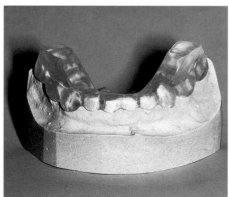

C

Figure 8.21 A Self-mutilation in a child with a peripheral sensory neuropathy. This child presented with exfoliation of the anterior teeth. She was investigated for many of the conditions described above until it was discovered that she herself was pulling out her teeth. Having no sensory nerve endings she could feel no pain. **B** Finger-biting can also be a manifestation of neuropathies. **C** An appliance to disclude the teeth and prevent self-injury. All cases are different and an appliance that is successful in one patient may not prove to be appropriate in another.

The term 'indifference to pain' in these cases is a misnomer in that indifference implies a cerebral inattention or cognitive dysfunction. Those patients with 'indifference' correctly receive painful stimuli but fail to react in the usual defensive manner by withdrawal. In those patients with 'insensitivity to pain,' the deep tendon reflexes are preserved as these are controlled by large-diameter myelinated fibres. The lack of pain perception is due to a true peripheral neuropathy.

Diagnosis

The diagnosis of these conditions is often made by exclusion and by careful observation of the child. It is not uncommon for many months to pass before a correct diagnosis is made and, in the absence of other pathologies, parents or caregivers may incorrectly be suspected of child abuse or Münchhausen's syndrome by proxy. Because of an inability to recognize or feel pain, these children may avulse teeth and inflict extensive trauma to the gingivae, tongue or mucosa with their fingers or by biting and chewing.

Self-inflicted ulceration (factitious ulceration) may also occur as a habit (akin to nail biting) but may also be a manifestation of psychological disorders.

Management

- Selective grinding of tooth cusps or 'dome' build-ups of the occlusal table with composite resin to produce a smooth surface.
- Acrylic splints or cast silver splints to prevent gross laceration of the tongue or fingers.
- Extraction of teeth may be required as a last option in severe cases.

Initial management in young children often necessitates restraint to prevent these children from injuring themselves. Even for the most vigilant parents, constant supervision is impossible and invariably these children will continue to sustain injuries despite the best care. The involvement of occupational therapists is invaluable to support parents and institute protective measures in the home such as the use of padded clothing, arm splints, helmets and other protective devices. Where lacerations to the tongue and other soft tissues occur, mouthguards and other appliances which prevent the teeth from occluding are required. Lower appliances are generally more suitable than those placed in the upper arch. In severe cases where the mutilation is intractable, botulinum toxin A (Botox) has been used to selectively paralyse the major mandibular elevator muscles (medial pterygoid and masseter).

Prognosis

The prognosis for most children with peripheral sensory neuropathies is poor and, in one case managed by one of the authors, the child died of an undiagnosed pneumonia before 3 years of age. Children tend to have repeated hospital admissions, fractures of long bones, injuries to the extremities and recurrent chronic infections. This pattern of repeated traumatic injuries is characterized in one such patient:

- Premature loss of all lower anterior primary teeth.
- Chronic ulceration of the lower alveolus.
- Second degree burn to right forearm from a radiator.
- Fracture of left humerus (during hospital admission) with subsequent multifocal osteomyelitis.
- Fracture of left condyle and mandibular symphysis.
- Death from respiratory sepsis at 2 years of age.

Ehlers–Danlos type IV and type VIII

These inborn errors of metabolism present as disorders of collagen formation. Typically, there is hyperextensibility of skin with capillary fragility, bruising of the skin and hypermobility of the joints. Types IV and VIII may present with dental complications, mainly progressive periodontal disease leading to the loss of teeth.

Erythromelalgia

A very rare condition, characterized by sympathetic overactivity, causing an endarteritis and the extremities feeling hot. One case has been reported with loss of primary and permanent teeth at 4 years of age. The child had extreme hypermobility of joints and slept on a tiled floor in the middle of winter because of the heat in her legs. She also had an unexplained tachycardia of 200 beats per minute and presented a diagnostic dilemma for many months. The teeth exfoliated because of necrosis of alveolar bone.

Acrodynia (pink disease)

Mercury toxicity causes alveolar destruction and sequestration. Extremely rare now, although in the past it was not uncommon with the use of teething powders containing mercury.

Acatalasia

Autosomal recessive catalase deficiency in neutrophils leading to periodontal destruction. Extremely rare outside Japan.

Scurvy

Almost unknown today, this nutritional deficiency of vitamin C results in a connective tissue disorder. Tooth loss is due to a failure of proline hydroxylation and consequent reduced collagen synthesis.

Oral pathology in the newborn infant

Differential diagnosis

- Keratin cysts of the newborn:
  - Epstein's pearls
  - Bohn's nodules.
- Congenital epulis of the newborn.
- Granular cell tumour (granular cell myoblastoma).
- Melanotic neuro-ectodermal tumour of infancy.
- Natal/neonatal teeth.

Cysts in the newborn (Figure 8.22A)

Epstein's pearls

These hard, raised nodules are small keratinizing cysts arising in epithelial remnants trapped along lines of fusion of embryological processes. They appear in the midline of the hard palate, most commonly posteriorly.

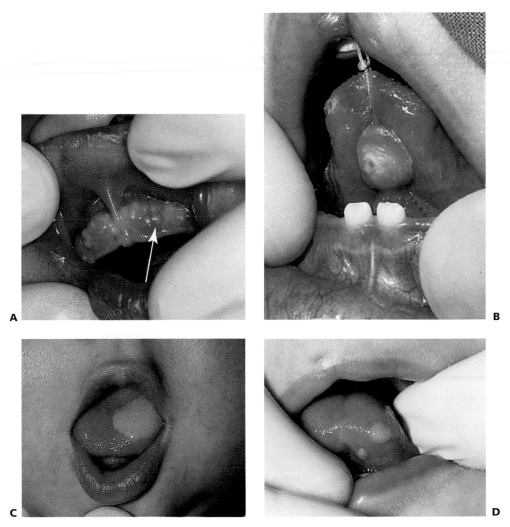

Figure 8.22 Oral pathology in infants. **A** Bohn's nodules in a newborn child (arrow).
B Fibroepithelial hyperplasia on the ventral surface of the tongue caused by trauma from the erupting mandibular incisors. **C** White sponge naevus of the tongue. **D** Granular cell tumour. (Continued)

Bohn's nodules

These are remnants of the dental lamina and usually occur on the labial or buccal aspect of the maxillary alveolar ridges.

Management

No treatment is required other than reassurance of the parents.

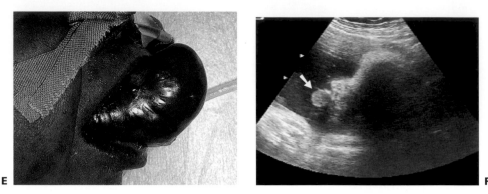

Figure 8.22 (cont.) E Congenital epulis measuring 4 cm in length. F The lesion was diagnosed prenatally on ultrasound (arrow).

Melanotic neuroectodermal tumour of infancy

A rare but important paediatric tumour derived from neural crest cells, this occurs predominantly in the maxilla. The condition may be present at birth and all recorded cases have been diagnosed by 4 months of age. Similar to a neuroblastoma, there may be high levels of vanillylmandelic acid (a catecholamine end-product) in the urine. Lesions may be multicentric with close approximation to, but not involving, dental tissues, reflecting their ectomesenchymal origin. Intra-orally, lesions appear as circumscribed swellings that may have the appearance of normal mucosal or have a blue–black hue and may be associated with premature eruption of the primary incisors.

Diagnosis

Computed tomography followed by excisional biopsy because of the extremely rapid growth of the lesion. This condition is usually so unique, at this age and at this site, that diagnosis is not difficult.

Management

- Enucleation of the tumour and involved primary teeth.
- Curettage of the bony floor of the multiple cavities.
- Radiotherapy is contraindicated.
- Recurrences are extremely rare.

Diseases of salivary glands

Differential diagnosis

- Mucocoele.
- Ranula.
- Sialoliths.
- Mumps.
- Autoimmune parotitis.

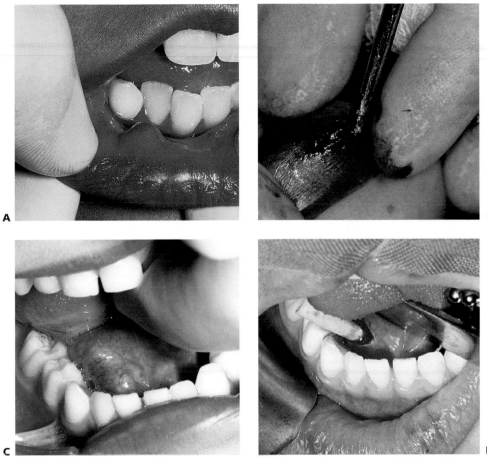

Figure 8.23 A Typical presentation of a mucocoele on the lower lip. Most lesions require removal. **B** Semilunal incision with exposure of cyst which may be removed with blunt dissection. **C** A mucous cyst of the floor of the mouth – a ranula. **D** Insertion of a Penrose drain lateral to Wharton's duct to marsupialize the cyst.

- Bilateral parotitis associated with bulimia.
- Aplasia (or hypoplasia) of major salivary glands

Mucocoele (Figure 8.23A, B)
Mucous extravasation cyst
The most common mucous cyst in the oral cavity, the mucous extravasation cyst arises from damage to the duct of one of the minor salivary glands in the (lower) lip or cheek. Often caused by lip biting or other minor injuries, mucus builds up in the connective tissue to be surrounded by fibrous tissue. Most mucocoeles are well-circumscribed bluish swellings, although traumatized lesions may have a keratinized surface.

Management
- Some cysts heal spontaneously.
- Surgical excision, ideally together with the associated minor salivary glands.

Mucous retention cyst
Less common than the mucous extravasation cyst, this cyst has a similar or identical clinical appearance but is lined by epithelium.

Ranula (Figure 8.23C)
A mucous (extravasation) cyst of the floor of the mouth caused by damage to the duct of either the sublingual or submandibular glands. A soft, bluish swelling presents on one side of the floor of the mouth. A plunging ranula occurs when the lesion herniates through the mylohyoid muscle to involve the neck.

Management
- Surgical excision.
- Large lesions may require marsupialization in the first instance.

Sialadenitis
Inflammation of the major salivary glands may result from:
- Viral infection:
  - Mumps or cytomegalovirus infection. Present with bilateral non-suppurative parotitis, usually epidemic.
  - Human immunodeficiency virus (HIV) infection and AIDS; 10–15% of children with AIDS will manifest bilateral parotitis.
- Bacterial infections:
  - Suppurative, usually retrograde infection.
- Autoimmune:
  - Sjögren's syndrome (usually seen in older patients).
  - Bilateral autoimmune parotitis. Punctate sialectasis appearance on sialogram.
- Bulimia:
  - Salivary gland enlargement is a common presentation of bulimia nervosa.
- Chronic sialadenitis:
  - Usually caused by unilateral obstruction of a major salivary gland, either by stricture, epithelial plugging or a sialolith (calculus) causing obstruction and inflammation. Pain occurs during eating and if there is acute exacerbation of infection.

Clinical Hint

A periodontal probe is useful for **gently** exploring the terminal part of a major salivary gland duct. This can identify a small calculus or dislodge an epithelial plug. This should not be attempted in younger and/or anxious patients.

Management

- Massage of the gland/milking of the duct for cases of recurrent epithelial plugging.
- Antibiotics to control infection in the acute phase.
- Removal of sialolith. Note – a suture should be passed under the duct behind the sialolith to prevent it being displaced backwards.
- In long-standing cases of obstructive sialadenitis, removal of the gland may be necessary.

Salivary gland tumours

Most tumours of the salivary glands in children are vascular malformations. Pleomorphic adenomas are uncommon. Malignant neoplasms such as mucoepidermoid carcinoma, adenocarcinoma and sarcoma are extremely uncommon and affect mainly older children and adolescents. The parotid is the most common site for such tumours.

Diagnostic imaging of the salivary glands

Radiology

Mandibular occlusal films are useful for imaging salivary calculi in the submandibular duct. These may also be seen on panoramic radiographs, albeit with the mandible superimposed.

Sialography

Used to demonstrate a stricture of the duct and gland architecture.

Computed tomography, magnetic resonance imaging, ultrasound

If neoplasms are suspected. Can be combined with sialography.

Nuclear medicine

Demonstrates salivary gland function. A technetium pertechnetate (^{99m}Tc) tracer seeks major protein-secreting exocrine and endocrine glands. The isotope is readily taken up by the major salivary glands. Lemon juice then administered orally to assess function and clearance of the glands.

Aplasia of salivary glands (Figure 8.24)

A number of cases of congenital salivary gland agenesis have been reported. Major salivary gland hypoplasia is an uncommon presentation of a child with gross caries in unusual sites. Caries of the lower anterior teeth should be regarded with suspicion in a young child as it may indicate aplasia of the submandibular glands. It is uncommon for children to be on medication that will cause severe xerostomia and so aplasia/hypoplasia should always be considered.

Diagnosis

Reduced uptake of technetium pertechnetate.

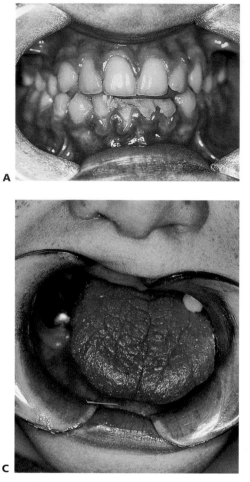

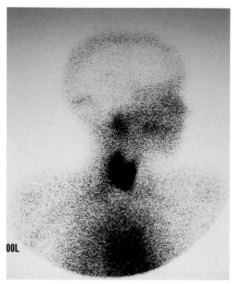

Figure 8.24 A Gross carious destruction of the mandibular anterior teeth. These are the only affected teeth. **B** The lateral nuclear medicine scan shows normal uptake of tracer in the parotid glands and thyroid but no function in the submandibular gland. A CT scan revealed that only rudimentary glands were present. **C** A 4-year-old boy who, after three procedures under general anaesthesia to treat gross caries in his primary dentition, was subsequently diagnosed with aplasia of his major salivary glands.

References and further reading

Infections

Doson TB, Perrott DH, Kaban LB 1989 Pediatric maxillofacial infections: a retrospective study of 113 patients. Journal of Oral and Maxillofacial Surgery 47:327–330

Flaitz CM, Baker KA 2000 Treatment approaches to common symptomatic oral lesions in children. Dental Clinics of North America 44:671–696

King DL, Steinhauer W, Garcia-Godoy F et al 1992 Herpetic gingivostomatitis and teething difficulty in infants. Pediatric Dentistry 14:82–85

Heggie AA, Shand JM, Aldred MJ et al 2003 Juvenile mandibular chronic osteomyelitis: a distinct clinical entity. International Journal of Oral and Maxillofacial Surgery 32:459–468

Oral ulceration

Challacombe SJ 1997 Oro-facial granulomatosis and oral Crohn disease: are they specific diseases and do they predict systemic Crohn disease? Oral Diseases 3:127–129

Field EA, Brooks V, Tyldesley WR 1992 Recurrent aphthous ulceration in children: a review. International Journal of Paediatric Dentistry 2:1–10

Flaitz CM, Baker KA 2000 Treatment approaches to common symptomatic oral lesions in children. Dental Clinics of North America 44: 671–696

Fridh G, Koch G 1999 Effect of a mouth rinse containing amyloglucosidase and glucose oxidase on recurrent aphthous ulcers in children and adolescents. Swedish Dental Journal 23:49–57

Harris JC, Bryan RA, Lucas VS et al 2001 Dental disease and caries related microflora in children with dystrophic epidermolysis bullosa. Pediatric Dentistry 23:438–443

Léauté-Labrèze C, Lamireau T, Chawki D et al 2000 Diagnosis, classification and management of erythema multiforme and Stevens-Johnson syndrome. Archives of Disease in Childhood 83:347–352

Scully C 1981 Orofacial manifestations of chronic granulomatous disease of childhood. Oral Surgery, Oral Medicine and Oral Pathology 57:148–157

Sedano HO, Gorlin RJ 1989 Epidermolysis bullosa. Oral Surgery, Oral Medicine and Oral Pathology 67:555–563

Tay Y-K, Huff JC, Weston WL 1996 Mycoplasma pneumoniae infection is associated with Stevens–Johnson syndrome, not erythema multiforme (von Hebra). Journal of the American Academy of Dermatology 35:757–760

Weston WL, Morelli JG, Rogers M 1997 Target lesions on the lips: childhood herpes simplex associated with erythema multiforme mimics Stevens–Johnson syndrome. Journal of the American Academy of Dermatology 37:848–850

Vascular lesions

Kaban LB, Mulliken JB 1986 Vascular anomalies of the maxillofacial region. Journal of Oral and Maxillofacial Surgery 44:203–213

Epulides

Kaiserling E, Ruck P, Xiao JC 1995 Congenital epulis and granular cell tumour: a histologic and immunohistochemical study. Oral Surgery, Oral Medicine and Oral Pathology 80:687–697

Welbury RR 1980 Congenital epulis of the newborn. British Journal of Oral Surgery 18:239–243

Gingival overgrowth

Miranda J, Brunet L, Roset P et al 2001 Prevalence and risk of gingival enlargement in patients treated with nifedipine. Journal of Periodontology 72:605–611

Pernu HE, Pernu LMH, Huttunen KE et al 1992 Gingival overgrowth among renal transplant recipients related to immunosuppressive medication and possible local background factors. Journal of Periodontology 63:548–553

Ross PJ, Nazif MM, Zullo T et al 1989 Effects of cyclosporin A on gingival status following liver transplantation. Journal of Dentistry for Children 56:56–59

Premature exfoliation of teeth

Erturk N, Dogan S 1991 Distribution of *Actinobacillus actinomycetemcomitans* and *Porphyromonas gingivalis* by subject age. Journal of Periodontology 62:490–494

Frisken KW, Higgins T, Palmer JM 1990 The incidence of periodontopathic micro-organisms in young children. Oral Microbiology and Immunology 5:43–45

Littlewood SJ, Mitchell L 1998 The dental problems and management of a patient suffering from congenital insensitivity to pain. International Journal of Pediatric Dentistry 8:47–50

Hartman KS 1980 Histiocytosis X: a review of 114 cases with oral involvement. Oral Surgery, Oral Medicine, and Oral Pathology 49:38–54

Macfaflane JD, Swart JGN 1989 Dental aspects of hypophosphatasia: a case report, family study and literature review. Oral Surgery, Oral Medicine and Oral Pathology 67:521–526

Meyle J, Gonzales JR 2000 Influences of systemic diseases on periodontitis in children and adolescents. Periodontology 26:92–112

Preus HR 1988 Treatment of rapidly destructive periodontitis in Papillon–Lefèvre syndrome. Clin Periodontol 15:639–643

Rasmussen P 1989 Cyclic neutropenia in an 8-year-old child. Journal of Pediatric Dentistry 5:121–126

Slayton RL 2000 Treatment alternatives for sublingual traumatic ulceration (Riga–Fedé disease). Pediatric Dentistry. 22:413–414

Watanabe K 1990 Prepubertal periodontitis: a review of diagnostic criteria, pathogenesis and differential diagnosis. Journal of Periodontalal Research 25:31–48

Salivary gland agenesis

Whyte AM, Hayward MWJ 1989 Agenesis of the salivary glands: a report of two cases. British Journal of Radiology 62:1023–1028

General

Hall RK 1994 Pediatric orofacial medicine and pathology. Chapman and Hall Medical, London

Worldwide web database

Online Mendelian Inheritance in Man, OMIM (TM). McKusick-Nathans Institute for Genetic Medicine, Johns Hopkins University (Baltimore, MD) and National Center for Biotechnology Information, National Library of Medicine (Bethesda, MD), 2000 (www.ncbi.nlm.nih.gov/omim/)

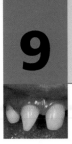

9 Dental anomalies

Contributors
Michael J Aldred, Peter J M Crawford, Angus Cameron, Nigel M King, Richard Widmer

Introduction

The diagnosis and management of dental anomalies constitute important areas of paediatric dentistry. Most dental anomalies will present in childhood, yet many are misdiagnosed or left untreated, perhaps because of lack of experience, or because the case is perceived to be 'too difficult'. In some cases, genetic consultation is desirable, not merely to put a name to the condition but also to give appropriate advice on the prognosis and the risk of recurrence in future generations. In many cases the presence of an inherited dental disorder would not stop a family from having children, but it is important to give parents and the affected children themselves appropriate advice. Genetic services are usually available at most paediatric hospitals.

In this chapter, reference to particular inherited conditions is made to entries in Online Mendelian Inheritance in Man (OMIM). This online database (see References and further reading for details) is a catalogue of genetic disorders developed by Dr Victor McKusick of the Johns Hopkins University and the National Center for Biotechnology Information.

Considerations in the management of dental anomalies

- Informing and supporting child and parent.
- Establishing a diagnosis.
- Genetic counselling.
- Interdisciplinary formulation of definitive treatment plan.
- Elimination of pain.
- Restoration of aesthetics.
- Provision of adequate function.
- Maintenance of occlusal vertical dimension.
- Use of intermediate restorations in childhood and adolescence.
- Planning for definitive treatment at an optimal age.

Treatment planning for children with dental anomalies
Treatment planning should be multidisciplinary. Decisions made must involve the child and the parents, and should consider the present and future needs and development of the child. While children will cope with a range of appliances and treatments during childhood, early adolescence represents a period of social adjustment as well as the

217

transitional changes in the dentition. It is perhaps the most difficult time in which to formulate a long-term plan. Teenagers are most concerned about aesthetics, yet it may be too early to provide definitive restorations; extensive orthodontic treatment may be required, or later orthognathic surgery. In institutions, various teams exist to treatment plan and/or manage these cases and a list is suggested below. Note the involvement of the child's local general dental practitioner.

The team approach
- Paediatric dentist.
- Orthodontist.
- Prosthodontist.
- Surgeon.
- Speech pathologist.
- Clinical psychologist.
- Local general dental practitioner.

It is essential to seek advice from colleagues in the management of children with uncommon dental conditions. Local and international collaboration provide the best opportunities to increase our knowledge and improve the outcomes for these children.

Dental anomalies at different stages of dental development

It is convenient to consider dental anomalies by the development stage at which they arise.

Migration of neural crest cells (ectomesenchyme) into branchial arches
- Duplication of dental arches.

Dental lamina formation stage
Induction and proliferation
- Hypodontia/oligodontia/anodontia (which may be associated with other features of an ectodermal dysplasia).
- Supernumerary teeth.
- Double teeth (geminated or fused teeth).
- Odontomes (complex and compound).
- Odontogenic tumours.
- Ameloblastic fibroma/fibrodentinoma/fibro-odontome (dependent on differentiation and the presence and type of calcification within the lesion).
- Odontogenic keratocysts.

Histodifferentiation
Developmental defects of multiple dental tissues
- Regional odontodysplasia.

Morphodifferentiaton
Abnormalities of size and shape
- Macrodontia.
- Microdontia (isolated or as part of a syndrome).
- Invaginated odontome (dens invaginatus).
- Evaginated odontome (dens evaginatus).
- Carabelli trait.
- Talon cusp.
- Hutchinson's incisors and mulberry molars in congenital syphilis.
- Taurodontism.

Matrix deposition
Organic matrix deposition and mineralization
- Enamel:
  - amelogenesis imperfecta
  - chronological enamel hypoplasia
  - molar–incisor hypoplasia
  - enamel opacities
  - fluorosis.
- Dentine:
  - dentinogenesis imperfecta
  - dentinal dysplasia
  - vitamin D-resistant rickets
  - pre-eruptive intracoronal resorptive lesions.

Eruption and root development
- Premature eruption.
- Natal and neonatal teeth.
- Delayed eruption.
- Ectopic eruption.
- Eruption cysts.
- Transposition of teeth.
- Impactions.
- Arrested root development from systemic illness (or treatment of systemic illness).
- Failure of eruption in amelogenesis imperfecta.
- Failure of eruption in cleidocranial dysplasia.
- Failure of eruption in cherubism.
- Failure of eruption associated with inflammatory follicular cysts.

Formation of dental lamina

Hypodontia
Alternative terminology: Hypodontia, oligodontia, anodontia.

Hypodontia, oligodontia and anodontia are terms that can be interpreted to refer to progressive degrees of missing teeth, though the term hypodontia is preferred because it is inclusive of any number of missing teeth (Figure 9.1A). Oligodontia refers to six or more missing teeth, and anodontia to the complete absence of teeth. It is implicit in all cases that the teeth are missing because of failure of development. The term 'congenitally missing teeth' is a misnomer when applied to the permanent dentition because these teeth do not commence development until after birth (and with regard to the primary dentition one cannot usually determine this clinically at birth); 'partial anodontia' is obviously a nonsense. Some degree of hypodontia is not uncommon, occurring sporadically or with a hereditary component. The teeth most commonly absent are the last teeth in each series (i.e. the lateral incisor, the second premolar and the third molar). Clinically, it is not so important how many, but rather which types of tooth are absent. It is particularly unusual to be missing central incisors, canines or first permanent molars. Multiple missing teeth in particular should lead to questioning regarding other affected family members. The presence of a rudimentary

Figure 9.1 A The teeth most commonly missing are the last teeth in each series, namely the upper lateral incisors, the second premolars and the third molars.
B Panoramic radiograph of a boy with autosomal dominant ectodermal dysplasia with absence of both primary and permanent teeth.

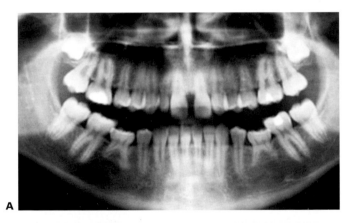

A

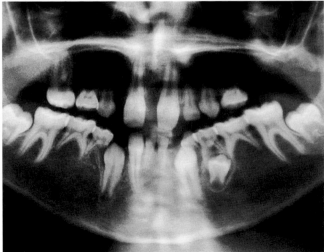

B

or conical tooth may be associated with the absence of the same tooth on the opposite side of the arch. A common example of this is the peg lateral incisor. Furthermore, that lateral incisor itself may be absent in subsequent generations. Missing teeth are also a manifestation of many syndromes of the head and neck.

Frequency

Primary teeth	~0.1–0.7%	male : female	ratio unknown
Permanent teeth	~2–9%	male : female	1 : 1.4

Third molars > maxillary lateral incisors > second premolars > mandibular central incisors.

Major conditions manifesting hypodontia

Hypodontia is a major clinical feature of over 50 syndromes. These include:

- Ectodermal dysplasias.
- Clefting.
- Trisomy 21 (Down's syndrome).
- Chondroectodermal dysplasia (Ellis–van Creveld syndrome).
- Rieger syndrome.
- Incontinentia pigmenti.
- Oro-facial-digital syndrome.
- Williams' syndrome.
- Craniosynostosis syndromes.

Ectodermal dysplasias

Ectodermal dysplasia describes a group of developmental, often inherited, disorders involving the ectodermally derived structures, i.e. the hair, teeth, nails, skin and sweat glands. The most common is the X-linked hypohidrotic form (OMIM 305100, EDA1, Xq12-q13.1 (short arm of X chromosome)). In this condition the usual presentation is a male child with:

- Multiple missing teeth (Figure 9.1B).
- Fine, sparse hair (Figure 9.2A, B).
- Dry skin (Figure 9.2A).
- Maxillary hypoplasia.
- Eversion of the lips.
- Pigmentation around the mouth and eyes.

Teeth are small and conical, often with a large anterior diastema (Figure 9.3). Heterozygous females are often identified by dental examination and their manifestations may be limited to a single missing tooth or to a peg lateral incisor (see the Lyon hypothesis below).

In the group of ectodermal dysplasias, autosomal dominant and recessive modes of inheritance are also seen. In such families there will not be such a striking difference in the degree of the disorder between males and females compared with X-linked hypohidrotic ectodermal dysplasia (Figures 9.2A, 9.4). Mutations in the MSX1 gene (4p16.1) have been identified in families with missing third molars and second premolars with or without clefting, as well as in families with tooth-nail (Witkop) syndrome. PAX9 (14q12-q13) gene mutations have been found in other families with autosomal dominant missing teeth.

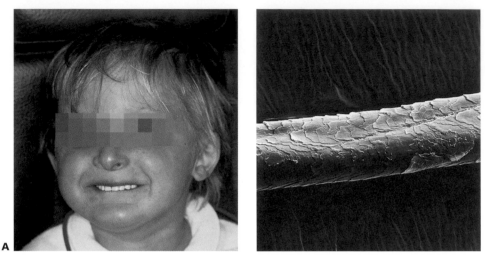

Figure 9.2 A Typical appearance of a boy with X-linked hypohidrotic ectodermal dysplasia (wearing a denture). The skin around the eyes is dry and wrinkled and may be pigmented. **B** The hair is fine and sparse and often displays longitudinal grooves on the surface, as demonstrated under the scanning electron microscope.

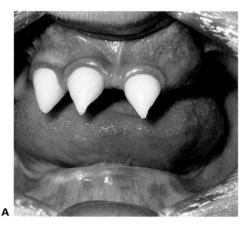

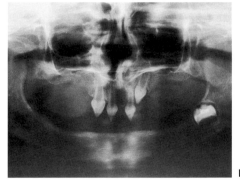

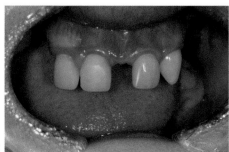

Figure 9.3 A, B Typical intra-oral and radiographic presentations in a boy with ectodermal dysplasia with multiple missing teeth; the teeth that are present are small and conical in shape. Where teeth are absent, alveolar bone does not develop. **C** Composite build-ups of the conical teeth have provided great improvement in aesthetics, however, the question of the diastema remains, given that there are few teeth for orthodontic anchorage.

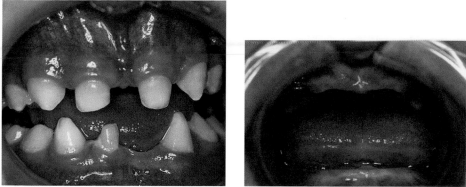

Figure 9.4 A This child is a heterozygous female with the X-linked form of ectodermal dysplasia and is less severely affected than her brother who has anodontia (**B**).

In some countries, dental care (including prevention, orthodontics and prosthetics) for affected children may be provided under government-funded schemes.

Management
The aim of treatment is to provide adequate function, maintain the vertical dimension and restore aesthetic appearance. Ideally, for social reasons, treatment should begin at around 2–3 years of age. A first step is often the placement of composite restorations to mask the 'fang-like' appearance of the caniniform anterior teeth (Figure 9.3A). There is often considerable parental pressure to 'normalize' the appearance and later steps may involve the provision of dentures to reduce the likelihood of teasing, often at about the time that the child starts school. This can begin as soon as the child will allow an adequate impression to be taken. Often, however, the first set of dentures is initially worn in the pocket(!), but as the child grows there is often a desire to have a more ordinary appearance. With encouragement and positive reinforcement, most children will soon try their new appliances.

Treatment planning for children with hypodontia
Treatment planning should be multidisciplinary and should consider the present and future needs and development of the child, being cognizant of the concerns of the individual and parents.

Treatment options
- Acid-etch retained, composite build-ups of conical teeth.
- Composite resin or bonded orthodontic buttons can also be added to provide undercuts for denture clasps and retainers (Figure 9.5)
- Partial dentures: conventional or overdentures (Figure 9.6).
- Surgical exposure of impacted teeth.
- Orthodontic management of spaces.
- Laboratory-fabricated composite veneers, crowns and bridges.
- Osseo-integrated implants (usually after the cessation of growth).

> **Clinical Hint   Provision of dentures for young children**
>
> Generally, children will tolerate dentures well. Provision of the upper denture before the lower may be one way of increasing acceptance. The aim is for these children to be wearing appliances that give them a dentition similar to their peers, to enhance their self-esteem and promote normal speech development and masticatory function by the time they are at kindergarten or primary school. Dentures need to be re-made at regular intervals and a same-age model from an unaffected child should be used as a template for the occlusion.
> - Use fast-setting alginate impression material and sit the child upright with the head forwards.
> - Use Adams' clasps on molars and ball retainers between upper canines and first molars.
> - Use overdentures when there are multiple missing teeth and/or irregular spacing.
> - Daily fluoride mouthrinses should be used with overdentures.
> - Resilient or soft liners aid retention.
> - Make dentures with irregular, even partly erupted, teeth during the mixed dentition stage.
> - Summer holidays are often a good time for provision of new dentures.

The Lyon hypothesis (X chromosome inactivation)

During cellular differentiation, one of the two X chromosomes in each female somatic cell is inactivated. This means that in families with X-linked disorders, approximately 50% of the cells of heterozygous females will express the mutant gene disorder whereas the remainder will express the normal gene. In the tissues affected by the condition, such females have a mosaic of affected and normal cells. This is of particular importance in conditions such as haemophilia, X-linked hypohidrotic ectodermal dysplasia, vitamin D-resistant rickets and X-linked amelogenesis imperfecta. Thus, heterozygous females with X-linked hypohidrotic ectodermal dysplasia may have missing teeth, although they are invariably less severely affected than males. Similarly, in haemophilia A, heterozygous females do not usually have a clinical bleeding abnormality but this can occur if lyonization is severely skewed so that there is a preponderance of cells producing factor VIII under control of the mutant gene.

Clefting

In patients affected by dentoalveolar clefting, because of disruption of the dental lamina at that site, there may be abnormal induction or proliferation. This may give rise to either missing teeth, usually the maxillary lateral incisor, and/or supernumerary teeth adjacent to the cleft. It is extremely rare for the canine tooth to be affected in the same way.

Solitary median maxillary central incisor syndrome (OMIM 147250)

Solitary median maxillary central incisor syndrome (SMMCI) (Figure 9.7) is very rare. It presents with a midline symmetrical maxillary central incisor. The condition may also

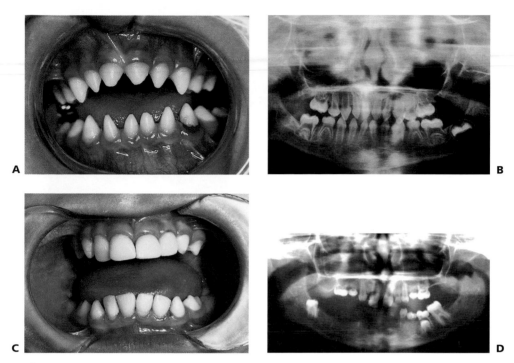

Figure 9.5 A, B Conical primary teeth are often associated with missing permanent teeth. This child had an autosomal recessive form of ectodermal dysplasia and was missing almost all of the permanent dentition. **C** The teeth have been built up with composite resin strip crowns. **D** Radiographic appearance of the same child at 15 years of age. Most of the primary teeth have exfoliated in the absence of a permanent successor. There has also been loss of bone in the region of the tuberosity due to pneumatization of the sinus that will complicate implant placement.

be associated with other midline disturbances such as cleft palate, choanal stenosis or atresia, imperforate anus or umbilical hernia and is probably part of the spectrum of the holoprosencephaly malformation complex. Of importance in some cases is the association with hypoplasia of the sella turcica, pituitary dysfunction, growth hormone deficiency and subsequent short stature. The syndrome is usually diagnosed on the basis of the dental manifestations. A mutation in the SHH gene (7q36) has been identified in one family but it is probable that there is genetic heterogeneity in the condition.

Ultimately, management of the dental anomaly is by orthodontic and prosthodontic means, determined by space considerations. In most cases, the single central incisor is moved to one side of the midline with either creation of space for a prosthodontic replacement or the adjacent lateral incisors are recontoured.

Osseo-integrated implants in children
There has been much controversy about the timing of placement of osseo-integrated implants in young children. To date, there has been only limited published material about early placement and any long-term consequences. It is generally understood

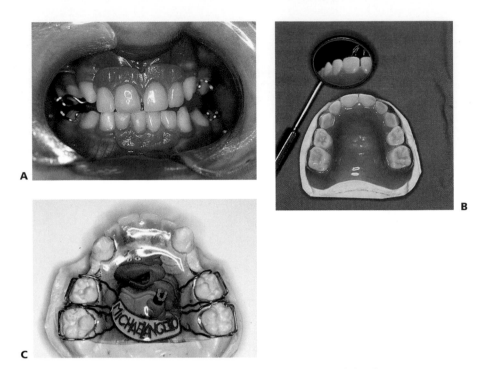

Figure 9.6 A, B, C Dentures for young children with ectodermal dysplasia. **A** Young children tolerate dentures extremely well and Adams' cribs and ball retainers provide ideal retention around primary molars. In this case an overdenture covers two conical, widely spaced incisors. **B** A full upper denture for a child of 30 months will require periodic relining and re-making as the child grows. Stock teeth are sometimes difficult to obtain but paediatric denture teeth may be made freehand from acrylic.

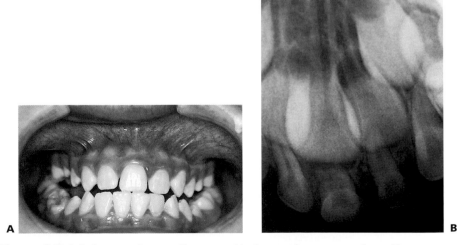

Figure 9.7 A Solitary median maxillary central incisor syndrome presenting with a symmetrical incisor in the midline. This child had a mild growth hormone deficiency, with his height on the 10th centile. **B** Periapical radiograph of the same patient in the primary dentition showing the single primary and permanent central incisors.

that implants act similarly to ankylosed teeth and do not move occlusally with growing bone around adjacent natural teeth. Recent animal research has confirmed that most fixtures do become osseo-integrated in growing jaws; however, there was no evidence from this research that the fixtures behaved like normal teeth during development. In the mandible the fixtures came to lie lingual to the natural teeth; in the maxilla they came to lie palatal and superior to the adjacent teeth and did not follow the normal downwards and forwards growth of this bone. This latter point is important when considering the placement of implants in the anterior maxilla. Furthermore, placement of fixtures retarded alveolar growth locally and changed the eruptive path of distally positioned tooth buds. Implants should, in most cases, not be considered before the cessation of growth. It should be noted, however, that in children with conditions such as ectodermal dysplasia, alveolar bone does not develop where teeth are not present. Consequently it may be considered appropriate, particularly where there are multiple missing teeth, to place implants much earlier in these children than in those with a normal alveolus. Recent research suggests that in cases of anodontia, implants are best placed in the mandibular canine region at around 8–10 years of age (following the period of maximal mandibular transverse growth) to facilitate lower denture construction.

Disorders of proliferation

Supernumerary teeth (Figure 9.8)
- Supernumerary teeth arising as a result of budding of the dental lamina can occur sporadically or be inherited, such as in cleidocranial dysplasia.
- The shape may resemble a tooth of the normal series (a supplemental tooth), in which case it can be incisiform, caniniform or molariform; otherwise it may be conical or tuberculate.
- Most often present as a result of failure of eruption of one or more permanent teeth. Usually appear as conical or tuberculate forms.
- Supernumerary teeth have been considered to be manifestations of a separate dentition (occurring between the primary and permanent dentitions), and consequently it may be possible to predict when and where supernumeraries may form (Jensen & Kreiborg 1990).

Alternative terminology
Mesiodens (a term restricted to supernumerary teeth in the midline of the maxilla), paramolar, distomolar, hyperdontia, polydontism, supplemental teeth.

Frequency

Primary teeth	~0.3–0.8%	male : female	ratio unknown
Permanent teeth	~1.0–3.5%	male : female	1 : 0.4

- 98% occur in the maxilla, 75% of which are mesiodens.

Diagnosis
- Failed or ectopic eruption of permanent tooth (Figure 9.8B).
- Routine radiographic survey.
- As part of a syndrome such as cleidocranial dysplasia (Figure 9.9).

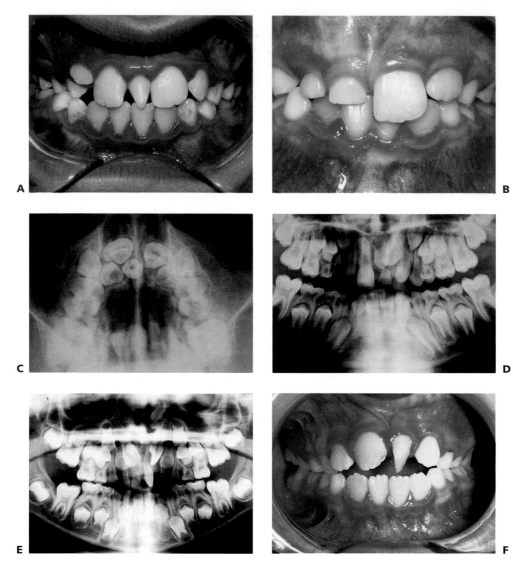

Figure 9.8 Common presentation of supernumerary teeth. **A** Conical teeth often erupt, except when inverted. **B** The late eruption of a permanent central incisor is most commonly caused by a supernumerary tooth. **C** A vertex occlusal radiograph showing the true anteroposterior position of the supernumerary tooth. This radiograph was taken by an extra-oral technique (modified submentovertex projection) using intensifying screens, thus significantly reducing the entrance radiation dose to approximately one-fifth of that using a conventional intraoral occlusal film. **D** A panoramic radiograph is useful in determining the vertical orientation of the extra tooth and the degree of displacement of the permanent central incisor. In this case, after removal of the supernumerary, an upper denture was used as a space maintainer and the impacted tooth subsequently erupted into a normal position. **E, F** Dependent on the degree of displacement, given adequate space, most impacted incisors will normally erupt once an obstruction such as a supernumerary is removed. The rotation can be corrected later.

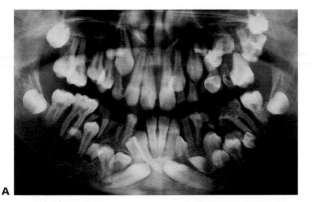

Figure 9.9 A A case of cleidocranial dysplasia with 18 supernumerary teeth. **B** A boy with cleidocranial dysplasia showing the characteristic absence of the clavicles.

A

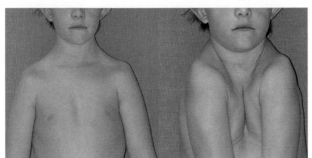

B

Management

- Conical teeth often erupt and are easily extracted (Figure 9.8A).
- Tuberculate and/or inverted conical teeth require surgical removal (Figure 9.8D) as early as possible to allow uninhibited eruption of the permanent tooth.
- It is essential to localize the position of the tooth to be removed *prior to* surgery. Periapical films using a tube-shift technique can be used to locate the tooth, however, this is always open to errors and misinterpretation. Panoramic and standard maxillary occlusal films may be used in the same way. The vertex occlusal radiograph gives a more precise indication of the horizontal and anteroposterior location and is therefore preferred (Figure 9.8C) to assist in determining the optimal surgical approach. Some centres prefer not to use this path due to increased cranial radiation.
- Digital imaging techniques using cone beam tomography provide high definition, three-dimensional imaging of the head and neck with much reduced radiation exposure than traditional computed tomography (CT) (see Figure 9.18 later).
- During surgical removal, care should be taken to avoid disturbing the developing permanent teeth.
- Before 10 years of age: if the unerupted central incisor is correctly aligned the treatment of choice is to remove the supernumerary surgically and allow normal

eruption of the permanent tooth. Gingival exposure may be required later because of surgical scar formation that can inhibit final soft-tissue emergence. Some authorities recommend the simultaneous removal of primary canines to counteract this tendency. Inverted supernumeraries, particularly when placed in the apical region of the incisors, may be left until the apices of the latter have formed to minimize the risk of damage.

- After 10 years of age, or if the central incisor is misaligned: surgical exposure with or without bonding of brackets or chains and subsequent orthodontic traction may be required (Figure 9.10).

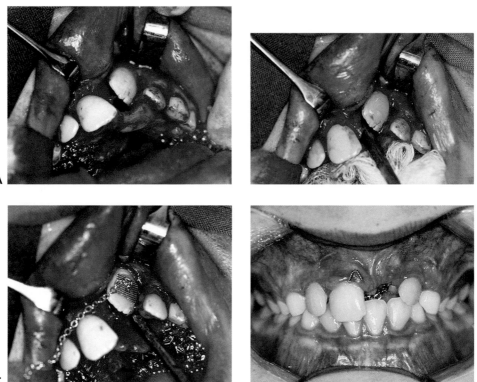

Figure 9.10 Surgical exposure and bonding of a gold chain to a central incisor which was impacted by a supernumerary tooth. **A** Elevation of the labial and palatal flap and removal of the supernumerary. **B** Acid-etch applied to the labial surface of the incisor to allow bonding of a stainless steel mesh and spot-welded gold chain, which was then spot-welded to a stainless steel mesh. **C** The flap is closed and the chain is ligated to the adjacent tooth. **D** The chain will be attached to an archwire and traction will be applied to orthodontically align the tooth.

Clinical Hint	Removal of supernumerary teeth

- Most maxillary supernumerary teeth are best removed surgically via a palatal approach. The only exceptions are those that are inverted, conical in shape and positioned between the roots of the central incisors. Usually the crown is found lying adjacent to the anterior nasal spine and is best approached via a labial flap.
- Supernumerary teeth may be also found in the midline of the palate as far back as the line of the first molars. These appear to be placed very high in the maxilla on radiographs but are usually quite superficial and simple to remove with a wide palatal flap.

Cleidocranial dysplasia (OMIM 119600) (Figure 9.9)

This condition has an autosomal dominant mode of inheritance, with a high frequency of spontaneous mutations. The condition has been mapped to 6p21 with mutations found in the CBFA1 gene.

Manifestations
- Short stature.
- Aplasia or hypoplasia of one or both clavicles (Figure 9.9B).
- Delayed ossification of fontanelles and sutures.
- Frontal bossing.
- Hypertelorism and maxillary hypoplasia.
- Wormian bones in cranial sutures.
- Multiple supernumerary teeth (Figure 9.9A).
- Delayed eruption of teeth.
- Dentigerous cyst formation.
- Absent or altered cellular cementum.

Management
- Early diagnosis and documentation.
- Planned removal of non-resorbing primary teeth.
- Surgical removal of supernumerary teeth.
- Surgical exposure of permanent teeth.
- Orthodontic alignment and consideration of orthognathic surgery when growth complete.

Note that extraction of the primary dentition without surgical exposure of the permanent teeth will not result in eruption of these teeth. A two-stage surgical procedure is usually required. The first procedure involves exposure of the anterior segments with removal of the anterior primary teeth and any supernumeraries that may be present. The permanent teeth are surgically exposed, either with primary apically repositioned flaps or with bonded gold chains attached for orthodontic traction. The anterior teeth are then aligned orthodontically. The second stage involves extraction of the primary molars, surgical removal of remaining supernumerary teeth and exposure of the pre-molars and molars in the buccal segments. Definitive orthodontics follows; orthogna-thic surgery may be required in cases with severe skeletal Class III malocclusion. Treatment obviously extends over many years and clinicians should be aware of the potential problems relating to the child's compliance.

Cherubism (OMIM 118400)

Cherubism is an autosomal dominant condition caused by mutations in the SH3BP2 gene on chromosome 4.

Patients may present in childhood with facial swelling and/or failure of eruption of teeth, typically the mandibular molars. Radiographs will reveal multilocular radiolucen-cies, typically involving the angles of the mandible (Figure 9.11). A biopsy will reveal multinucleate giant cells in a fibrous tissue stroma. Developing teeth in the affected area tend to be displaced and fail to erupt at the normal time. The maxillae can also be affected, as can the ribs. The facial swelling reflects the involvement of the under-lying bone. In some patients the sclera in the lower part of the eyes may be exposed to give the cherubic or heavenward gaze which gives the condition its name. In some cases there is no discernible facial swelling and the condition is identified as a result of routine radiographic studies such as for orthodontic treatment planning, or because of delayed eruption of teeth.

The condition progresses into adolescence and then tends to resolve, so that by the third or fourth decade radiographic changes may no longer be found. In some families more affected males than females may be identified – this is a result of reduced pen-etrance in females and needs to be taken into account in genetic counselling. A subset of patients with cherubism is more severely affected with the multilocular radiolucen-cies affecting the whole of the mandible and maxillae. In mildly affected cases regular review may that all is necessary, in more severely affected cases surgical reduction may be considered if the patient is distressed by their appearance.

Inflammatory follicular cysts

Some children may present with failure of eruption of a mandibular premolar associ-ated with a radiolucency involving the roots of the deciduous molar and crown of the unerupted premolar (see Figure 6.2B). There is controversy as to whether such cases

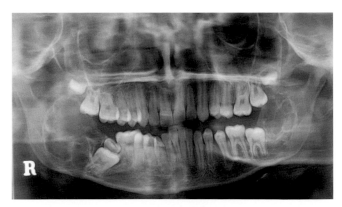

Figure 9.11 Dental panoramic radiograph showing multilocular radiolucencies in the right and left angles of the mandible of a 12-year-old boy. The displacement of developing molars is often seen in cherubism.

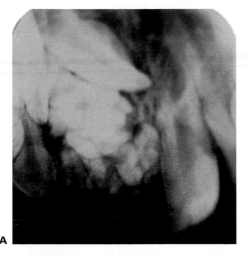

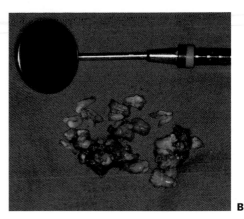

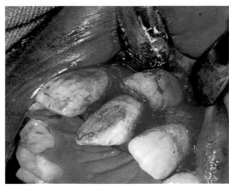

Figure 9.12 Odontomes. **A** Compound odontome with multiple denticles causing displacement of the maxillary right central incisor. **B** Macroscopic specimen of a compound odontome from the anterior maxilla showing the numerous denticles surrounded by a well-defined capsule. **C** Complex odontome.

are due to radicular cyst formation associated with the roots of the deciduous tooth (which is considered by some to be a rare occurrence) or dentigerous cyst formation around the crown of the premolar. The common characteristics of such cases tend to be:

- Prior endodontic treatment of the primary molar.
- A radiolucency involving the roots of the primary molar and crown of the permanent successor.
- Displacement of the permanent successor inferiorly.

Histopathological examination tends to show intense acute and chronic inflammation of the curetted tissue which is lined by hyperplastic stratified squamous epithelium. Such cases have been designated 'inflammatory follicular cysts', with persistent inflammation from the endodontically treated deciduous molar leading to an inflammatory enlargement of the follicle of the underlying permanent tooth.

Odontomes (Figure 9.12)

Odontomes lesions occur because of disordered differentiation and often present because of failure of eruption of a permanent tooth. In compound odontomes, masses of irregular denticles are found in a circumscribed soft-tissue stroma. Complex odont-omes are disordered lesions with a discrete, haphazard mass of calcified tissue containing all dental elements. There is either a normal complement of teeth or the odontome replaces a tooth of the normal series.

Management
- Enucleation.
- Depending on the time of diagnosis, permanent teeth may be ectopically positioned and may require surgical exposure and orthodontic alignment.

Odontogenic tumours

The ameloblastic fibroma, fibrodentinoma and fibro-odontome are uncommon benign odontogenic mixed tumours. All are seen as altered differentiation of the tooth bud: in an ameloblastic fibroma no hard tissue is formed, in an ameloblastic fibrodentinoma only dentine-like tissue is recognizable and in an ameloblastic fibro-odontome enamel is also formed. The lesions tend to be well demarcated.

Management
- Surgical enucleation.
- Follow-up of erupting permanent dentition if teeth are displaced by the lesion.

Odontogenic keratocysts

Odontogenic keratocysts may arise in place of a tooth of the normal series or from the dental lamina in addition to a normal complement of teeth. They constitute 5–15% of odontogenic cysts.

Basal cell naevus syndrome

Basal cell naevus syndrome ('Gorlin' or 'Gorlin–Goltz' syndrome) is an autosomal dominant condition characterized by multiple basal cell naevi, odontogenic keratocysts and a range of developmental abnormalities including frontal and parietal bossing, calcification of the falx cerebri, bifid ribs and palmar pitting. The gene responsible is the PTC ('patched') gene on chromosome 9. The odontogenic keratocysts may be the first manifestation of the condition, presenting as one or more unilocular or multilocular radiolucencies of the jaws. The tendency of odontogenic keratocysts to recur has implications for the management of patients with basal cell naevus syndrome.

Regional odontodysplasia (Figure 9.13)

Regional odontodysplasia is a sporadic defect in tooth formation with segmental involvement, usually localized to one or part of one quadrant but may cross the midline to affect the contralateral central incisor. All dental tissues are involved in a bizarre dysplasia with hypoplastic teeth which are slow to erupt and which typically show a ghostly radiographic appearance. The aetiology is unclear.
- Usually presents initially with abscessed primary teeth before or soon after eruption.
- Some cases are associated with superficial vascular anomalies.

Alternative terminology
Ghost teeth.

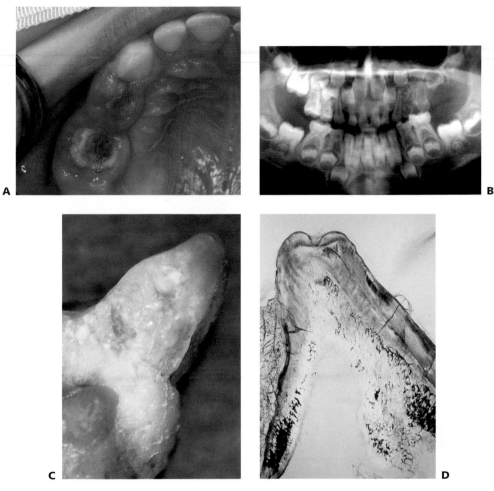

Figure 9.13 A Regional odontodysplasia presenting with abscessed primary molars in the maxillary left quadrant, soon after eruption. **B** The panoramic radiograph shows involvement of all the teeth in this quadrant including the permanent teeth. **C** Grossly abnormal enamel in an affected tooth, and **D** the hard-tissue section demonstrates the disruption of odontogenesis. (Courtesy Dr N Pai.)

Management

- In spite of attempts to restore teeth with stainless-steel crowns or composite resin, most affected teeth require extraction. Permanent successors of affected primary teeth are invariably affected, though sometimes to a lesser degree. There is no justification for bony excision at the time of tooth removal. There are reports of successful autologous tooth transplantation into the sites of removal of affected teeth.
- Partial dentures are required to restore the lost teeth.
- Implants may be appropriate.

Abnormalities of morphology (Figures 9.14–9.16)

Macrodontia (Figure 9.15)
- Any tooth or teeth larger than normal for that particular tooth type.
- True macrodontia involving the whole dentition is extremely rare. More commonly, single teeth are abnormally large because of an isolated disturbance of development (Figure 7.15A).

Aetiology
- Unknown for a single tooth, but generalized macrodontia may be caused by a hormonal imbalance, as this has been described in pituitary gigantism. It should be remembered that an illusion of generalized macrodontia will occur if the jaws are small relative to the size of the teeth.
- May also be associated with hemi-facial hyperplasia.
- True macrodontia should not be confused with the fusion or gemination of adjacent tooth units or a supernumerary to form a single tooth.
- Generalized macrodontia is also associated with KBG syndrome (the initials are taken from the surnames of families first reported with the condition). These children present with short stature, intellectual disability, skeletal abnormalities, syndactyly, a broad face with microcephaly and other facial anomalies (Figure 9.15B).

Alternative terminology
Megadontia, megalodontia and gigantism.

Frequency
Primary dentition   unknown
Permanent dentition   ~1.1%
More common in males.

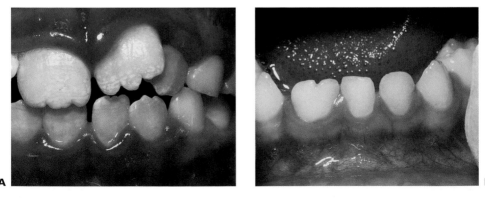

A   **B**

Figure 9.14 Morphological anomalies. **A** Mamelons, which are variations of normal anatomy. **B** Double tooth involving the right mandibular incisor, probably caused by fusion of the lateral and central incisor tooth germs.

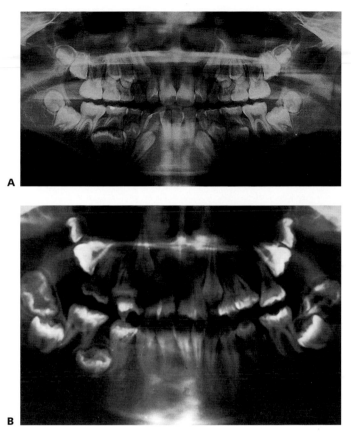

Figure 9.15 Macrodontia. **A** Isolated macrodontia in a mandibular second premolar tooth. **B** Generalized macrodontia associated with the KBG syndrome. These children presented with intellectual disabilities, broad facies, short stature and skeletal abnormalities.

Management

- Stripping to reduce tooth size; however, usually only a small change can be achieved.
- Can be combined with build-up of antimere if only one tooth affected.
- Extraction and replacement by a prosthesis.
- Aesthetic adjustment of an isolated macrodont tooth by incisal edge 'notching' and the generation of a labial groove to break up reflections may be helpful in some cases.

Microdontia

- One or more teeth that are smaller than normal for the tooth type.
- The most common form of microdontia affects only one or possibly two teeth; it is much rarer in the primary than in the permanent dentition.

- This anomaly most often affects the maxillary third molars and lateral incisors. It is noteworthy that the teeth affected are usually the ones that are also most often missing.
- Supernumerary teeth are frequently microdont.
- Patients with ectodermal dysplasia often present with microdontia.

True generalized microdontia
All of the teeth are of a normal form but they are smaller than normal teeth. This condition is exceedingly rare but can occur in pituitary dwarfism.

Generalized relative microdontia
The teeth are of normal size but appear relatively small with respect to the jaws which are larger than normal.

Alternative terminology
Peg-shaped laterals.

Frequency
Most data are available only for maxillary lateral incisors.
Primary dentition   <0.5%.
Permanent dentition   ~2.0% (maxillary lateral incisors).
More common in females.

Management
- Composite resin or (eventually) porcelain veneers to improve shape.
- The profile of the tooth is narrower at the gingival margin than a normal-sized tooth, and there is therefore a limit to how large the tooth can be made without producing an overhang in the gingival region or an unsightly interdental shadow.
- Orthodontic alignment and extraction of the tooth may be required and other techniques such as autotransplantation and implants should also be considered.

Clinical Hint   Acid-etch composite build-ups

In patients with missing teeth, the central incisors are often conical in form. When closing an anterior diastema, it is often preferable to add composite to the distal aspect of the crown rather than the mesial. The diastema can be closed orthodontically to avoid a 'flared' appearance of the tooth crown which tends to look artificial. A more vertical mesial proximal surface and the addition of composite to the distal surface gives a better appearance with a more normal distal angle and arch form.

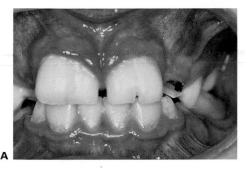
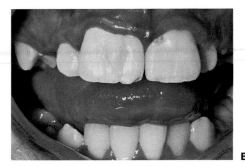

A B

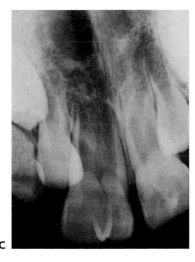

C

Figure 9.16 A Double tooth formed by fusion of the maxillary central incisors with two supernumerary teeth. Two root canals were present. **B** Bilateral double teeth in the maxillary central incisor region with single root canals (**C**). These teeth were extracted and the lateral incisors moved mesially with orthodontics.

Double tooth (Figure 9.16)

This anomaly is manifest as a structure resembling two teeth that have been joined together. In the anterior region, the anomalous tooth usually has a groove on (at least) the labial surface and a notch in the incisal edge. Although rarer in the posterior region, the cuspal morphology is suggestive of two teeth that are joined together. Radiographs are necessary to determine if there is a union of the pulp chambers, and even then it may be speculative. If the 'double tooth' is present together with a normal complement of teeth in the same quadrant then it is presumed to have arisen as a result of gemination; if the number of teeth is reduced then fusion of tooth germs is assumed. If teeth have been extracted or exfoliated, the use of the neutral term 'double tooth' avoids the need to arbitrarily decide if this is due to gemination or fusion.

Alternative terminology

Fusion, gemination, connation, schizodontia, dichotomy.

Fusion

Joining of two teeth of the normal series or a normal tooth and a supernumerary tooth by pulp and dentine. Two canals are usually present. The tooth has arisen from two tooth germs and so the number of teeth in the dentition is normally reduced by one unit. If, however, the normal tooth is fused to a supernumerary, the number of teeth in the arch will be normal. This fusion is assumed to occur between normal and supernumerary teeth because of the close proximity of the tooth buds.

Gemination
Budding of a second tooth from a single tooth germ. Usually one root canal is present.

Management
- The central groove on the labial and palatal surfaces of a double tooth is prone to caries; therefore early application of a fissure sealant is recommended.
- In the permanent dentition, surgical separation of fused teeth may be possible with subsequent orthodontic alignment and restorative treatment as needed to reshape the crown.
- Reshaping or reduction of a double tooth with a single canal (geminated tooth) may be attempted by modifying the appearance of the labial groove and the use of composite resin but is often impossible and extraction may be the only alternative. Orthodontic treatment and/or prosthetic replacement is then required. Implants may be an option for adolescents.
- Deliberate extraction and surgical separation outside the mouth with replantation might also be considered, though this is not always successful because of resorption subsequent to reimplantation.

Clinical Hint   Fused and geminated teeth

Large geminated teeth present great difficulties in management. It is essential to diagnose whether a single canal or separate canals are present. Plain films are often of little benefit, especially when the abnormal tooth is in the central incisor region and there is superimposition of the lateral incisor which erupts palatal to the double tooth due to a lack of space. We have used CT scans (Figure 9.17) and cone beam tomography (Figure 9.18) to determine the morphology of the root canal.

Concrescence
Joining of two teeth, one of which may be a supernumerary, by cementum. Concrescence most commonly affects maxillary second and third permanent molars in older adults. Apart from when involving supernumeraries, this is rarely seen in children.

Frequency
Primary dentition   ~2.5%
Permanent dentition   ~0.2%
    Fusion, gemination or a 'double tooth' in the primary dentition should alert the clinician to the possibility of the same condition in the permanent dentition.

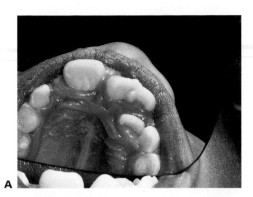

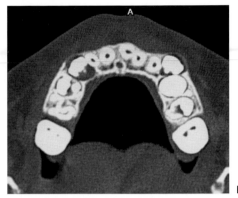

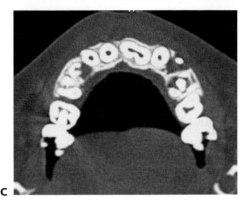

Figure 9.17 A It is often very difficult to determine the root canal anatomy of double teeth when using periapical films due to superimposition of the lateral incisor that has usually erupted palatally. CT can be used to determine the true internal anatomy of the root canal. **B** Apically, it appears that there are two distinct canals; however, a more coronal section shows that there is communication between the canals. **C** This contraindicates surgical separation of the roots. The diagnostic value of this radiography must be weighed against the radiation exposure.

Dens invaginatus (Figures 9.19, 9.20)

Maxillary lateral incisors may have a developmental invagination of the cingulum pit with often only a thin hard-tissue barrier between the oral cavity and the pulp. Pulp necrosis often occurs soon after the eruption of the affected tooth and may lead to a canine fossa abscess or cellulitis. This anomaly may occur in other teeth such as the maxillary central incisors and canines.

Alternative terminology

Invaginated odontome, dens in dente (used to describe the extreme variant, but is a misnomer), dilated odontome.

Frequency

Primary dentition   ~0.1%
Permanent dentition   ~4%
Has been reported to be more common in males.

Management

- If newly erupted, the palatal fissures should be sealed as a preventive measure.
- If caries is evident, then place an acid-etched retained composite resin.

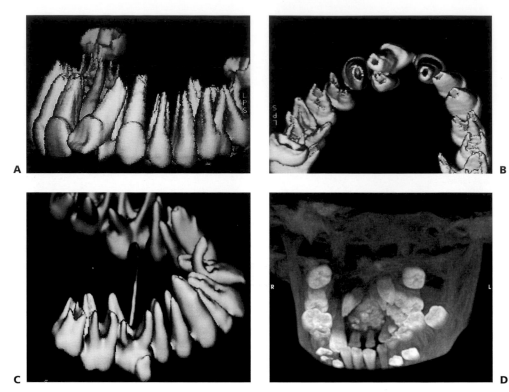

Figure 9.18 Further use of three-dimensional CT to determine positioning and morphology of teeth. In these projections the bone has been removed by software thresholding revealing an image of the teeth alone. **A, B** It was impossible to determine the relationship of the lateral root to the rotated and impacted maxillary left central incisor on plain films. Rotation of the image demonstrates the proximity of the root and the extent of the ectopic positioning of the central incisor. **C** A severely dilacerated maxillary left central incisor. Such images are invaluable to the surgeon. **D** Three-dimensional imaging of a maxillary compound odontome identifying the positions of the maxillary left central and lateral incisors in relation to the lesion.

- If symptomatic and the root canal morphology is favourable, endodontic treatment of the root can be undertaken.
- If the internal anatomy is complex and the root canal is not negotiable then, in the event of infection, extraction is necessary. The presence of this anomaly should be carefully considered during orthodontic treatment planning.

Dens evaginatus (Figure 9.20C)
- An enamel-covered tubercle usually projecting from the occlusal surface of a premolar tooth.
- Usually bilateral and more common in the mandible.
- There is evidence of pulp tissue within the tubercle in 43% of cases.
- Radiographs may show occlusal extension of the pulp chamber.

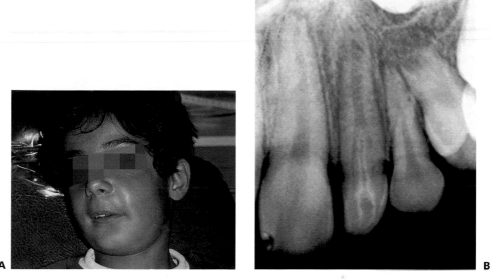

Figure 9.19 A, B Maxillary canine fossa cellulitis from an infected dens invaginatus.
B Because of root canal morphology and the severity of the infection the tooth was removed.
The patient required hospital admission with high-dose intravenous antibiotics and surgical
drainage of the abscess under general anaesthesia.

Alternative terminology
Leong's premolar, tuberculated premolar, axial core type odontome, occlusal enamel
pearl, composite dilated odontome, cone-shaped supernumerary cusp, evaginated
odontome, interstitial cusp.

Frequency
Primary dentition   almost unknown
Permanent dentition   ~4% (almost exclusively in people of Asian extraction)
Reportedly more common in females.

Management
- The tubercle can easily fracture because of occlusal interference, therefore grinding
  of the tubercle followed by fissure sealing can be of assistance. An alternative
  prophylactic measure is to support the sides of the tubercle with composite resin
  and then to recontour the occlusal surface to produce a central ridge. Ideally, this
  should be performed before the tooth comes into complete occlusion.
- If fractured or subject to attrition, pulp exposure commonly occurs. Because this
  exposure occurs soon after eruption, the apex of the tooth is often open and the
  long-term prognosis is less certain. Extraction of the tooth may be considered after
  orthodontic consultation. If the tooth is to be retained, a calcium hydroxide dressing is appropriate with an apexification procedure (see Chapter 6) to stabilize the

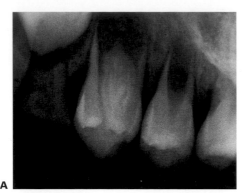

A

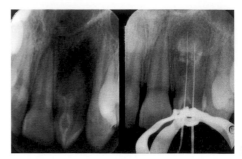

B

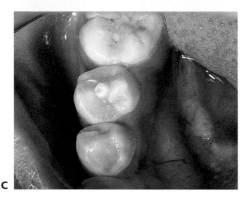

C

Figure 9.20 A Dens invaginatus in a maxillary first premolar tooth. **B** Ultimately, the prognosis is related to the ability to adequately instrument and obturate the canals of these teeth. Temporary endodontic dressings can be placed in such teeth to relieve symptoms and treat infection but it is almost impossible to obturate such canals. **C** Dens evaginatus.

tooth if orthodontics is to commence later (and subsequent definitive endodontic treatment).
- If diagnosed early, an elective (Cvek) pulpotomy can be performed in an attempt to allow normal root formation.

Talon cusp (Figure 9.21)
This is a horn-like projection of the cingulum of the maxillary incisor teeth. It may reach the incisal edge of the tooth.

Alternative terminology
T cingulum, Y-shaped cingulum.

Frequency
Primary dentition almost unknown
Permanent dentition ~1–2%

Management
- If there is no interference with the occlusion no treatment is required.
- Fissure sealants to prevent caries in the grooves between the various parts of the tooth.

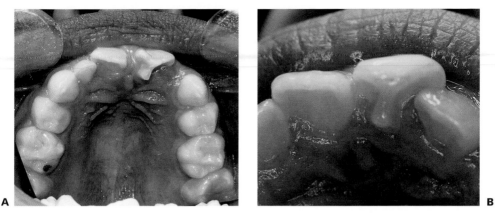

Figure 9.21 A Talon cusp. **B** T cingulum. The cingulum cusp has pulp horns and removal of the cusp will often result in an exposure of the pulp.

- If occlusal interference is present, small progressive reduction of enamel only to avoid pulp exposure, or elective pulpotomy to allow root completion.

Taurodontism

Used to describe molar teeth with a pulp chamber that is vertically enlarged at the expense of the roots. The distance from the cementoenamel junction to the furcation of the root may be greater than the distance from the furcation to the apices. The tooth, therefore, has a long body and short roots, with a tendency towards a single root or apical displacement of the furcation. The anomaly appears to be caused by delay or failure of invagination of Hertwig's epithelial root sheath. Taurodontism may have a genetic basis. Several syndromes and conditions such as ectodermal dysplasias, X-chromosome aneuploidies and some families with (autosomal dominant) amelogenesis imperfecta have this anomaly. The appearance may also be reflected in single-rooted teeth, with the pulp canals being wider than usual.

Frequency

Unknown, uncommon rather than rare.
Enlarged pulp chambers may also be seen in:
- X-linked vitamin D-resistant rickets (hypophosphataemic rickets).
- Vitamin D-dependent rickets.
- Hypophosphatasia.
- Dentinogenesis imperfecta (some cases).
- Regional odontodysplasia.
- Klinefelter's syndrome.
- Shell teeth.

Congenital syphilis

Although now very rare in most parts of the world, congenital syphilis presents with several important diagnostic dental manifestations. Both primary and permanent incisors have tapering crowns and central notching of the incisal edge. This tapering or screwdriver-like appearance is important in the differential diagnosis as there are other causes of non-syphilitic notching of the incisal edge (e.g. trauma). This screwdriver morphology is also seen in Nance–Horan syndrome. Crowns of the molar teeth have a 'cobbled' or 'mulberry' appearance in congenital syphilis.

Developmental defects of enamel

Developmental defects of enamel can be acquired or inherited.

Chronological disturbances

Any severe systemic event during the development of the teeth (i.e. from 3 months in utero to 20 years) may result in some dental abnormality. Many of these anomalies are subclinical and can only be observed in hard-tissue sections as changes in incremental deposition lines. The neonatal line is manifest in all primary teeth, but unless there is severe physiological disturbance or fetal distress the disturbance may not be clinically evident. Different teeth will show defects at different levels of the crown depending on the stage of crown formation at the time the disturbance occurred. The resulting enamel may be reduced in quantity (hypoplasia) and/or quality (usually hypomineralization).

A defect is described as localized when one or more teeth are affected, in an asymmetrical way, and generalized when there is a symmetrical disturbance on teeth of the same type on both left and right sides (and in both maxillary and mandibular teeth).

More than 100 aetiological agents have been reported to cause developmental defects of enamel. Those causing localized defects are listed in Table 9.1 and those causing generalized defects are listed in Table 9.2.

Developmental defects of enamel can be considered according to their clinical appearance:

- Discoloration.
- Opacity.
- Hypoplasia.

Table 9.1 Aetiological agents shown to produce developmental defects of enamel with a localized distribution

Acute osteomyelitis	Gunshot wounds to jaws
Acute trauma to primary teeth	Irradiation
Ankylosis	Jaw fracture
Cleft palate	Laryngoscopy
Congenital epulis	Periapical infection of primary teeth
Electrical burn to mouth	Periodontal ligament injection
Extraction of primary teeth	

Table 9.2 Environmental aetiological agents shown to produce developmental defects of enamel and discoloration with a generalized distribution

Prenatal	Perinatal	Postnatal	
Anaemia	Bile duct defects	Adrenal hyperfunction	Mumps
Cardiac disease	Breech presentation	Cytotoxic medications	Nephrotic syndrome
Congenital allergies	Caesarean section	Bulbar poliomyelitis	Neurological disorders
Congenital syphilis	Erythroblastosis fetalis	Candida-endocrinopathy syndrome	Otitis media
Cytomegalovirus	Haemolytic disorder	Chickenpox (varicella)	Pneumonia
Diabetes	Hepatitis	Cholera	Pseudohypothyroidism
Fluoride	Intrapartum haemorrhage	Congenital cardiac disease	Renal dysfunction
Hypoxia	Low birth weight	Diphtheria	Scarlet fever
Pregnancy toxaemia	Neonatal asphyxia	Encephalitis	Sickle cell anaemia
Malnutrition	Neonatal hypocalcaemia	Fluoride	Small pox
Renal disease	Placenta praevia	Gastrointestinal disturbances	Stress
Rubella	Prematurity	Hyperpituitarism	Tetracyclines
Stress	Prolonged labour	Hyperthyroidism	Tuberculosis
Thalidomide	Respiratory distress syndrome	Hypogonadism	Typhus
Urinary tract infection	Tetanus	Hypoparathyroidism	Vitamin A deficiency
Vitamin A deficiency	Tetracyclines	Hypothyroidism	Vitamin C deficiency
Vitamin D deficiency	Traumatic birth injuries	Intestinal lymphangiectasia	Vitamin D deficiency
	Twinning	Lead intoxication	Vitamin D intoxication
		Measles	

In general, the aims of management are to treat pathology and pain, provide adequate aesthetic appeal, maintain occlusal function and maintain the vertical dimension.

Tooth discoloration
Tooth discolouration may be extrinsic or intrinsic in nature. Extrinsic staining is superficial and occurs after tooth eruption. Intrinsic discoloration may result from a

developmental defect of enamel or internal staining of the tooth (Figure 9.22). Although such internal staining is manifest as a change in tooth colour, the intrinsic defect may affect the dentine primarily or exclusively. See Table 9.3 for the differential diagnosis of tooth discoloration.

Opacity

Opacities result from a defect in the quality of the enamel, affecting the lucency of the tissue. Hypomineralization results in a change in the porosity of the enamel, causing opacity. This may be located below the enamel surface, which otherwise remains intact.

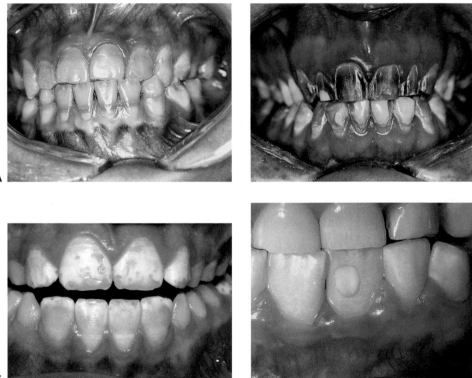

Figure 9.22 Tooth discoloration. **A** Tetracycline staining in a child from South East Asia. Tetracyclines are still available over the counter in some countries (and may be included in some homoeopathic preparations in some Asian countries) and this staining is primarily seen in this population group. **B** A severe case of tetracycline staining in a boy with cystic fibrosis. The anterior teeth have been prepared for porcelain veneers, which were unsatisfactory. In these cases, intentional devitalization and non-vital bleaching with hydrogen peroxide may be a more conservative option than crowning every tooth. **C** Fluorosis – uniform opacity throughout the crown. Some of the hypomineralized enamel has been lost on the incisal edge revealing normal enamel underneath. **D** Localized enamel opacity caused by the root apex of a traumatized primary incisor.

Table 9.3 Causes of tooth discoloration

Colour	Aetiology	Comments
Extrinsic discoloration		
Green	Chromogenic bacteria	Usually cervical and gingival areas
Yellow	Bile pigments from gingival crevicular fluid	Biliary atresia and jaundice
Black	Ferrous sulphate	Iron supplementation
Brown	Chromogenic bacteria	Arrested caries
Intrinsic discoloration with localized staining on one or several teeth		
Yellow/brown	Developmental defects	Usually after trauma or infection
White	Developmental defects	Subsurface decalcification in permanent teeth, after trauma or infection
Pink	Internal resorption	Seen before exfoliation or after trauma
Grey/Black	Amalgam staining	Leakage of old amalgam restorations causing discoloration at the periphery
Chronological staining of dentition		
Bright yellow	Tetracycline	Unoxidized fluorophore, seen in newly erupted teeth
Yellow/grey-brown	Tetracycline	Erupted teeth, oxidized fluorophore (UV light)
Yellow-brown	Systemic illness	Developmental defect of enamel affecting all teeth forming during illness
Generalized intrinsic staining of teeth, either single of complete dentition		
Grey-brown	Necrotic tooth	Usually after trauma
Yellow-brown to dark yellow	Amelogenesis imperfecta	Both dentitions are affected
Green-blue	Hyperbilirubinaemia	Seen in children with end-stage liver disease and premature infants
Blue-brown (opalescent)	Dentinogenesis imperfecta	All teeth uniformly affected, may be associated with osteogenesis imperfecta
Red-brown	Congenital porphyria	All teeth affected
White	Fluorosis/non-fluorotic	Usually only permanent dentition

Fluorosis (Figure 9.22C, see also Chapter 4)

In its mildest forms, fluorosis is manifest as hypomineralization of the enamel, leading to opacities. These can range from tiny white flecks to confluent opacities throughout the enamel, making the crown totally lacking in translucency. Hypoplasia occurs at higher concentrations of fluoride. When the tooth first erupts, the surface of even the most severely affected enamel may be intact; however, with wear, areas of enamel are lost and stains are taken up into the porosities. At 1 ppm of fluoride in public water supplies, up to 10% of the population will show very mild opacities attributable to fluorosis (though this may depend on individual water consumption); interestingly, this seems to be a minimum value and the proportion of opacities increases as fluoride levels either fall below 1 ppm or rise above 2 ppm. Severely affected cases may require microabrasion or restoration with composite resin, either in a localized or a more generalized manner, or porcelain veneers. Many opacities are incorrectly labelled as fluorosis without adequate justification or investigation of fluoride history.

Management of stains and opacities

- Extrinsic stains can be removed with abrasives.
- Mild discoloration may be improved using professionally or home-applied peroxide-based bleaching agents.
- Intrinsic stains, if superficial, may be removed with microabrasion techniques.

Microabrasion

It must be understood that microabrasion techniques involve removal of the surface opaque layer of enamel. The opaque but often bright white layer of enamel is removed and children and parents are often disappointed at the appearance of the normal 'yellow' colour of the permanent crown. It is important to make an initial decision whether to attempt to alter the entire dentition to this darker colour, or to continue with the piecemeal adjustment of darker areas to match the overall 'paper-white' appearance. In present-day society, the latter decision may prove to be satisfactory, or even desirable. Acid-based techniques may create more porosity in the enamel, which may accumulate more stains over time.

18% hydrochloric acid (with or without the use of pumice)

Rubber dam should always be used and must be secured by ligating around individual teeth and sealing with copal ether varnish. Orabase paste applied to the gingival margin prior to dam placement can be used to protect the soft tissues from any acid leakage. An aqueous slurry of sodium bicarbonate may be laid on the dam around the teeth to neutralize any inadvertent excess acid. A hydrochloric acid/pumice slurry is applied to the affected area using a slowly rotating rubber cup for 10 seconds only, and then rinsed thoroughly with water. Application is repeated a maximum of 10 times. This technique is potentially destructive to enamel and soft tissues, and must be used with caution.

Alternatives, particularly where rubber dam cannot be used

- Abrasion with a mixture of pumice and 37% phosphoric acid (etchant).
- Polishing labial surfaces with a multi-fluted tungsten-carbide bur.

- Application of a neutral 2% sodium fluoride, followed after a short time by polishing with a fine polishing paste (non-coloured toothpaste is suitable) in a rotating rubber cup is advisable after use of each of these techniques.
- Recent research has shown that mild fluorosis can also be remineralized and the opacity reduced by casein phosphopeptide-amorphous calcium phosphate (CPP-ACP) or casein phosphopeptide-amorphous calcium phosphate fluoride (CPP-ACPF). The enamel should be pretreated with sodium hypochlorite to denature protein.

Deep intrinsic stains require removal of the affected enamel and rebuilding, usually with composite resin. Although localized marks may be dealt with by this method, treatment using composite resin or porcelain as full-face veneers, or the use of crowns, should ideally be delayed in adolescents until the gingival attachment is established at the cementoenamel junction. The longevity of hybrid composite resins has improved substantially, along with their colour stability, strength and translucency. These materials may be placed quickly and more cost-effectively than porcelain and other complex restorations such as crowns. Modern materials generally provide for densely white shades that make matching possible. It is important always to keep treatment options open. Involvement in contact sports may be another reason for delaying placement of complex restorations.

Enamel hypoplasia (Figure 9.23)

A defect in quantity that causes a defect of contour in the surface of the enamel. This is usually caused by initial failure of the deposition of enamel protein, but the same clinical effect could also result if there is a mineralization defect which leads to loss of enamel substance after eruption. In the former case the enamel is often hard and glassy, in the latter it will usually pit on probing. In some trauma cases, tissue may be lost after formation and is not regarded as a true hypoplasia. Examples of hypoplastic defects following trauma are shown in Figure 7.18.

Management

- Localized hypoplastic defects may be restored with composite resin. Pitting defects may need initial localized debris or stain removal with either rotary instruments or amine peroxide bleaching systems.
- It is important to maintain posterior support, and stainless steel crowns may be required to restore grossly hypoplastic molars. These teeth may be exquisitely sensitive to thermal and osmotic stimuli and treatment is made difficult by an inability to achieve good isolation of teeth which are only partially erupted. Glass ionomers may be used temporarily to restore hypoplastic occlusal defects and prevent caries.
- A realistic assessment of the likely longevity of affected first molars is important from an early age. Consideration should be given to the elective loss of these teeth as part of an occlusal developmental plan for the child. A pre-assessment with orthodontic advice not later than 8 years of age is recommended.
- Complex restorative treatment involving onlays, veneers and crowns should generally be delayed until late adolescence but the selective use of metal, adhesively retained onlays may provide a long-term solution in some molar cases.

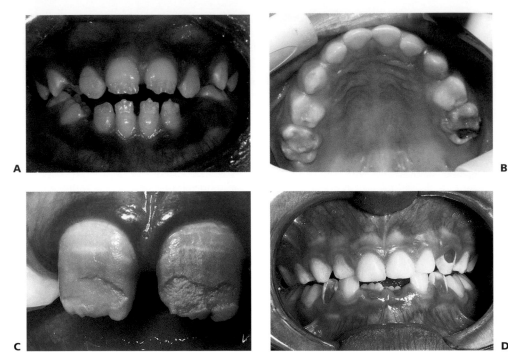

Figure 9.23 A Chronological enamel hypoplasia after a childhood illness up to 10 months of age. The maxillary lateral incisors are unaffected and there is little hypomineralization of the teeth, making the dentition more easily restored with composite resin. **B** Chronological hypoplasia may affect the primary dentition, in this case with a child who suffered fetal distress and meconium aspiration at delivery. It is possible that the tips of the cusps of the first permanent molars are similarly affected. **C** Another form of chronological hypoplasia. Note that there is normal enamel at the cervical region and the primary tooth is not affected. **D** Localized hypoplasia of primary canines. These anomalies present as defects on the labial surface of primary canine teeth and often become carious. A minute area of hypoplasia is visible on the maxillary right canine, and all the other canine teeth are carious while the remainder of the mouth is caries free.

Molar–incisor hypomineralization (Figure 9.24)

Molar–incisor hypomineralization (MIH) is a condition which, although recognized as a clinical entity for some time, is still a subject of considerable study. It presents as a change in enamel quality, ranging from localized opacity through opacity with discoloration and obvious poor quality to enamel loss, probably due to post-eruptive breakdown. These findings affect one or more first permanent molars in a quasi-chronological but inconsistent manner, together with (usually lesser) effects on one or more incisor teeth. The presentation is puzzling since as few as one molar or as many as all four may be affected. Many possible aetiological factors, from the presence of environmental pollutants in breast milk to childhood disease, have been suggested. Work is under

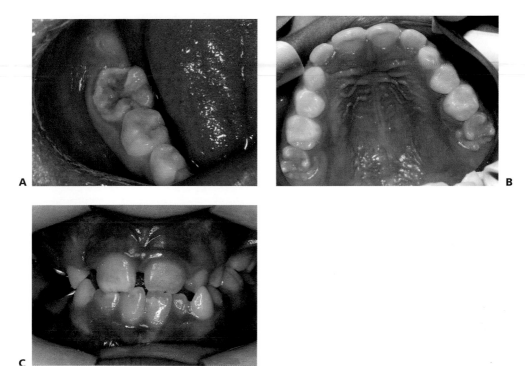

Figure 9.24 MIH. Teeth may be variably affected in the one mouth. **A** Severe tooth loss with caries secondary to the hypomineralization affected the first permanent molar. **B** An otherwise intact dentition shows typical MIH. The incisors (palatal surface) are less severely affected than the molars. **C** Hypomineralization of the incisors associated with MIH and rampant caries in the primary dentition. Note that the crowns of the second primary molars and first permanent molars form at similar times, and this may explain the high rate of caries seen in the primary dentition in some of these patients. (Courtesy Dr E Alcaino.)

way in many centres to define the risk factors, since a knowledge of aetiology would permit early preventive and restorative interventions.

A familial tendency to the condition has been recognized by some authors. Irrespective of the exact aetiology of MIH, it is important to recognize that this condition represents a chronological disturbance in tooth formation between birth and 12 months of age. Teeth that calcify after this time are unaffected, namely canines, premolars and second permanent molars. This is a consideration in long-term treatment planning.

Management
- The ideal restorative approach for these cases has yet to be determined. Adhesive restorations are often attempted but retention is unpredictable and the stainless steel crown option is generally preferred. Trimming the length of the stainless steel crown for partly erupted first permanent molars so as to obtain a fit just apical to

the maximum convexity of the crown makes such placement easier in many cases.
- There is a clear association between repeated, well-meaning attempts by practitioners to place 'minimal', adhesive or other treatments for these molars, without adequate local anaesthesia, and a real antipathy to dental treatment on the part of the affected children. Local analgesia should be used for the treatment of these cases but is should be noted even under these conditions, pain control will not always be adequate and treatment may be compromised.

Clinical Hint   Questions regarding severely hypoplastic first permanent molars

Always consider the long-term implications of your treatment.
- Is it preferable to extract the first molar at 8 years of age and allow the second molar to migrate mesially? (See Chapter 11.)
- Once a stainless steel crown has been placed – what are your options at age 20? A clear record of the state of the underlying tooth at crown placement is essential for the later restorative dentist.
- Does it matter if a third molar is not present – does this affect your decision?
- Is it preferable to leave a child free of disease – but also free of any restoration what will require multiple replacements throughout life?

Amelogenesis imperfecta

The term amelogenesis imperfecta (Figure 9.25) is usually applied to inherited defects of the enamel of both primary and permanent teeth. Although the definition implies a family history, for practical purposes it seems reasonable to extend this to include sporadic cases and also to those cases where the enamel defects are associated with extra-oral features, as found in some syndromes (i.e. focal dermal hypoplasia or the tricho-dento-osseous syndrome).

Frequency
- Estimated 1 : 14 000 in the USA.
- Up to 1 : 800 in northern Sweden.
  (Few studies of prevalence have been carried out and there may be marked differences according to the gene pool involved.)

Diagnosis
- Based on a combination of the mode of inheritance and clinical and radiographic appearances.

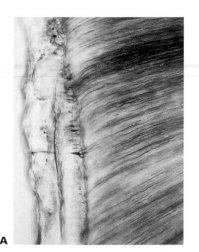
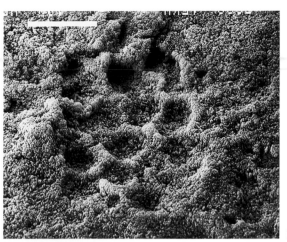

A

B

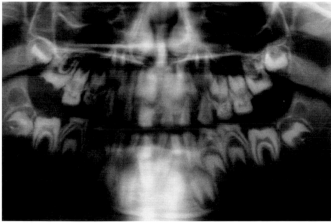

C

Figure 9.25 A Hard-tissue section of autosomal dominant amelogenesis imperfecta showing extremely thin enamel in this particular patient. **B** Scanning electron micrograph of similar patient with abnormal etching pattern of enamel. **C** Panoramic radiograph showing absent or very thin enamel in this form of amelogenesis imperfecta.

Amelogenesis imperfecta variants with Mendelian inheritance

- X-linked (Xp22.3-p22.1) (OMIM 301200): The AMELX gene on the short arm of the X chromosome which codes for amelogenin, the major enamel matrix protein, has been shown to be mutated in several families with X-linked amelogenesis imperfecta. Another locus for X-linked amelogenesis imperfecta (OMIM 301201) has been identified on the long arm of the X chromosome (Xq22-q28).
- X-linked (Xq22-q28) (OMIM 301201): Another locus for X-linked amelogenesis imperfecta has been identified on the long arm of the X chromosome.

- Autosomal dominant (OMIM 104500): Linkage analysis has shown that a gene in the 4q11-q21 region causes autosomal dominant amelogenesis imperfecta in some families. Mutations in the enamelin gene, which maps to the same region, have been identified. Families with autosomal dominant amelogenesis imperfecta with taurodontism (ADAIT) as part of the trichodentoosseous (TDO) syndrome have mutations in the DLX3 gene; one family with ADAIT without other features of TDO has also been found to have a mutation in the same gene, whereas in other ADAIT families mutations in the DLX3 gene have been excluded. With time it is expected that this area will be better understood as it is probable that as yet unknown genes are involved in the disorder in some families.
- Autosomal recessive (OMIM 204650): Mutations in the matrix metalloproteinase-20 (MMP-20) or kallikrein-4 (KLK-4) gene appear to cause autosomal recessive amelogenesis imperfecta.
- Sporadic cases.

Phenotypes

Phenotypes range from markedly hypoplastic (thin) enamel (either uniformly with spacing between adjacent teeth or irregularly giving rise to pits or grooves) to varying degrees of hypomineralization (poorly formed enamel) with altered colour and translucency. In many cases both hypoplasia and hypomineralization are seen together. The colour of the teeth is presumed to reflect the degree of hypomineralization of the enamel – the darker the colour the more severe the degree of hypomineralization.

In X-linked amelogenesis imperfecta, females exhibit vertical bands of altered enamel (manifesting lyonization – see Lyon hypothesis earlier in this chapter). There may be vertical grooves (because of hypoplasia) and/or vertical bands of enamel of altered colour or lucency (because of hypomineralization), or a combination of the two. In such families there will be no male-to-male transmission, whereas the heterozygous females may pass on the trait to children of either sex.

In some patients affected by amelogenesis imperfecta the teeth fail to erupt, presumably due to a disturbance of the enamel organ, and may undergo resorption of their crowns. In some cases (up to 50%), a skeletal anterior open bite is seen.

Classification of amelogenesis imperfecta

There has been great controversy and confusion created with nomenclature and different classifications. Indeed, in some texts up to 14 different forms of the condition are described. It should be noted that all of these different manifestations are based on a clinical appearance. It is essential that diagnosis and classification be based on the mode of inheritance and phenotype. Understanding the mode of inheritance is essential for genetic counselling. However, setting aside questions of inheritance for our present purposes, from a clinical treatment planning perspective, two clinically distinct basic forms are considered here.

Predominantly/exclusively hypoplastic forms (Figure 9.26A–E)

- Thin enamel.
- Lack of contact points between teeth.
- Enamel may be rough, smooth, or randomly pitted.

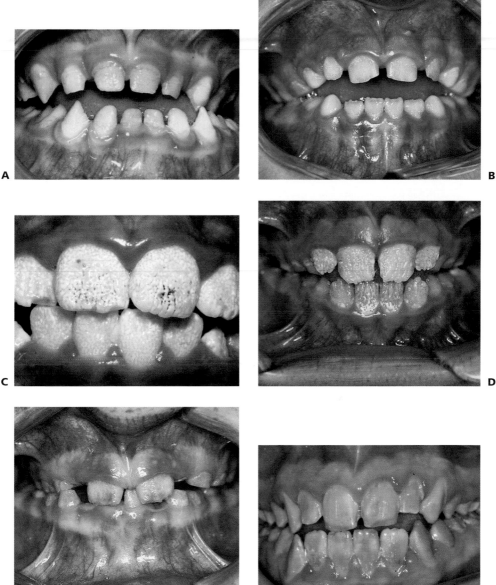

Figure 9.26 Different forms of amelogenesis imperfecta. **A** Autosomal recessive with a rough hypoplastic phenotype. **B** Autosomal dominant with smooth hypoplasia with a marked anterior open bite. Note the open contact points in these two cases. **C** Autosomal dominant amelogenesis imperfecta with pitting hypoplasia. **D** X-linked inheritance with hypoplastic vertical grooves in a female. These represent enamel derived from different clones of ameloblasts that have undergone Lyonization (X chromosome inactivation). **E** Stained rough hypoplastic amelogenesis imperfecta. **F** Apparently sporadic case of amelogenesis imperfecta characterized by severe hypomineralization. Note the discoloration and gross build-up of calculus on all surfaces.

- Heterozygous females with X-linked amelogenesis imperfecta manifest Lyonization (*see above*) with vertical banding of normal and abnormal enamel.
- Teeth may be delayed in eruption.
- Unerupted teeth may undergo resorption.
- Anterior open bite associated in about 50% of cases.
- Radiographically may be difficult to distinguish enamel from dentine if the former is extremely thin.

Predominantly/exclusively hypomineralized forms (Figure 9.26F)

- May be normal thickness of enamel, at least initially.
- Yellow to brown in colour.
- Enamel may be softer than normal, tends to chip and can be penetrated with an explorer. In severely hypomineralized cases the enamel may be scraped away with a scaler.
- Teeth may erupt with normal thickness but enamel can be quickly lost, exposing rough, highly sensitive dentine.
- Large masses of supragingival calculus may be present.
- Radiographically, can be difficult to distinguish between enamel and dentine because of decreased degree of mineralization of enamel.
- Unerupted teeth may undergo resorption; radiographic review is needed to monitor this.

Management

- Appropriate diagnosis, taking into account the mode of inheritance and phenotype.
- Continued commitment to and support of both children and families. These are disfiguring, painful conditions and children may be badly teased.
- Offer genetic counselling if appropriate.
- Early orthodontic assessment.
- Preservation of molar teeth with full coverage restorations to maintain vertical dimension. Overdentures may be an option in children with small, hypoplastic teeth (Figure 9.27E, F).
- Stainless steel crowns or gold onlays on molars (Figure 9.28). Laboratory made, composite crowns may be useful.
- Care is required when trial fitting crowns, because defective enamel can be easily scraped or flaked off the tooth in some cases.
- Composite resin veneers over anterior teeth for aesthetics. It is possible to bond composite resin successfully to hypoplastic and hypomineralized enamel (Figures 9.27 and 9.28).
- Adequate margins may be difficult to achieve because of the poor quality of the enamel (Figure 9.28C).
- Ideally, delay definitive treatment with porcelain and precious metals until late adolescence. However, some people in their forties have commented that, had they known that their dentition was going to 'fail' at that stage, they would have

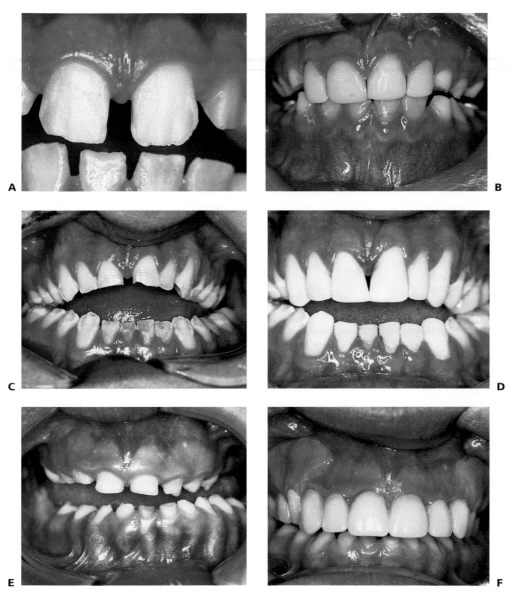

Figure 9.27 Different management options for amelogenesis imperfecta. **A, B** Composite bonding in a case with rough hypoplasia of the enamel. Etching times should be slightly longer than usual; however, the roughness of the enamel surface aids in mechanical retention. **C, D** A case with smooth hypoplasia of the enamel with a severe anterior open bite and posterior open bites. The patient did not want orthodontics or orthognathic surgery and so the posterior occlusion was built up with composite resin, as were the anterior teeth. Because of the open bite, crown lengthening was easily achieved and the restorations have lasted for over 7 years without replacement. **E, F** A patient with autosomal recessive dystrophic epidermolysis bullosa with enamel defects. The posterior teeth failed to erupt and underwent spontaneous replacement resorption within the alveolus. Because of the small crown length and the prominent alveolus, an overdenture without a labial flange was constructed.

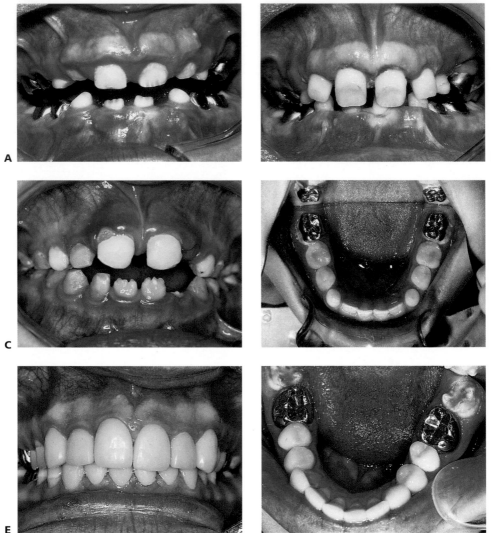

Figure 9.28 A, B A case of autosomal dominant amelogenesis imperfecta with failure of eruption of the anterior teeth. Many of the posterior teeth are unerupted and undergoing resorption. Initial surgical exposure of the anterior segments did not aid their complete eruption. The gingivae contained small islands of calcification which be significant in the failure of eruption. Periodontal surgery with apically repositioned flaps was used to fully expose the crowns. **C** Not all cases using composite resin are successful. With progressive eruption of the teeth it is difficult for the patient to keep the gingival margins clean and the restoration may therefore fail. **D** Cast gold onlays are useful to protect the occlusal surfaces. No preparation of the crown was performed. Onlays were cemented with composite luting cement. **E, F** Use of gold onlays and indirect composite resin veneers on anterior teeth and onlays on premolars. These composite restorations provide can provide good aesthetics during adolescence.

preferred their practitioner to have been less 'conservative' in their teenage years and to have provided more conventional restorative care. Two points arise:

- modern composites have improved greatly and 'adolescent' treatment now is hopefully more aesthetic and longer lasting than previously
- there is evidence of a clear association between these conditions and lack of self-esteem. It is as important here as anywhere in dentistry to treat the whole patient, and not only the teeth.
- Orthodontic and possible orthognathic surgery to correct anterior open bite in hypoplastic forms.

Clinical Hint   Bonding to abnormal enamel

- Acid-etch composite resin seems to bond more successfully to hypoplastic enamel than to hypomineralized enamel.
- In severely affected dentitions it is preferable to place stainless steel crowns on primary molar teeth very early (e.g. at around 3–4 years of age) to preserve the vertical dimension, prevent caries and allow maximal eruption of the first permanent molar.
- Cast metal (precious or base-metal) onlays on suitable permanent posterior teeth have the best long-term clinical success.
- Regular radiographic examination is required to detect early caries.

Disorders of dentine

Dentinogenesis imperfecta (OMIM 125490) (Figure 9.29)
Dentinogenesis imperfecta is an inherited disorder of dentine, which may or may not be associated with osteogenesis imperfecta. The term 'hereditary opalescent dentine' is sometimes used for the isolated condition. Both osteogenesis imperfecta and dentinogenesis imperfecta are transmitted as autosomal dominant traits and are clinically indistinguishable dentally, although they have a different genetic basis. Osteogenesis imperfecta is caused by mutations in the type I collagen genes and dentinogenesis imperfecta to mutations in the dentine sialophosphoprotein I gene. Some individuals and families with osteogenesis imperfecta may have clinical evidence of dentinogenesis imperfecta but in other families there may be variable expression of the trait. Within these families, some individuals may have abnormal dentine while others are clinically unaffected as far as the teeth are concerned. However, because of the same collagen defect, all such children with osteogenesis imperfecta may have abnormal dentine, albeit at a subclinical level. The possibility of osteogenesis imperfecta should be considered in children presenting with dentinogenesis imperfecta and investigated by measurement of bone density if necessary. The presence of blue sclera or a history of bone fractures should alert the clinician to osteogenesis imperfecta.

Dental manifestations
- Amber, grey to purple-bluish discoloration or opalescence (Figure 9.29)
- Pulpal obliteration (Figure 9.29D).

- Relatively bulbous crowns.
- Short, narrow roots.
- Enamel may be lost after tooth eruption, exposing the soft dentine, which rapidly wears. This is probably due to inherent weakness in the dentine rather than because of an enamel defect or abnormality at the dentinoenamel junction.
- Mantle dentine appears normal.
- Circumpulpal dentine has poorly formed dentine with abnormal direction of tubules. Small soft-tissue inclusions represent remnants of pulpal tissue.

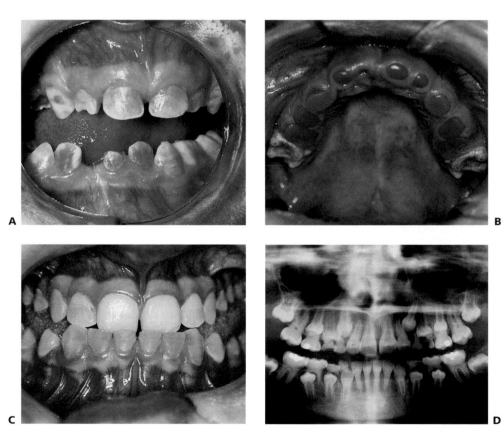

Figure 9.29 Manifestations of dentinogenesis imperfecta. **A** Dentinogenesis imperfecta associated with osteogenesis imperfecta. Dark discoloration of the crowns which appear normal in size and shape. **B** Severe attrition in the primary dentition in a case of dentinogenesis imperfecta. An overdenture was used to restore the vertical dimension and provide function as well as aesthetic appeal. **C** The permanent dentition may not be as severely affected when associated with osteogenesis imperfecta. In this case, the severe skeletal Class III malocclusion and the posterior open bite required a surgical solution. **D** Radiographic manifestations of dentinogenesis imperfecta showing pulpal obliteration and short, bulbous crowns. Periapical pathology is fortunately rare.

Management

- Preservation of the vertical dimension of the occlusion.
- Continued commitment to and support of both children and families. These are disfiguring conditions and children may be badly teased.
- Protection of posterior teeth from attrition using full coverage restorations.
- Provision of aesthetic appeal.
- Stainless steel crowns for posterior teeth.
- Initially composite resin to build up anterior teeth, possibly followed later by porcelain crowns. (These teeth will remain or even become increasingly brittle throughout life. Conventional crowns requiring tooth preparation may never be the treatment of choice, but see above under 'Management of amelogenesis imperfecta.')
- Overdentures or even full dentures may be required in severe cases.

We have followed cases over many years into adulthood. The initial optimism over retaining these teeth for a life-time has been tempered by the eventual failure of complex restorative work and the loss of teeth in early adulthood. Clinicians must be sensitive to the implications of long-term failure and the aesthetic, functional and indeed financial legacy with which the patient is left.

Osteogenesis imperfecta (OMIM 166200)

Osteogenesis imperfecta is caused by mutations in the collagen type I genes on chromosomes 7 (7q22.1) and 17 (17q21.3-q22). Previous classifications listed several variants of osteogenesis imperfecta with either autosomal dominant or autosomal recessive modes of inheritance. More recently it has been realized that most or all cases represent autosomal dominant osteogenesis imperfecta with variable expression. The essential features are:

- Bone fragility (Figure 9.30).
- Blue sclera.
- Progressive hearing loss.
- Dentinal changes.

Dentinal dysplasia – radicular dentinal dysplasia (Shields type I DD) (OMIM 125400)

- Originally described as rootless teeth, this appears to be a distinct entity from dentinogenesis imperfecta. Both dentitions are equally affected. The teeth may be lost early due to periapical infection or spontaneous exfoliation caused by the short roots.
- Autosomal dominant transmission.
- Very short or absent roots but clinically normal crowns.
- Total or partial obliteration of radicular pulp prior to eruption but with demilune of coronal pulp shown on the radiographs of molar teeth.
- Mantle and coronal dentine are histologically normal.

Management

- In spite of excellent preventive care, these affected teeth are commonly lost due to loss of enamel, pulp necrosis or periodontal disease.

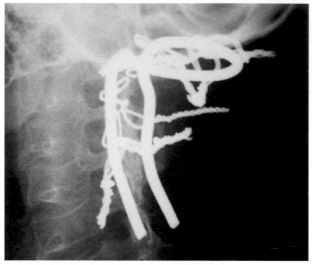

A

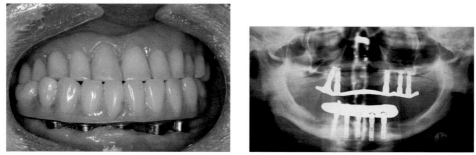

B

C

Figure 9.30 A The 'Ransford Loop' used to stabilize the vertebral column in a child with type IV osteogenesis imperfecta and basilar compression. This life-saving procedure is performed by an anterior approach through the pharynx, splitting the palate and sectioning the odontoid process of C2. The vertebral column is then wired to the occipital bone. This child initially presented with trigeminal neuralgia caused by pressure from C2 on the pons. **B** In spite of the bone pathology, osseointegrated implants can be successfully placed in patients with osteogenesis imperfecta. The same patient as in Figure 9.30A was rehabilitated with implant supported dentures following his surgery. **C** The panoramic radiograph shows the survival of the implants at 9-year follow-up.

- Prophylactic stainless steel crowns.
- Endodontic therapy may be successful if there is minimal pulpal obliteration.
- Long-term prognosis for the dentition is poor.

Dentinal dysplasia – coronal dentinal dysplasia (Shields type II DD) (OMIM 125420)

- The consensus now is that this is a variant of dentinogenesis imperfecta rather than a distinct entity. The primary teeth have a typical amber discoloration and

undergo tooth wear associated with loss of the enamel and the appearance of shell teeth radiographically.
- Normal crown and root form.
- Varying degrees of pulp canal obliteration.
- Altered pulp morphology resembling a 'thistle shaped' pulp chamber.
- Intrapulpal calcifications (pulp stones).

Management
Similar to management of dentinogenesis imperfecta, however some authors suggest that no treatment is required as there are few sequelae. If there is enamel loss in the primary dentition, then full coverage restorations should be placed (stainless steel crowns). If the permanent dentition is clinically normal, then no special care may be needed.

Different classification of dentine anomalies
Many texts describe up to four different forms of dentinogenesis imperfecta. All these dentine anomalies are autosomal dominant in inheritance. Dentinogenesis imperfecta has been mapped to 4q13-21. Recently, linkage studies of families with coronal dentine dysplasia (Shields type II DD) have shown that the candidate mutation occurs in a region on 4q that overlaps the most likely location of the dentinogenesis imperfecta locus. Further, a similar locus has been determined in that of dentinogenesis imperfecta Shields type III (Brandywine isolate – OMIM 125500). These results suggest that dentinogenesis imperfecta (Shields type II), Shields type III and DD type II (coronal dentine dysplasia) are allelic or the result of mutations in tightly-linked genes. Radicular dentine dysplasia may be a separate entity.

X-linked vitamin D-resistant rickets
(OMIM 307800) (Figure 9.31)
- Also termed X-linked rickets (Xp22) or hereditary hypophosphataemic rickets.
- X-linked disorder with rachitic changes in long bones associated with a failure of distal tubular reabsorption of phosphate in the kidneys. The rickets is unresponsive to vitamin D.
- Short stature.
- Bowing of legs.
- Males severely affected, females may show milder features (typically short stature with bowing of legs), often not affecting the teeth.
- Low serum phosphate.
- Elevated alkaline phosphatase.

Dental manifestations
- Attrition of incisal and occlusal enamel exposes elongated pulp horns, which often extend up to the dentinoenamel junction.
- In males (and some females), typically presents with multiple abscesses in the absence of caries.
- Large pulp chambers and delayed apical root closure.
- May be reduced radiodensity of dentine on radiographs. Enamel may be spared or show some evidence of hypoplasia and/or hypomineralization.

- These patients may have repeated orthopaedic procedures and indwelling mechanics to promote bone straightening or lengthening. The avoidance of sepsis is essential. Treatment planning should include collaboration with orthopaedic colleagues and may demand the regrettable removal of infected teeth at times of particular infection risk.

Pre-eruptive intracoronal resorptive defects (Figure 9.32)

These defects are dentine lesions found on unerupted teeth, usually detected on routine dental radiographs. They are often erroneously been referred to as 'pre-

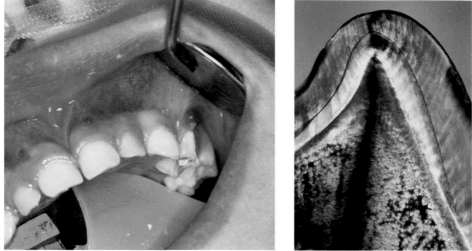

A **B**

Figure 9.31 A X-linked vitamin D-resistant rickets presenting with multiple abscessed teeth in the absence of caries. **B** Under polarized light, the hard-tissue section demonstrates globular dentine and a pulp horn that extends to the dentinoenamel junction, resulting in early exposure caused by attrition and subsequently pulpal necrosis.

Figure 9.32 Pre-eruptive intracoronal resorptive defect in an unerupted mandibular second molar.

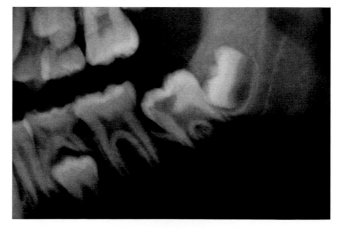

eruptive caries' or 'dentine cysts'. They are often located adjacent to the dentino-enamel junction in the occlusal aspect of the crown. There is evidence that these defects develop as a result of coronal resorption. On opening into the lesion, it is often empty or filled with an amorphous tissue comprising small particles of tubular dentine and crystalline material. Resorptive cells such as osteoclasts and macrophages may be found. When the tooth erupts, the lesion is likely to be rapidly colonized by oral flora and the lesion becomes similar to a carious lesion.

Management
The cavity should be restored conservatively. It has been proposed that these lesions may be responsible for many of the lesions that are clinically undetected in molar teeth that progress to rapid carious breakdown and, ultimately, loss of the tooth.

Dental effects of prematurity and low birth weight

Normal birth weight for gestational age	>2500 g
Low birthweight	>1500–2500 g
Very low birthweight	<1500 g
Extremely low birthweight	<1000 g

Problems in extreme prematurity
- Hyaline membrane disease and respiratory insufficiency.
- Hyperbilirubinaemia (Figure 9.33D)
- Necrotizing enterocolitis.
- Cerebral intraventricular haemorrhage.
- Oxygen retinopathy.

The limiting factor in survival is based on lung development and infants weighing less than 400 g at birth or those born before 24 weeks rarely survive. Hyaline membrane disease is now treated with synthetic surfactant, although very young babies often develop pneumothoraces caused by the prematurity and fragility of the alveoli. Cerebral intraventricular bleeding and necrotizing enterocolitis with the resulting sepsis are common causes of mortality and morbidity. Surviving children may be left with problems of growth retardation, delayed cognitive development and a range of other abnormalities.

Dental implications
- Hypoglycaemia.
- Hypocalcaemia with reactive pseudohyperparathyroidism.
- Hyperbilirubinaemia, causing intrinsic staining of the teeth.
- Intubation trauma, causing enamel hypoplasia/hypocalcification. The maxillary (most commonly the left) central incisors are most often affected (Figure 9.33E) If the baby is intubated orally, palatal grooving may occur. Tooth eruption may be delayed, although it is often normal for the 'corrected' age after adjustment for prematurity.
- Chronological opacities or hypoplasia.

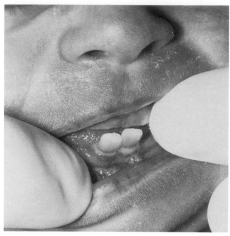
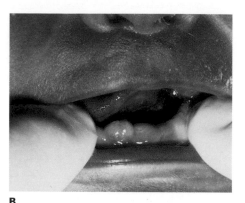

A   B

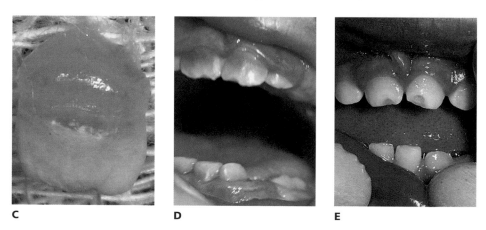

C   D   E

Figure 9.33 A Natal teeth in a 36-week premature infant. The teeth were extremely loose and, because of the respiratory difficulties experienced by the child, the teeth were removed. **B** A newborn infant with two mandibular incisors soon to erupt. The reduced enamel epithelium has fused with the gingivae and teeth will probably erupt within a few days. **C** A neonatal tooth from a 27-week premature infant. Note the extent of the crown formation consistent with age. **D, E** Dental effects of prematurity: hyperbilirubinaemia staining of the enamel (**D**) and hypoplastic defects on the incisal edges of the central incisors caused by laryngoscopy (**E**).

Disorders of eruption (Figure 9.34)

Eruption of teeth is not always correlated with somatic development. Children with growth disturbances may exhibit delayed eruption or the delay may be due to other causes such as gingival overgrowth due to medication such as phenytoin. More importantly, premature exfoliation of teeth is invariably associated with severe systemic disease (see Chapter 8) and requires investigation.

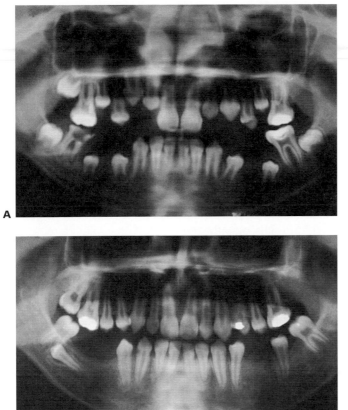

A

B

Figure 9.34 Teeth require guidance for normal eruption. **A** In this case the mandibular right first permanent molar was removed because of gross caries and pulpal necrosis. **B** While the second molar has drifted slightly mesially, the second premolar has rotated and drifted distally and impacted against the second molar. Had the second primary molar not been removed it is unlikely that this premolar would have drifted.

Delayed eruption of the primary dentition requires no treatment other than determining that all teeth are present. It is uncommon for children to require surgical exposure of the teeth in infancy. Parents should be reassured that there is very considerable variability in the eruption of teeth (plus or minus 6 months for primary teeth, plus or minus 1 year for permanent teeth). In the permanent dentition, delayed eruption should be investigated for the presence of supernumeraries and other pathology. Although the actual timing of tooth eruption is variable, evidence of progress in tooth crown and root development and the eruption sequence are of much more relevance. In contrast, the failure of eruption of a contralateral tooth more than six months after the appearance of its partner requires investigation.

Natal and neonatal teeth (Figure 9.33)
A neonatal tooth is one that erupts within 30 days of birth. A natal tooth is present at birth and in almost all cases is simply the early eruption of a normal primary incisor tooth. The development of this tooth is consistent with the expected stage of development of a primary incisor at birth (i.e. only five-sixths of the crown is formed without any root being present). This lack of root development accounts for the mobility of

the tooth. Babies with posterior natal teeth should be carefully investigated for other systemic conditions that may be associated with syndromes or other diseases.

Management

- The most important point to consider is whether the nursing mother can adequately establish breastfeeding. If either the nipples or the ventral surface of the infant's tongue are getting traumatized, the tooth should be removed.
- If the tooth is not too mobile it should be retained as it can become firm with time as the root continues to develop.
- If the tooth is excessively mobile then it may spontaneously exfoliate; however, because of the theoretical risk of aspiration or ingestion it should be electively removed.
- If tooth removal is indicated care should be taken to extract the entire tooth, as the crown only may be removed leaving behind the pulpal tissue. If this is the case, the dentine and a root will form subsequently; the root will then require removal at a later date.
- The permanent teeth should be unaffected by extraction of the primary tooth.

Clinical Hint   Extracting natal and neonatal teeth

- Always protect the airway when removing these teeth by placing a gauze in the back of the mouth. The teeth are easily dislodged or dropped. A pair of Spencer Wells forceps or similar will provide a firm grip on the tooth to be removed.
- Check the medical history for significant jaundice which may predispose to postoperative bleeding.

Ankylosed (submerged) primary molars (Figure 9.35)

It is quite common for primary molars to become ankylosed. If this occurs before eruption the teeth will fail to appear in the mouth. If this occurs post-eruption, the tooth will appear to submerge into the alveolus (in fact, the tooth remains stationary while the alveolar bone grows around it and adjacent teeth erupt). The timing of the removal of these teeth is based on the position of the first permanent molar and the extent of deciduous root resorption.

Management

- If there is radiographic evidence of resorption of the roots, then removal should be delayed as the vast majority of these teeth will exfoliate normally.
- Orthodontic consultation (see Chapter 11).
- If the premolar is congenitally absent early removal might be indicated.
- Surgical removal of the ankylosed tooth is to be avoided before eruption of the first permanent molar as this latter tooth will migrate mesially and space loss is likely to occur together with impaction of the second premolar. Once the

permanent tooth has erupted, the primary tooth may be removed and a space maintainer inserted.
- Retain space and use orthodontic treatment to align the permanent molar as required.

Clinical Hint Submerged teeth

- Submerged primary molars are difficult to remove intact surgically and there may be significant comorbidity associated with surgery.
- Where space has been lost due to migration or tipping of the first permanent molar, consider orthodontic uprighting in the first instance. Space can be maintained to await normal root resorption or facilitate more conservative surgical removal later.

Failure of eruption of first permanent molars (Figure 9.36)
Failure of eruption of first permanent is an uncommon finding, however, no one has yet been able to explain the mechanism as to why these teeth do not erupt. During surgically intervention it is invariably noted that these teeth are not ankylosed.

Root development (Figure 9.37)
Just as enamel can be affected by systemic illness, so too can root development be delayed, altered or arrested by systemic disease. This is most commonly seen when

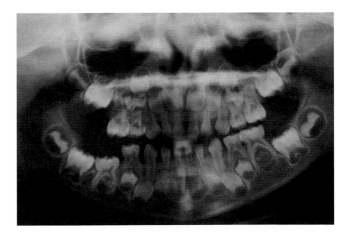

Figure 9.35 Failure of eruption of the mandibular right second primary molar. It is questionable whether these teeth are truly ankylosed. It is important to wait until the first permanent molar has erupted before surgical removal to avoid impaction of the second premolar. These teeth are often difficult to remove, especially if there is space loss and they should therefore be sectioned and elevated to minimize excessive bone loss.

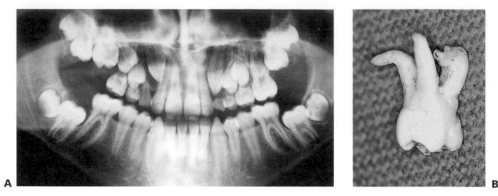

A   B

Figure 9.36 A, B Failure of eruption of first permanent molars is not uncommon. Surgical exposure of the crown may be sufficient to allow these teeth to erupt. Note that root development will continue in spite of a failure of tooth eruption and deviation of the roots will occur when the roots reach the cortical bone, in this case the antral floor. This root deviation may not be evident on radiographs, especially in the maxilla, and extraction of these teeth may prove extremely difficult.

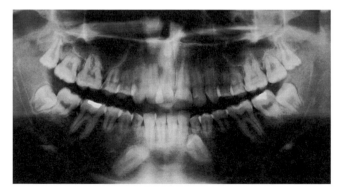

Figure 9.37 Arrested root development in a child who developed Stevens–Johnson syndrome at 10 years of age. Root development ceased at that time (probably as a result of the treatment as much as the disorder itself) and all teeth except the third molars were affected. It is interesting that these molars, which were not undergoing calcification, were unaffected.

radiotherapy causes shortening and tapering of the roots of premolars (see Chapter 10). Excessive orthodontic forces may also cause root resorption.

Dental age (maturity) determination

The paediatric dentist is often asked to help in age assessment, either at necropsy or for orphaned children. It is important to take into consideration ethnicity and variation in somatic growth potential.

Tooth emergence is not as important as tooth crown calcification and root development. The most widely used and accepted method is that developed by Demirjian and co-workers (1978) based on the panoramic radiographic appearance of tooth calcification at different ages.

Although there remains little doubt that peak height velocity, skeletal development and sexual maturation are associated, dental development seems to be independent of general somatic development.

Loss of tooth structure

- Attrition:
  - from wear of one or more teeth in one arch against one or more teeth in the opposing arch.
- Erosion:
  - exogenous from diet, habits or environment
  - gastro-oesophageal reflux
  - bulimia.
- Abrasion.
- Exogenous tooth substance loss from diet, habits or environment.

Enamel erosion

The prevalence of erosion in children and adolescents has been reported recently as very high, with over half of 14-year-olds in a UK population having moderate erosion, with an increased prevalence seen in lower socioeconomic groups. The aetiology of erosion in children and adolescents is varied and it has been suggested that the increased consumption of fruit juices and carbonated drinks is the most important factor, with the sale of soft drinks increasing by 56% over the past decade.

The erosive potential of acidic drinks is related to:

- Titratable acidity (TA).
- pKa.
- Type of acid.
- Calcium chelation ability.
- Method and temperature of consumption.

Carbonated soft drinks contain carbonic acid and often organic acids (commonly citric acid) are added to improve taste and 'mouth feel'. Citrate ions strongly chelate calcium in both acidic and basic environments decreasing the amount of free ionic calcium available in both saliva and at the enamel surface and thereby enhancing demineralization. The erosive potential of 'diet' soft drinks is similar to that of sugared drinks; however their potential to increase caries risk is decreased markedly. The method of drinking can also affect the extent of erosion, with the decrease in intra-oral pH becoming greater as the beverage is held in the mouth or is drunk by 'long sipping'; when the beverage is gulped, intra-oral pH does not decrease significantly.

The long-term and short-term consequences of dental erosion are marked, with the need for extensive and costly dental care and potential loss of teeth. The concomitant dental sensitivity can be severe and debilitating. It has been shown that even few intakes of acidic drinks on a regular basis may be associated with considerable dental erosion. It is important to question the child and parent(s) carefully as to total family usage of such drinks (fruit squashes, fresh fruit juices, particularly citrus juices, carbonated drinks, colas) in the first instance. The taking of study models and the institution of an exclusion diet for 3 months may show a diagnostic 'tide mark' of unattacked tooth substance at a later review.

Prevention of erosion

- Cessation or restriction of exposure to the aetiological factor.
- Modification of beverage erosivity seems to have the most future potential for reducing tooth structure loss. Recent research has concentrated on the addition of calcium and/or phosphate and pH alteration of soft drinks.
- Families are bombarded with advice on healthy eating. They may find advice to limit intake of fruit juices confusing and careful explanation is required.

Gastro-oesophageal reflux (Figure 9.38A)

When loss of enamel by erosion cannot be explained by dietary factors, reflux must be considered. Children with reflux will show enamel erosion, which is a smooth loss

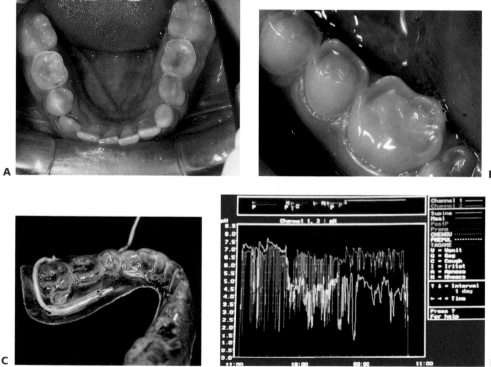

Figure 9.38 A Enamel erosion with asymptomatic gastro-oesophageal reflux. The first presentation of this child was to a dentist because of the erosion. **B** Severe erosion in a 12-year-old boy showing the outline of enamel with exposed dentine. **C** A mouthguard containing a micro pH probe was worn in the mouth for a 24-hour period to measure the intra-oral pH. Another is placed in the lower oesophageal sphincter. **D** In some children an intra-oral pH of <1 has been recorded.

of tooth structure, characteristically with amalgam restorations standing proud. Some children have undiagnosed, asymptomatic reflux that presents first with enamel erosion.

Diagnosis
- Barium swallows may not demonstrate reflux.
- 24-hour pH manometry is required to assess the extent of reflux (Figure 9.38D).

Management
- Diagnosis and treatment of reflux condition before definitive restoration of the teeth.
- Histamine blockers (H$_2$ antagonists) such as ranitidine and cimetidine.
- Anti-emetics (prokinetic agents) such as metoclopramide.
- Composite resin, stainless steel crowns, glass ionomer cement coverings or other onlays over the posterior teeth.
- Onlays on posterior teeth to protect occlusion and maintain vertical height.
- Professional application of fluorides. Nocturnal mouthguards with fluoride toothpaste as mechanical barriers against acid attack and fluoride to promote remineralization.

References and further reading

Oligodontia
Bergendal T, Eckerdal O, Hallonsten A-L et al 1991 Osseointegrated implants in the oral habilitation of a boy with ectodermal dysplasia: a case report. International Dental Journal 41:149–156

Fleming P, Nelson J, Gorlin RJ 1990 Single maxillary central incisor in association with mid-line anomalies. British Dental Journal 168:476–479

Freire-Maia N, Pinheiro M, eds 1984 Ectodermal dysplasias: a clinical and genetic study. Alan R Liss, New York

Hall RK 1983 Congenitally missing teeth – diagnostic feature in many syndromes of the head and neck. Journal of the International Association of Dentistry for Children 14:69–75

Hall RK, Bankier A, Aldred MJ et al 1997 Solitary median maxillary central incisor, short stature, choanal atresia/midnasal stenosis (SMMCI) syndrome. Oral Surgery, Oral Medicine, Oral Pathology, Oral Radiology, and Endodontics 84:651–662

Lai PY, Seow WK 1989 A controlled study of the association of various dental anomalies with hypodontia of permanent teeth. Journal of Pediatric Dentistry 11:291–295

Rappaport EB, Ulstrom R, Gorlin RJ et al 1977 Solitary maxillary central incisor syndrome and short stature. Journal of Pediatrics 91:924–928

Supernumerary teeth
Hogstrom A, Andersson L 1987 Complications related to surgical removal of anterior supernumerary teeth in children. Journal of Dentistry for Children 54:341–343

Jensen BL, Kreiborg S 1990 Development of the dentition in cleidocranial dysplasia. Journal of Oral Medicine and Pathology 19:89–93

Jensen BL, Kreiborg S 1992 Dental treatment strategies in cleidocranial dysplasia. British Dental Journal 172:243–247

Von Arx T 1992 Anterior maxillary supernumerary teeth. A clinical and radiographic study. Australian Dental Journal 37:189–195

Morphological anomalies

Nazif MM, Laughlin DF 1990 Dens invaginatus in a geminated central incisor: case report. Journal of Pediatric Dentistry 12:250–251

Rakes GM, Aiello AS, Kuster CG 1998 Complications occurring resultant to dens invaginatus: a case report. Pediatric Dentistry 10:53–56

Tsai SJJ, King NM 1998 A catalogue of anomalies and traits of the permanent dentition of southern Chinese. Journal of Clinical Pediatric Dentistry 22:185–194

Regional odontodysplasia

Aldred MJ, Crawford PJM 1989 Regional odontodysplasia: a bibliography. Oral Pathology and Medicine 18:251–263

Enamel hypomineralization

Cullen C 1990 Erythroblastosis fetalis produced by Kell immunisation: dental findings. Journal of Pediatric Dentistry 12:393–396

Fleming P, Witkop CJ, Kuhlmann WH 1987 Staining and hypoplasia caused by tetracycline Journal of Pediatric Dentistry 9:245–246

Enamel hypoplasia

Croll TP 1990 Enamel microabrasion for removal of superficial dysmineralisation and decalcification defects. Journal of the American Dental Association 129:411–415

Eli H, Sarnat H, Talmi E 1989 Effect of the birth process on the neonatal line in primary tooth enamel. Journal of Pediatric Dentistry 11:220–223

Pendrys DG 1989 Dental fluorosis in perspective. Journal of the American Dental Association 122:63–66

Molar–incisor hypomineralization (MIH)

Beentjes VE, Weerheijm KL, Groen HJ 2002 Factors involved in the aetiology of molar–incisor hypomineralisation (MIH). European Journal of Paediatric Dentistry 3:9–13

Fayle SA 2003 Molar–incisor hypomineralisation: restorative management. European Journal of Paediatric Dentistry 4:121–126

Weerheijm KL 2003 Molar–incisor hypomineralisation (MIH). European Journal of Paediatric Dentistry 4:114–120

Weerheijm KL, Duggal M, Mejare I et al 2003 Judgement criteria for molar–incisor hypomineralisation (MIH) in epidemiologic studies: a summary of the European meeting on MIH held in Athens, 2003. European Journal of Paediatric Dentistry 4:110–113

Amelogenesis imperfecta

Bäckman B, Ammeroth G 1989 Microradiographic study of amelogenesis imperfecta. Scand J Dent Res 97:316–329

Seow WK 1993 Clinical diagnosis and management strategies of amelogenesis imperfecta variants. Pediatric Dentistry 15:384–393

Dentine anomalies

Cole DEC, Cohen MM 1991 Osteogenesis imperfecta: an update. Journal of Pediatrics 115:73–74

Gage JP, Symons AL, Roumaniuk K et al 1991 Hereditary opalescent dentine: variation in expression. Journal of Dentistry for Children 58:134–139

O'Carroll MK, Duncan WK, Perkins TM 1991 Dentin dysplasia: review of the literature and a proposed sub-classification based on radiographic findings. Oral Surgery, Oral Medicine, and Oral Pathology 72:119–125

Seow WK, Latham SC 1991 The spectrum of dental manifestations in vitamin D-resistant rickets: implication for management. Pediatric Dentistry 8:245–250

Seow WK, Brown JP, Tudehope DA et al 1984 Dental defects in the deciduous dentition of premature infants with low birth weight and neonatal rickets. Pediatric Dentistry 6:88–92

Eruption disorders

Friend GW, Mincer HM, Carruth KR et al 1991 Natal primary molar: case report. Journal of Pediatric Dentistry 13:173–175

Masatomi Y, Abe K, Ooshima T 1991 Unusual multiple natal teeth: case report. Journal of Pediatric Dentistry 13:170–172

Sauk JJ 1988 Genetic disorders involving tooth eruption anomalies. In: Davidovitch Z, ed. The biological mechanisms of tooth eruption and root resorption. EBSCO Media, Birmingham; 171–179

Shaw W, Smith M, Hill F 1980 Inflammatory follicular cysts. ASDC Journal of Dentistry for Children 47:97–101

Erosion

Jarvinen V, Muerman JH, Hyvarinen H et al 1988 Dental erosion and upper gastrointestinal disorders. Oral Surgery, Oral Medicine, and Oral Pathology 65:298–303

General

Hall RK 1994 Pediatric orofacial medicine and pathology. London: Chapman and Hall Medical

Worldwide web database

Online Mendelian Inheritance in Man, OMIM (TM). McKusick-Nathans Institute for Genetic Medicine, Johns Hopkins University (Baltimore, MD) and National Center for Biotechnology Information, National Library of Medicine (Bethesda, MD), 2000. http://www.ncbi.nlm.nih.gov/omim/

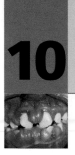

10 Medically compromised children

Contributors

Kerrod B Hallett, Angus Cameron, Richard Widmer, Wendy J Bellis,
Meredith Wilson

Introduction

Comprehensive dental care of a medically compromised child requires consideration of their underlying systemic condition and coordination of their dental treatment with their medical consultant. Although dental problems are common in this group, their oral health is frequently overlooked by the medical profession. The term used to identify this particular group, 'medically compromised children', has been replaced recently by the more general term 'children with special needs'. However, the older term is still relevant because it reminds the dentist that these children often have medical conditions that can affect dental treatment or that they can present with specific oral manifestations of a systemic disease. This chapter discusses the common paediatric medical conditions that require consideration in the provision of optimal dental treatment. The prevention of oral diseases is important in children with chronic medical problems (Figure 10.1) as oral complications can severely compromise a child's medical management and overall prognosis.

Cardiology

Congenital heart disease

Congenital heart disease (CHD) has an incidence of approximately 8–10 cases per 1000 live births and represents the largest group of paediatric cardiovascular diseases. Although most lesions occur individually, several form major components of syndromes or chromosomal disorders such as Down's syndrome (trisomy 21) (Figure 10.2A) and Turner's syndrome (XO chromosome) with over 40% of children being affected. However, in the majority of cases, no cause can be determined and a multifactorial aetiology is often assumed. Known risk factors associated with CHD include maternal rubella, diabetes, alcoholism, irradiation and drugs such as thalidomide, phenytoin sodium (Dilantin) and warfarin sodium (Coumadin).

Turbulent blood flow is caused by structural abnormalities of the heart anatomy and presents clinically as an audible murmur. The degree of clinical morbidity is determined by the haemodynamics of the lesion. Congenital heart disease can be classified into acyanotic (shunt or stenotic) and cyanotic lesions depending on clinical presentation. Eight common conditions account for 85% of all cases.

Acyanotic conditions

The acyanotic group of conditions is characterized by a connection between the systemic and pulmonary circulations or a stenosis (narrowing) of either circulation. Infants

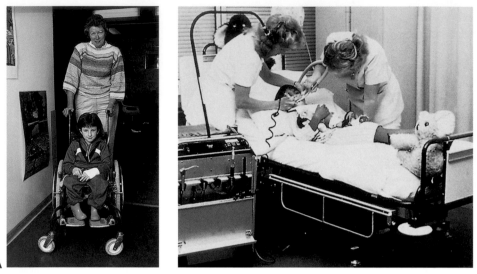

A   B

Figure 10.1 A Children with medical problems may have conditions with a dental manifestation such as this child with osteogenesis imperfecta or may present with a medical co-morbidity that complicates their general dental care. **B** Not all children with medical problems require hospital admission, although treatment of such patients is often challenging. Mobile dental equipment is invaluable in providing quality dental care. The majority of hospital inpatients are treated in the dental surgery and usually only those who may be in traction or in intensive care units require bedside treatment.

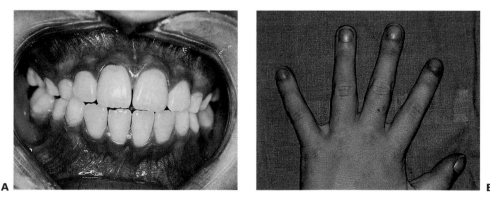

A   B

Figure 10.2 A Intra-oral photograph of a child with complex cyanotic cardiac disease associated with trisomy 21. Note the cyanosis of the gingival tissues. Of importance is to note that he has no dental disease. His oral hygiene is exceptional and there is no caries. Treatment would have been extremely difficult due to his intellectual disability. **B** Clubbing of the fingers associated with complex cyanotic cardiac disease. The nail beds also show cyanosis.

often present with feeding difficulties, breathlessness and failure to thrive. Shunts are from the left to right. The most common anomalies and their specific sites are:

- **Atrial septal defect** (ASD) – usually located near foramen ovale.
- **Ventricular septal defect** (VSD) – in the membranous septum of the ventricular wall.
- **Patent ductus arteriosus** (PDA) – caused by failure of closure of the ductus connecting the pulmonary artery with the aorta (normally closes soon after birth). If cardiac failure develops the infant is digitalized and prescribed diuretics if necessary. Hospitalization, oxygen, nasogastric tube feeding and antibiotic therapy for chest infection may also be required. If the lesion does not close spontaneously, surgery to reduce torrential pulmonary flow or repair of the defect is indicated.
  Acyanotic defects with obstruction include:
- **Coarctation or localized constriction of the aorta** – usually in the area related to the insertion of the ductus.
- **Aortic stenosis** or narrowing of the aortic central orifice – due to fusion of the aortic valve cusps.
- **Pulmonary stenosis** – due to narrowing of the pulmonary valve which may also involve the pulmonary arteries.

Cyanotic conditions (Figure 10.2)
All cyanotic conditions exhibit right-to-left shunting of desaturated blood. Cyanotic defects become clinically evident when 50 g/L of desaturated haemoglobin is present in peripheral arterial blood. Infants with mild cyanosis may be pink at rest but become very blue during crying or physical exertion. Children with cyanotic defects are at significant risk for desaturation during general anaesthesia and preoperative consultation with the paediatric cardiologist and anaesthetist is essential.

The most common cyanotic lesions are:

- **Tetralogy of Fallot** – which includes a VSD, pulmonary stenosis at valve or sub-valve levels, a large overriding aorta and right ventricular hypertrophy.
- **Transposition of great vessels** – when the aorta exits the heart from the right side and the pulmonary artery exits from the left. Although the internal heart anatomy is normal, the systemic blood circulation cannot be resaturated with oxygen and immediate management of transposition by opening the ductus arteriosus and corrective surgery is required.
- **Eisenmenger's syndrome** – this refers to cyanosis from any right-to-left shunt caused by increased pulmonary resistance through a VSD or PDA.
- **Tricuspid atresia** – due to absent tricuspid valve and may present with an absent right ventricle and pulmonary valve. The pulmonary circulation is maintained through a PDA in the neonate.
- **Pulmonary atresia** – which is similar to tricuspid atresia except that the tricuspid valve is patent.

Other cardiovascular diseases
Other common paediatric cardiovascular disorders include cardiomyopathies such as myocardial disease and pericardial disease, cardiac arrhythmia, infective endocarditis and rheumatic heart disease (RHD). Both CHD and RHD can predispose the internal

lining of the heart to bacterial or fungal infection (infective endocarditis) and lead to the formation of friable vegetations of blood cells and organisms. Vegetations may embolize and cause renal, pulmonary or myocardial infarcts or cerebrovascular accidents. *Streptococcus viridans*, a common commensal organism in the oral cavity, is most frequently responsible for chronic infective endocarditis, whereas *Staphylococcus aureus* is often implicated in the acute fulminating form of infective endocarditis.

Dental management

Several important principles need to be followed when managing children with cardiac disease. Transient bacteraemia can occur following invasive dental procedures and potentially cause infective endocarditis in a susceptible patient. Therefore all children with CHD or previous RHD require antibiotic prophylaxis to reduce the risk of infective endocarditis (see Appendix E). Those children who have been previously taking long-term antibiotics should be prescribed an alternative medication as per the protocol to avoid development of resistant oral organisms. In addition, a preoperative oral antiseptic mouthwash, such as 0.2% chlorhexidine gluconate, is recommended to reduce the oral bacterial counts.

Children with CHD have a higher prevalence of enamel anomalies in the primary dentition and concomitant risk of early childhood caries. Some cardiac medications may contain up to 30% sucrose and dietary prescription with high-caloric supplements (Polyjoule) further potentiate caries risk. Meticulous oral hygiene and preventive dental care, such as fissure sealants and topical fluoride therapy is recommended to reduce the risk of dental caries in susceptible children.

Dental disease in children with cardiac disorders can seriously complicate their medical management. Children with advanced cardiovascular disease should receive only palliative dental care until their medical condition has been stabilized. Aggressive treatment of pulpally involved primary teeth is recommended. Pulpotomy or pulpectomy is contraindicated in these children due to the possibility of subsequent chronic bacteraemia. Although routine treatment in the dental surgery environment is possible, it is often preferable to manage children with multiple carious teeth under general anaesthesia in the hospital environment. This protocol allows completion of treatment with one invasive procedure and negates the risk of infective endocarditis with further operative procedures. If multiple visits are planned, there is a need to prescribe alternative antibiotics or wait for a month between appointments to reduce bacterial resistance.

A thorough preoperative assessment of the child's regular medication (including anticoagulants, antiarrhythmics, and antihypertensives) is essential to avoid any potential drug interactions during treatment. There is no contraindication to the use of vasoconstrictors in local anaesthetic solutions. If conscious sedation is used, vital signs and oxygen saturation during the procedure should be carefully monitored. Avoid the use of electrosurgery, electronic pulp testers and ultrasonic cleaning devices in children with cardiac pacemakers, in case of potential interference.

Haematology

Disorders of haemostasis

Primary haemostasis is initiated after injury to a blood vessel with the formation of a primary platelet plug. This process is mediated by interactions between the platelets and coagulation factors in the plasma and the vessel wall. Secondary haemostasis or coagulation is also triggered by the initial injury and reaches its greatest intensity after the primary platelet plug is formed. Fibrin deposition provides the framework for the formation of a stable blood clot.

Prolonged bleeding can occur when either phase of haemostasis is disturbed. The clinical manifestations of a haemostasis disorder vary depending on the phase affected. Defects in primary haemostasis generally result in bleeding from the skin or mucosal surfaces, with the development of petechiae and purpura (ecchymoses). These disorders include von Willebrand's disease as well as defects in platelet function. In contrast, defects in secondary haemostasis, such as haemophilia, lead to bleeding that tends to be more deep-seated in muscles and joints. In both disorders, uncontrolled prolonged oral bleeding can occur from innocuous insults such as a tongue laceration or cheek biting.

Children with haemostasis disorders can be identified from a thorough medical history, examination and laboratory tests. Questions should reveal episodes of spontaneous bleeding or bruising; the occurrence of prolonged bleeding in other family members and prescription of anticoagulant medication. A physical examination of skin, joints and oral mucosa should be undertaken for evidence of petechiae, ecchymoses and haematoma. If a haemostasis disorder is suspected, referral to a haematologist is recommended for evaluation and laboratory blood tests.

Laboratory tests

- **PFA 100** (platelet function analysis) may be used as a screening test for von Willebrand's disease and platelet dysfunction. If it is prolonged, specific testing for these disorders may be required
- **Full blood count** (FBC) is required to determine platelet levels (normal range $150–400 \times 10^9$ /L) and platelet function tests may be necessary in selected cases. Adequate haemostasis can usually be maintained by no less than 40×10^9 platelets/L.
- Coagulation tests include **prothrombin time** (PT) which is a test of the extrinsic coagulation pathway (normal range 11–17 seconds) and **activated partial thromboplastin time** (APTT) which is a test of the intrinsic coagulation pathway (normal range 24–38 seconds). Test results greater than 2 seconds compared with control values should be considered abnormal.

Classification
Vascular disorders
Vascular disorders are characterized by increased capillary fragility and include the purpuras, hereditary haemorrhagic telangiectasia, haemangiomas, vitamin C deficiency and connective tissue diseases such as Ehlers–Danlos syndrome.

Platelet disorders
Platelet disorders can be either a deficiency (thrombocytopenia) or dysfunction.

Thrombocytopenia
Thrombocytopenia is defined as a platelet count $<150 \times 10^9$/L. Clinical signs and symptoms associated with decreased platelet counts are as follows:

$<75 \times 10^9/L$ May exhibit post-surgical haemorrhage
$<25 \times 10^9/L$ Spontaneous haemorrhage, easy bruising
$<15 \times 10^9/L$ Petechiae appear on the skin
$<5 \times 10^9/L$ Oral petechiae, submucosal and mucosal bleeding

Thrombocytopenia may occur as an isolated entity of unknown cause (idiopathic thrombocytopenic purpura (ITP)), as a result of marrow suppression by drugs or from other haematological diseases such as aplastic anaemia. Marrow replacement by neoplastic cells in haematological malignancies will also result in thrombocytopenia. Children undergoing chemotherapy will have decreased platelet counts.

Thrombocytosis

Thrombocytosis is an increased number of platelets ($>500 \times 10^9/L$) and may be associated with prolonged bleeding due to abnormal platelet function. Myeloproliferative disorders may present with thrombocytosis.

Platelet function disorders

These may be congenital or acquired. The most common cause of acquired platelet dysfunction is the use of non-steroidal anti-inflammatory drugs (e.g. aspirin). Administration of cyclo-oxygenase inhibitors will result in blockage of the production of thromboxane A_2 for the life of the platelet (7–9 days). This results in a decrease in platelet aggregation. Some metabolic diseases such as Gaucher's disease also manifest as defects of platelet function.

A decrease in the number of platelets or platelet dysfunction will result in failure of initial clot formation. Children with thrombocytopenia will bleed immediately after trauma or surgery, unlike those with haemophilia, who usually start to bleed 4 hours after the incident. The most common oral manifestations are petechiae and ecchymoses. There may also be spontaneous gingival bleeding and prolonged episodes of bleeding after minor trauma or tooth brushing.

Inherited coagulation disorders

Coagulation disorders result from a decrease in the amount of particular plasma factors in the coagulation cascade. The most common disorders are haemophilia A and von Willebrand's disease, both manifesting a decrease in factor VIII levels. The factor VIII is produced by endothelial cells and is composed of two portions. The largest part of the molecule is the von Willebrand's factor and is responsible for initial platelet aggregation. The factor VIII part of the complex and factor IX are responsible for activation of factor X in the intrinsic pathway of the coagulation cascade. Other disorders of coagulation include vitamin K deficiency, liver disease and disseminated intravascular coagulation usually from overwhelming (Gram-negative) infection.

Coagulation disorders are classified according to the defective plasma factor; the most common conditions are factor VIII (haemophilia A) and factor IX (haemophilia B or Christmas disease). von Willebrand's disease occupies a unique position in that both platelet and factor VIII activity is decreased, therefore both bleeding time and APTT are prolonged.

Haemophilia A

This is inherited as an X-linked recessive disorder with deficiency of factor VIII, and occurs 1 in 10 000 live male births. Spontaneous mutation occurs in 30% of cases. The disease is classified as:

- Severe (<1% factor VIII) – with spontaneous bleeding into joints and muscles.
- Moderate (2–5% factor VIII) – with less severe bleeding usually following minor trauma.
- Mild (5–25% factor VIII) – which may not manifest until middle age following significant trauma or surgery.

Factor VIII assay is usually performed after the initial diagnosis of a coagulopathy. Affected children and their families require considerable medical support and may have an indwelling central line for regular factor VIII concentrate infusion.

Haemophilia B or Christmas disease
This disease has clinical features similar to factor VIII deficiency. It is also inherited as an X-linked recessive gene and results in prolongation of the APTT. It is diagnosed by specific assay of factor IX.

von Willebrand's disease
von Willebrand's disease is inherited as an autosomal dominant trait (gene locus 12p13). The most common clinical manifestations include epistaxis and gingival and gastrointestinal bleeding. von Willebrand's factor is found in the plasma, platelets, megakaryocytes and endothelial cells and circulates as a major component of the factor VIII molecule complex. This disease is divided into various subtypes, based on the platelet and plasma multimeric structure of the von Willebrand's factor.

Dental management
Dental management of children with suspected haemostasis disorders should begin with screening laboratory tests. If tests are abnormal, haematological consultation is required for a definitive diagnosis. Invasive dental procedures should be performed only after the extent of the problem has been determined. Extractions must never be performed without first consulting the haematologist. It is preferable to have platelet levels greater than 80×10^9/L before extractions. Endodontic procedures may be preferable to extractions to avoid the need for platelet transfusion.

Dental procedures
- Use an atraumatic technique. In the event that oral surgery is necessary, a sound surgical technique to minimize trauma and local measures to control bleeding such as careful atraumatic suturing and socket dressings are mandatory.
- Maxillary infiltration anaesthesia can generally be administered slowly without pretreatment with platelet or factor replacement. However, if the infiltration injection is into loose connective tissue or a highly vascular area, then factor replacement to achieve 40% activity levels is recommended.
- Avoid mandibular block injections as these may be complicated by dissecting haematoma and airway obstruction. In the absence of suitable factor replacement, intraperiodontal injections may be used, but with great caution. The anaesthetic solution is placed under moderate pressure along the four axial surfaces of the tooth by inserting the needle into the gingival sulcus and the periodontal ligament space.
- Nitrous oxide sedation can be effective for restorative procedures with the need for local anaesthesia; however, care must be taken when placing matrix bands.

- Use rubber dam to protect the soft tissues.
- Endodontic treatment can be safely carried out without factor cover.
- Periodontal treatment with deep scaling and subgingival curettage requires factor replacement.
- Multiple extractions require hospital admission and haematological work-up in conjunction with the haematology team.

Medical management
Haemophilia A
- All children and most adult patients are treated with recombinant factor VIII. A small number of adults continue to receive either recombinant or purified plasma derived factor VIII.
- Severe haemorrhage is treated to 100% replacement, although minor bleeds can be controlled with partial replacement between 30% and 50%.
- Minor trauma may also be life-threatening, especially with intracerebral bleeds.
- Some patients will form antibodies (inhibitors) to factor VIII, severely complicating medical management.
- A single unit of factor VIII concentrate per kg will raise blood levels by approximately 2% and has a half-life of 10–12 hours.

Haemophilia B
- Same as for haemophilia A but infused with either recombinant (monoclonal) factor IX or highly purified plasma derived factor IX.

von Willebrand's disease
- Type I may be treated with 1-deamino (8-D-arginine) vasopressin (DDAVP).
- Types II and III require treatment with purified plasma derived factor VIII concentrate (which contains both factor VIII and von Willebrand's factor).
- Avoid platelet transfusions, if possible, due to the development of antiplatelet antibodies and the risk of transmission of viral diseases such as hepatitis B and C.

Other factor replacements
- Recombinant activated factor VII for haemophilia A with inhibitors and genetic deficiency of factor VII.

Antifibrinolytics
- Tranexamic acid (Cyklokapron).

DDAVP
- Can be used for people with mild haemophilia and those with von Willebrand's disease.
- Can result in an up to twofold release of factor VIII from endothelial cells – this is adequate if levels of factor VIII are >10% and the patient is responsive to DDAVP.

Postsurgical administration of antifibrinolytic agents such as tranexamic acid (Cyklokapron) 25 mg/kg loading dose and 15–20 mg/kg three times daily for 5–7 days is helpful to prevent clot lysis. During the time that antifibrinolytics are given, the parent and child should be instructed not to use straws, metal utensils, pacifiers or baby bottle teats.

Characteristically, haemophilia bleeds are delayed 12–24 hours, as primary haemostasis is not impaired, and local pressure has little effect. It is worth noting that mild haemophilia can go undiagnosed. The APTT is not sensitive to detect mild deficiencies of FVIIIc and levels of FVIIIc 25–30 IU/dl can be associated with a normal APTT. In addition, FVIIIc values in mild haemophilia are temporarily increased (as occurs in unaffected persons) by stress, exercise, and bleeding. If there is a convincing history of a bleeding tendency always do a specific factor assay even if the initial screening tests are normal.

The normal regimen for DDAVP is 0.3 µg/kg intravenous infusion over 1 hour before surgery followed by tranexamic acid 15–20 mg/kg orally every 8 hours for 7 days. After 9–12 hours, if the FVIIIc levels are still low (50–60%), then the original dose of DDAVP may be repeated. If repeated doses are planned or required it is important to fluid restrict the patient and monitor electrolytes. Repeated doses of DDAVP may cause fluid retention and hyponatraemia. This regimen is useful in von Willebrand's disease and children on renal dialysis.

Clinical Hint

Questions commonly asked by parents are:
- Will my child's teeth erupt normally? Usually yes, but there is often more bleeding from a traumatized operculum that may require active intervention.
- Will my child's teeth fall out normally? Usually yes, unless continually traumatized there is normally no abnormal bleeding associated with exfoliating primary teeth. However, if there is prolonged mobility and oozing occurs, then extraction may be necessary under appropriate factor cover to reduce the risk of persistent bleeding (Figure 10.3).
- Can a child with a bleeding disorder have orthodontic treatment? Yes, provided extractions are performed after appropriate consultation with the haematologist and there is vigilant maintenance of the appliances.

Anticoagulant therapy
Management of children on anticoagulant therapy needs special consideration. Anticoagulants are usually prescribed for children with valvular heart disease and prosthetic

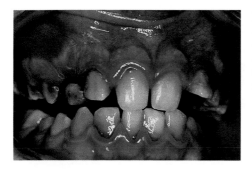

Figure 10.3 Gingival haemorrhage around an exfoliating maxillary right primary canine in a child with Christmas disease (factor IX deficiency). Normally, exfoliation of primary teeth is not of major concern and bleeding is locally controllable.

valves to reduce the risk of remobilization. If extractions or surgery are required, it is necessary to decrease the clotting times to facilitate adequate coagulation but not to such an extent so as to cause emboli or clotting around the valves. The dental management of these children is also complicated by their congenital cardiac defect and antibiotics are required for prophylaxis against infective endocarditis.

Therapeutic drugs used
- Oral warfarin sodium (Coumadin):
  - vitamin K antagonist depleting factors II, VII, IX and X
  - usually 3–4 days are required for full anticoagulation onset and its efficacy is assessed by PT level (factor VII levels).
- Heparin sodium (Heparin):
  - shorter acting and has an immediate onset (inhibits factors IX, X and XII)
  - can be administered either subcutaneously using a low-molecular-weight derivative or intravenously under the supervision of a paediatric haematologist.
- Enoxaparin sodium (Clexane):
  - low-molecular-weight heparin which inhibits factor Xa and thrombin
  - usually administered subcutaneously.

Children on anticoagulant therapy should stop taking warfarin 3–5 days prior to the surgery date. In those in whom there is a significant risk for thrombosis with subtherapeutic warfarin level, parenteral anticoagulation may be necessary. This is generally achieved with enoxaparin sodium (Clexane) 1.5 mg/kg subcutaneously once daily (mane) via Insuflon. This drug is omitted on the morning of surgery. With the use of this regimen the child may be admitted to hospital on the day of dental surgery. Warfarin is recommenced in normal dose on the evening of surgery. If further enoxaparin sodium prophylaxis is required, it should be given the morning after surgery and continued until the PT and international normalized ratio (INR) are therapeutic. Monitoring of enoxaparin sodium is rarely required. In emergency situations with prolonged bleeding from oral wounds post surgery, following recommencement of warfarin, FFP (fresh frozen plasma) may also be of benefit.

Local haemostatic measures
- Application of topical thrombin (Avitene).
- Packing of the socket with microfibrillar collagen haemostat (MCH or CollaTape), oxidized regenerated cellulose (Gelfoam or Surgicel).
- Suturing of attached gingivae to maintain pressure.
- Splints or stomo-adhesive bandages may also be of benefit.
- There have been recent reports of the efficacy of 'fibrin glue' in the management of coagulopathies, but its use on moist oral mucosa is limited.

Management of oral haemorrhage
Unexpected bleeding from the oral cavity can occur at any time. There may have been a slow ooze for several days or, in the other extreme, there may be a significant sudden oral bleed. Such bleeding can occur without warning and may not be associated with any prior investigative or operative work. As well, haemorrhage from the mouth can occur following such routine procedures as biopsy, restorative work or tooth extraction.

The initial management of such cases involves identifying the exact site of haemorrhage, controlling the bleeding and then preventing a recurrence. In the cases of haemorrhage from the mouth that has not been associated with any dental procedure, clinicians should take an accurate history of the bleeding, the duration, lost volume and any causative factors. Abnormal bleeding may occur around an erupting tooth, from an exfoliating tooth site, or may be associated with physical and sexual child abuse or congenital vascular anomalies such as arteriovenous malformations. The possibility of a childhood malignancy should also be considered.

In cases of oral haemorrhage following dental procedures, the following steps should be taken (it is important to prevent or minimize bleeding in the first instance):

- A sensible limitation of surgical trauma.
- Digital compression of the alveolus after tooth extraction.
- Packing of the socket with a resorbable gel.
- Adequate suturing of extraction sites to help reduce postoperative complications.
- Pressure application to the surgical site with gauze packs.
- Construction of a removable splint is recommended following more extensive surgery.
- Written postoperative instructions to ensure adequate rest, avoidance of hard foods and early mouth rinsing.
- Prescription of non-aspirin medication are necessary to avoid any parent misunderstanding.

In cases of severe uncontrollable haemorrhage following tooth extraction that can occur due to arteriovenous malformations, remember that the best method of controlling the bleeding is to replant the extracted tooth back into the socket and suture it well.

Red cell disorders

Anaemia

Anaemia is considered to be present if the haemoglobin level falls below 100 g/L. The cause of anaemia in children may be due to blood loss, iron, folate and vitamin B_{12} deficiency, bone marrow failure, haemolysis of red blood cells or anaemia of chronic disorders. It is usually an incidental finding in the routine dental management of children. A full blood count (FBC) is usually ordered when children present with pallor, lethargy, fever, bruising, undiagnosed systemic or oral pathology, after major trauma associated with excessive blood loss or on work-up before surgery for other medical conditions. When unexpected anaemia is discovered, follow-up by the paediatrician is required.

Haemolytic anaemia

Acute haemolytic disease of the newborn or erythroblastosis fetalis is caused by ABO incompatibility and Rhesus (Rh) iso-immunization. There will be discoloration of those primary teeth that are calcifying at the time of birth. The cusp tips of the first permanent molars may also be affected. A yellow to green staining is most commonly seen as a result of high levels of unconjugated bilirubin.

Glucose 6-phosphate dehydrogenase (G6PD)

G6PD deficiency also results in acute haemolytic anaemia when the child is exposed to certain drugs (sulphonamides, chloramphenicol, aspirin, antimalarials) or infection (hepatitis).

Aplastic anaemia

Aplastic anaemia is defined as a decrease or absence of haemopoiesis in the bone marrow that is not due to marrow involvement or recognised disease process. FBC and bone marrow aspirate confirms the diagnosis. Bone marrow transplantation is the treatment of choice for moderate to severe aplastic anaemia.

Haemoglobinopathies

Thalassaemia

The haemoglobinopathies are a group of genetic disorders involving the globin chains of the haemoglobin (Hb) complex. These diseases comprise two main groups: the structural haemoglobinopathies resulting in abnormal globin structure (HbE, HbS) and the thalassaemias, in which the genetic mutation results in the decreased production of the globin chain.

Adult blood contains haemoglobin A, which is composed of two globin chains (HbA) and a small amount of haemoglobin A_2 (HbA$_2$). Children also produce some fetal haemoglobin (HbF). Homozygous α-thalassaemia is incompatible with life, while the heterozygous phenotype has few clinically significant symptoms. Since there are many genes involved, the most likely combination is homozygotes of the same gene or double heterozygotes of different genes.

Of more significance is homozygous β-thalassaemia major (Cooley's anaemia). Due to the absence of the β chain, there is a compensatory increased production of HbA$_2$ and HbF. As erythropoiesis is inadequate, the bone marrow is reactive and there is compensatory intermedullary haemopoiesis in the maxilla and diploe of the skull. There may be severe haemolytic anaemia with marked hepatosplenomegaly and failure to thrive. Those children with sickle β-thalassaemia show evidence of vascular thrombosis with ischaemia to organs, especially bones.

Due to maxillary and zygomatic overgrowth there is often a severe Class II Division 1 malocclusion with separation of teeth and widening of the periodontal ligament space. Lateral skull radiographs demonstrate a 'hair on end' appearance. Children are given regular packed red cell hypertransfusions until the haemoglobin rises to 140–150 g/L and desferrioxamine, an iron-chelating agent, to increase iron excretion. When excessive haemosiderosis in the spleen adds significantly to the haemolysis rate, elective splenectomy is performed.

Sickle cell disease

This is different from the other haemoglobinopathies in that the red blood cells are more susceptible to haemolysis and have difficulty passing through small blood vessels causing infarcts and ischaemia of organs and bone. Blood transfusions, analgesics, antimicrobials, adequate hydration and other life-supportive measures are necessary.

Dental management

Consultation with the child's haematologist prior to treatment is essential to arrange haematological preparation and transfusion. It is important to schedule dental treatment shortly after blood transfusions and provide antibiotic prophylaxis, especially if the child has had splenectomy. Avoid elective treatment if haemoglobin level is less than 100 g/L. Minimize stress that might compromise the child's ability to oxygenate the tissue adequately. Respiratory depressants should be avoided and additional oxygenation during conscious sedation or general anaesthesia is desirable. Local anaesthesia is not contraindicated but the use of prilocaine (Citanest) is not advised due to the formation of methaemoglobin. Vasoconstrictors in the standard dose are not contraindicated. Orthodontic treatment may be undertaken but teeth will move quickly through the bone and relapse will most likely occur.

Immunodeficiency

Immunodeficiency may be caused by quantitative or qualitative defects in neutrophils, primary immunodeficiencies, involving T cells, B cells, complement, or combined defects and secondary immunodeficiency or acquired disorders.

Qualitative neutrophil disorders
Chemotactic disorders
- Chediak–Higashi syndrome.
- Lazy leukocyte syndrome.
- Leukocyte adhesion defects (Figure 10.4).

Phagocytic disorders
- Agammaglobulinaemia.
- Chronic granulomatous disease.

Quantitative neutrophil disorders
Neutropenia
This is defined as $<1.8 \times 10^9$ cells/L. Life-threatening sepsis is associated with a level of neutrophils $<0.5 \times 10^9$ cells/L. Neutropenia can occur in the following situations:

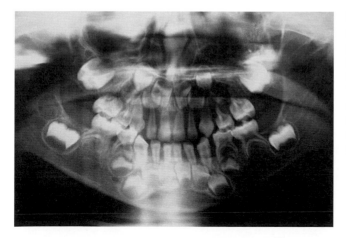

Figure 10.4 Leukocyte adhesion defect in a 4-year-old manifesting as severe periodontal disease and marginal bone loss. The maxillary and mandibular anterior teeth exfoliated within months of this radiograph being taken.

- Infiltration of bone marrow by neoplastic cells.
- After administration of cytotoxic drugs used for treatment of childhood malignancy.
- Cyclic neutropenia (21–28 day cycling).
- Agranulocytosis.
- Aplastic anaemia.
- Drug-induced neutropenia.

Primary immunodeficiencies
B-cell defects
- Selective IgA deficiency.
- Agammaglobulinaemia.

T-cell defects
- Di George syndrome with thymic aplasia.
- Chronic mucocutaneous candidiasis.

Secondary or acquired immunodeficiencies
Secondary or acquired immunodeficiencies include those conditions acquired during childhood such as:
- Human immunodeficiency virus (HIV) infection.
- Drug-induced immunodeficiency (cytotoxics, corticosteroids, ciclosporin A, tacrolimus).

  These can also occur in children who have undergone bone marrow transplantation and radiotherapy (radiotherapy-induced immunodeficiency).

Combined immunodeficiencies
- Severe combined immunodeficiency.
- Wiskott–Aldrich syndrome.
- Ataxia telangiectasia.

Dental implications
Both neutrophil and T-cell-mediated immunodeficiency predispose the child to infection by compromise of the host defence system. Opportunistic organisms that do not usually cause disease in a healthy child can proliferate in the oral cavity of the immunodeficient host. Common oral manifestations seen are:
- Acute pseudomembranous candidiasis (Figure 10.5B).
- Severe gingivitis.
- Generalized prepubertal periodontitis (Figure 10.4).
- Gingivostomatitis.
- Recurrent aphthous ulceration.
- Recurrent herpes simplex (HSV) infection.
- Premature exfoliation of primary teeth.

  Generally, B-cell deficiencies exhibit fewer oral complications but are often associated with chronic bacterial infections such as pneumonia, otitis media and skin lesions.

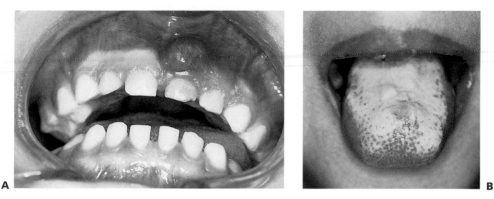

Figure 10.5 Two manifestations of immunodeficiency. **A** Abscess formation above the maxillary right primary lateral incisor tooth after administration of high-dose steroids for asthma, in an area that was previously quiescent. **B** Candidal infection of the tongue in an immunocompromised child.

Dental management

Regular review of the developing dentition, gingivae and mucosa and the institution of a preventive programme are essential for maintenance of healthy hard and soft tissues. Elimination of any potential oral focus of infection during the course of medical treatment is the primary goal.

The underlying deficiency must be fully assessed and the likelihood of oral complications endangering the child's medical status should be evaluated. An individual risk–benefit assessment of any oral lesion must be considered with regard to the overall management plan. A decision whether to extract or maintain carious teeth and exfoliating primary teeth must be based on the worst case scenario during the immunodeficiency period. If a carious lesion cannot be stabilized with an adequate interim restoration, then extraction is the preferred treatment. In a case being prepared for bone marrow transplantation, all mobile primary teeth should be removed at least 2 weeks prior to the conditioning phase.

Prophylactic antimicrobials specific for commensal oral organisms determined from culture and sensitivity tests are indicated during the course of medical treatment. Biopsy specimens may assist the diagnostic process. The antimicrobial protocol may include appropriate antibiotics (amoxicillin trihydrate and ampicillin), aciclovir sodium if HSV-positive, ganciclovir if cytomegalovirus-positive, antifungals (topical nystatin and amphotericin B) and twice daily 0.2% chlorhexidine gluconate (Curasept) mouthwashes during the active therapy phase.

Thorough dental scaling and prophylaxis and the provision of custom trays for delivery of medication (antiseptic or fluoride gels) prior to commencement of head and neck radiotherapy is also recommended to prevent oral sepsis and radiation-induced dental caries.

Acquired immunodeficiency syndrome (AIDS)/HIV

HIV infection has been identified in increasing numbers of children with otherwise unexplained immune deficiency and opportunistic infections of the type found in adults with acquired immune deficiency syndrome (AIDS). For the limited purposes of epidemiological surveillance, the Centers for Disease Control (CDC) characterizes a case of paediatric HIV infection as a reliably diagnosed disease in children that is at least moderately indicative of underlying cellular immunodeficiency, and with which no known cause of underlying cellular immunodeficiency or any other reduced resistance is reported to be associated.

Transmission
The main transmission media are body fluid, such as blood and semen. Saliva contains low and inconsistent levels of the HIV virus and is unlikely to provide a significant mode of transmission. Consequently, the two major routes of transmission in children are vertical (from an infected mother) and from blood products, with children with haemophilia being most at risk. Vertical transmission rates are up to 39% and occur before, during or after birth. Infection from breastfeeding may be up to 29%.

Risk factors
- The risk factors for paediatric HIV infection vary depending on the age group.
- Most children with AIDS are under 5 years of age.
- The primary risk factors are perinatal.
- Infants born to women who are intravenous drug users or who have bisexual partners comprise the largest group.
- About a third of the infants weigh less than 2500 g at birth and are small for gestational age. Of these babies, 25–30% of children develop AIDS in the first year of life.
- The presenting pattern of encephalopathy varies with age and significant growth failure occurs in early infancy.

Serodiagnosis and immune function
The screening ELISA test for HIV antibodies is liable to give false negatives and any apparently positive results must be confirmed by the western blot assay. Antigen assays are far more reliable, but a failure to detect virus or antigen in a young antibody-positive child does not exclude infection. A positive virus or antigen test is likely to indicate infection. Due to the long incubation period and the limitations of medical history and serodiagnosis, it must be assumed that all blood derivatives may be infectious.

The human immunodeficiency virus attaches to the CD4 variant of the T4 helper lymphocyte and remains within infected cells throughout their life, being transmitted to other cells mainly by cell to cell contact. Other cells that may be affected include macrophages, and possibly endothelial, neuroglial, epithelial and dendritic cells. The principal effect of HIV infection on the immune system is depletion of CD4 lymphocytes (helper cells) which results in a drop in the absolute CD4 count and a reversal of the CD4/CD8 ratio. These are immune indicators of disease progression.

Oral manifestations (Figure 10.6)
Oral lesions are often early warning signs of HIV infection. Common disorders may manifest in different ways in the presence of HIV. In children, the most common lesions are:

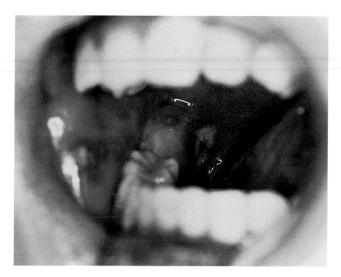

Figure 10.6 Severe oral ulceration in a child in the terminal stages of HIV/AIDS. The ulceration was most likely due to disseminated HSV infection to which the child succumbed 7 days after this photograph was taken.

Candidosis

The most common oral lesion in HIV infection is acute pseudomembranous candidiasis. It is an early lesion and suggests the presence of other opportunistic infections. The severity of the candida infection may be related to the T4/T8 ratio and occurs when CD4 counts are less than 300/mL. Oesophageal candidiasis occurs when CD4 counts drop below 100/mL. Fungal infections can be related to reduced salivary flow and S-IgA. It responds well to treatment with systemic antifungals and an improvement in oral hygiene.

Ulceration

Recurrent herpes simplex infections are frequent and are typically intra-oral and circumoral. Other parts of the body may also be affected. Aphthous-type ulcers are persistent and very common in children. Treatment is palliative with adequate hydration and analgesia.

Atypical gingivitis

HIV-related gingivitis manifests as red erythematous gingival tissues and can extend to the free gingival margin. There is often spontaneous gingival haemorrhage and petechiae within the gingival margin, either localized or generalized. Consideration must be given to a fungal component. Treatment involves improved tooth brushing and flossing and the use of daily 0.2% chlorhexidine gluconate (Curasept) mouthwashes and gels.

Salivary gland enlargement

Parotitis occurs in both paediatric and adult patients and is similar to the presentation of mumps. It may be unilateral or bilateral and results in xerostomia and pain. Reduced salivary flow may lead to pseudomembranous candidiasis and dental caries.

Hairy leukoplakia

This is uncommon in children, with only a few reported cases in children. It occurs predominantly on the lateral border of the tongue and occasionally on the buccal mucosa and the soft palate.

HIV-related periodontitis

HIV-related periodontitis presents with deep pain and spontaneous bleeding, interproximal necrosis and cratering, and intense erythema more severe than acute necrotizing ulcerative gingivitis (ANUG). HIV periodontitis appears more frequently in HIV-infected patients who have reduced T4/T8 ratios and symptomatic opportunistic infection. Organisms such as black-pigmented bacteroides and Gram-positive bacilli, which are similar to those found in adult periodontitis, have been identified in HIV periodontitis.

Kaposi's sarcoma

Uncommon in children and adolescents. The lesion mainly affects the palate, and also the gingivae and the tongue. Treatment is by chemotherapy, radiotherapy or laser excision.

Outcomes

Primary colonization by commensal organisms rather than reactivation of opportunistic infections usually occurs (cytomegalovirus, retinitis and toxoplasmosis are rare). Bacterial infections are also rare, although *Streptococcus pneumoniae* and *Haemophilus influenzae* are common respiratory complications. Kaposi's sarcoma is seen infrequently but lymphomas (especially with central nervous system (CNS) involvement) can occur. The progression of disease process can vary and in many instances, oral and physical symptoms do not often present for years after infection with the immunodeficiency virus. Lymphocytic interstitial pneumonitis is frequently the cause of death for children with AIDS, but is often asymptomatic. There have been major advances in the management of HIV/AIDS with antiretroviral medications and consequently, many children may lead a normal and effective life.

Oncology

Childhood cancer accounts for about 1% of all cancer cases in the population. In Australia, the annual incidence of malignant tumours in children under 15 years is approximately 11 per 100 000 children. Approximately 600–700 children between birth and 15 years develop cancer each year. Whereas most adult cancers are carcinomas with strong aetiological associations, childhood cancers are a wide range of different histological types of tumour with less aetiological connection.

The incidence, either in childhood cancer as a whole or in individual types of cancer, varies little from one country to the next and no racial group is exempt. Among more than 50 types of childhood cancers, the most common forms include leukaemias, lymphomas, CNS tumours, primary sarcomas of bone (Figure 10.7A) and soft tissues, Wilms' tumours, neuroblastomas and retinoblastomas. Acute leukaemias and tumours of the CNS account for approximately one-half of all childhood malignancies. Multimodal therapy (chemotherapy, radiotherapy and surgery) has resulted in an overall 5-year survival rate for childhood cancer of approximately 70%.

Leukaemia

Leukaemia is a heterogeneous group of haematological malignancies caused by clonal proliferation of primitive white blood cells.

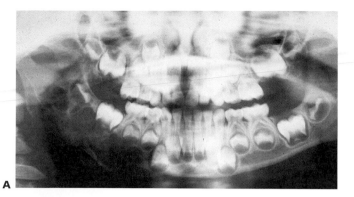

A

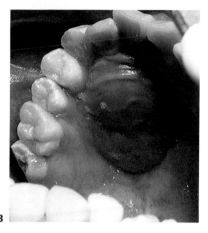

B

Figure 10.7 Neoplasms may arise as primary lesions within the jaws, invade from local tumours or may seed as metastases from distant primaries. **A** The panoramic radiograph shows an extensive primary neoplasm of the right mandible involving the infratemporal fossa. Histologically, this lesion was a desmoplastic fibroma and required a hemimandibulectomy. **B** Presentation of a lymphoma in the palate of a 15-year-old girl. The lesion was asymptomatic and the child had merely presented for a routine check-up.

Acute lymphoblastic leukaemia (ALL)

- Accounts for 80–85% of acute childhood leukaemias.
- Defined by the presence of more than 25% lymphoblasts in the bone marrow.
- Therapy is tailored to the risk of relapse dependent on cytogenetic markers and includes a combination of induction chemotherapy, CNS prophylaxis and maintenance chemotherapy for approximately 2 years' duration.
- Intrathecal therapy (commonly methotrexate) has been used to replace cranial irradiation.
- Cure rates for standard risk ALL are now over 90–92% on current protocols. If relapse occurs 40–50% can be cured with chemotherapy and/or haematopoietic stem cell transplantation.
- Prognosis depends on age of onset, initial white cell count, cytogenetic abnormalities and other features.
- Bone marrow transplantation is reserved for very high risk or patients with relapse.

Acute myeloid leukaemia (AML)
- Accounts for 15–20% of acute childhood leukaemias.
- In this disease, the bone marrow is infiltrated with primitive myeloid cells, classified by their morphological appearance (FAB subtypes M1–M7). The clinical features of AML are similar to other leukaemias.
- AML with monocytic morphology (M4/M5) can manifest gingival infiltration and promyelocytic morphology (M3) is associated with disseminated intravascular coagulation.
- Induction chemotherapy therapy is often followed by early allogenic bone marrow transplantation for high-risk patients.
- The cure rate is approximately 60% with modern therapy.

Chronic myeloid leukaemia (CML)
- Rare in childhood and accounts for less than 5% of leukaemic cases.
- Two types; one identical to adult CML and characterized by the presence of the Philadelphia chromosome (Ph) in malignant cells, the second or juvenile form (JCML) occurs earlier in infancy with a rapid course, infection, haemorrhage and poor survival rate.
- Bone marrow aspirate reveals granulocytic proliferation without an excess of lymphoblasts.
- The chronic phase of this disease is now effectively treated with specific bcr-abl tyrosine kinase inhibitors (imatinib or dasatinib) which can lead to remission lasting for years.
- Allogeneic bone marrow transplantation remains the only definitive curative therapy but is now generally reserved for patients relapsing on tyrosine kinase inhibitors or for children who have an HLA-matched sibling.

Clinical features of childhood leukaemia
- Fatigue and weight loss.
- Anaemia.
- Purpura.
- Infections and unexplained febrile episodes.
- Marked hepatosplenomegaly and lymphadenopathy.

Investigations
- FBC shows anaemia, neutropenia, thrombocytopenia and leukocytosis with circulating lymphoblasts
- Bone marrow aspirate is required to confirm diagnosis.
- Lumbar puncture to exclude CNS involvement.

Problems in medical management
The main problems in medical management are bone marrow suppression initially at diagnosis due to malignant infiltration and later due to chemotherapy, subsequent anaemia, infection and mucosal ulceration and bleeding. Infection in the immunocompromised child is a life-threatening condition and may be due to bacteria, viruses, fungi or parasites. Broad-spectrum triple antibiotic treatment is usually required. Disease relapse may occur in the marrow, CNS or other organs (e.g. testes).

Solid tumours in childhood
Brain tumours
- These are most frequent solid tumours of childhood.
- Approximately 70% are gliomas, mostly low-grade astrocytomas or medullo-blastoma.
- More than 50% of paediatric intracranial tumours occur in the posterior cranial fossa region. Surgical excision combined where possible combined with chemotherapy and radiotherapy is the standard approach to treatment.
- Chemotherapy can be used to delay or avoid cranial radiotherapy in infants.
- The overall survival rate is approximately 60% at 10 years.

Non-Hodgkin's lymphoma (Figure 10.7B)
- Arises from neoplastic B or T lymphocytes in lymph nodes and lymphoreticular tissue.
- The primary tumour may be abdominal (B cell) or in the mediastinum (T cell).
- Tumour spread is usually local or to bone marrow and CNS.
- The primary mode of therapy is chemotherapy.
- 90% cure rate for localized tumours.

Wilms' tumour
- Occurs in the kidney around 3–4 years of age.
- Usually presents as an asymptomatic abdominal mass.
- Often associated with aniridia and other congenital anomalies.
- The tumour responds well to combined therapy: chemotherapy with or without radiotherapy to reduce the tumour mass and surgical removal depending on disease stage. Commonly lung, hepatic and skeletal metastases occur.

Neuroblastoma
- Arises from neural crest cells anywhere along the sympathetic chain.
- Most common site is abdominal, either in the adrenal gland or paraspinal ganglia. Other sites include thorax, neck or pelvis.
- Tumour spread to lymph nodes, bone marrow, liver or subcutaneous tissues.
- Diagnosis is confirmed by raised levels of urinary catecholamines and tissue biopsy.
- Prognosis depends on patient age at diagnosis, tumour stage and biological features of the tumour, especially presence of amplification of the n-myc gene. Children with high-risk disease (approximately 50% of cases) have 25% survival rates even with aggressive chemotherapy, surgery, radiation and autologous bone marrow transplantation.

Rhabdomyosarcoma
- Arises from embryonal mesenchymal tissue with potential for differentiation to skeletal (striated) muscle.
- Children often present with a painless, usually rapidly enlarging subcutaneous lump, almost anywhere in the body.
- Common sites include head and neck, genitourinary tract and extremities.

- Large lesions in the head and neck invade bone and jaw lesions are quite common in advanced cases.
- Treatment involves surgery with adjuvant chemotherapy and radiotherapy.
- Prognosis is influenced by site, subtype of rhabdomyosarcoma, and stage at diagnosis.

Hodgkin's disease
- Lymphoid malignancy characterized by presence of Reed–Sternberg cells in the tumour.
- Usually affects teenagers and young adults.
- Presents most commonly as a painless enlargement of the lower cervical or mediastinal lymph nodes accompanied by unexplained fever and weight loss.
- Excellent response (cure rate approaches 90% for low stage disease) to chemotherapy.
- Radiotherapy is often required for more advanced disease.

Retinoblastoma
- Tumour of the retinoblasts in children under 5 years of age.
- Strong hereditary component.
- Diagnosis is usually a white or yellow pupillary reflex (normally red reflex).
- Treatment often requires enucleation of the globe and post-surgical radiotherapy. Occasionally adjunct chemotherapy is also required.

Osteosarcoma
- Rare malignant tumour of bone, mostly in the metaphyseal region of long bones, with the distal femur being the most common site.
- Teenagers are the most common age group affected.
- Frequently metastasizes to the lung and requires wide resection of primary tumour plus multi-agent chemotherapy.

Ewing's sarcoma
- Malignant tumour of bone in teenagers, commonly involving the midshaft of long bones, although any bone may be involved.
- Occurs most commonly in the proximal femur or pelvis and is characterized by densely packed small round cells.
- Treatment involves surgery, chemotherapy and local irradiation.
- The prognosis worsens with pelvic primary or metastatic disease.

Langerhans' cell histiocytosis (see Chapter 8)
- A rare neoplasm similar to ALL, often presenting with eczematous, purpuric rash on the hands, scalp and trunk.
- Osteolytic lesions of the skull and mandible can occur and premature exfoliation of primary teeth has been reported.
- Prognosis depends on the extent of disease at diagnosis and the progression of lesions.

Dental management

Close collaboration between the child's oncologist and the paediatric dentist is essential when planning appropriate dental care. At the time of diagnosis and during the initial stages of chemotherapy, dental care should be provided by the paediatric dentist at the hospital. Once the child has achieved remission, or has successfully completed chemotherapy, routine dental care can often be provided by the child's own dentist.

Where dental treatment is needed prior to or during chemotherapy, planning with the oncology team is essential. If extractions are required, a FBC including differential white cells and platelets is necessary. If the platelet count is less than 30×10^9/L, then platelet infusion is indicated and antifibrinolytic agents (doses similar to management of haemostatic disorders) may be helpful. As with immunocompromised children, if the neutrophil count is less than 1.8×10^9/L, specific antimicrobial prophylaxis should be administered. As many children have been receiving systemic corticosteroids, the possibility of adrenocortical suppression should be considered and additional steroid cover provided as appropriate.

Elective dental treatment should be delayed until the child is in remission or on maintenance chemotherapy. Children in full remission can be treated as normal for most routine dental treatment, although an FBC is prudent if an invasive procedure is planned. Pulpal therapy of primary teeth during the induction and consolidation phase of chemotherapy is contraindicated. When pulpal therapy of permanent teeth is needed, the risk of bacteraemia and potential septicaemia must be weighed against the potential benefits.

Oral hygiene and prevention

It is important to maintain meticulous oral hygiene by using a soft toothbrush during chemotherapy. Four times daily 0.2 % chlorhexidine gluconate mouthwashes or gel application to the mucosa helps reduce the symptoms of mucositis and topical and systemic antifungal agents (nystatin or fluconazole) help prevent candidiasis during immunosuppression. Topical lidocaine hydrochloride (Xylocaine Viscous 2%) is helpful during acute episodes of mucositis prior to eating (if possible) or drinking. Prophylactic parenteral antibiotics and antiviral medications, if indicated, are always given during febrile episodes and periods of severe neutropenia to prevent further medical complications.

Immediate oro-dental effects of childhood neoplasia and treatment

Dramatic advances in the treatment of childhood cancer in the past three decades have led to the long-term cure of 70% of the children diagnosed today. Since about 1 in 600 children develop cancer before the age of 15 years, almost 1 young adult in every 1000 will be a long-term survivor of childhood cancer.

As the number of survivors of a variety of paediatric cancers increases, the oro-dental sequelae of effective medical treatment in these patients are emerging. These effects are unique because of the impairment of active growth and development during the cancer therapy. Adverse sequelae caused by the cancer treatment can be grouped into postsurgical, post-radiotherapy, post-chemotherapy and combined effects.

Post surgery

Surgical removal of a solid tumour in the oral cavity can cause:

- Disfigurement (temporary or permanent) (Figure 10.8A)
- Loss of teeth and function.
- Stenosis and paraesthesia.

Post radiotherapy (Figure 10.8B)

Radiotherapy produces an initial mucosal inflammation that is often followed by surface sloughing and ulceration (mucositis). The extent of inflammation depends on the location and dosage of radiotherapy and whether fractionated versus whole-dose radiation is used. The most common symptoms following cranial irradiation are oral pain and difficulty in eating and drinking which are most severe 10–14 days following commencement of radiotherapy. The mucositis usually resolves in another 2–3 weeks after radiotherapy.

When radiotherapy involves the major salivary glands, xerostomia frequently occurs within a few days producing a viscous, acidic saliva. Loss or alteration of taste may also occur prompting the patient to change to a softer, more cariogenic diet to alleviate soreness and dryness of the oral cavity. This is probably the major factor in the aetiology of rapid dental caries that has been reported in these patients if they are not given adequate preventive therapy. Radiation-induced dental caries has a distinctive generalized cervical pattern and sometimes the complete dentition can be destroyed in a relatively short period.

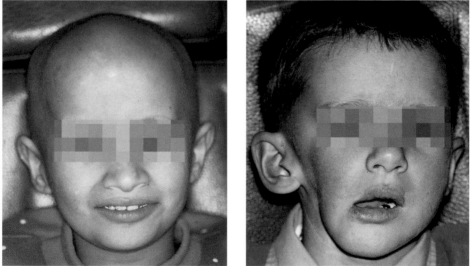

A B

Figure 10.8 A A child in remission from acute lymphoblastic leukaemia with typical alopecia resulting from chemotherapy. **B** Late effects of surgery and radiotherapy for a rhabdomyosarcoma of the right mandible involving the parotid, neck and infratemporal fossa. This child underwent a hemimandibulectomy and radical neck dissection, followed by reconstruction with a free vascular rib graft. Note the limited oral opening and the facial deformity. Access for restorative work on the carious molars was extremely difficult. Caries resulted from reduced salivary flow after removal of the parotid gland.

Progressive endarteritis is a complication that can occur in irradiated bone and can lead to osteoradionecrosis. The mandible is particularly prone to this complication and if such an area of dead bone should become infected following dental extraction, a refractory osteomyelitis may ensue. Endarteritis may also cause fibrosis in the masticatory muscles and subsequent trismus.

Chemotherapy

The cytotoxic drugs used during chemotherapy can cause damage to several organs:

- Liver.
- Kidney.
- Intestine.
- Germ cells of the testes and ovaries.
- Lung.
- Heart.
- Brain.

Direct stomatotoxicity is caused by the cytotoxic action of the chemotherapeutic agents on oral mucosal cells leading to inflammation, thinning and ulceration of the mucosa (mucositis). Saliva function may also be diminished although this response has not been reported as common in children. These problems are commonly encountered in the induction and consolidation phases of chemotherapy when relative high doses of multi-agent therapy are employed. Recent case reports suggest that the incidence and severity of stomatotoxicity is reduced with the concomitant administration of granulocyte colony-stimulating factor (G-CSF) during chemotherapy.

The effects of chemotherapy and radiotherapy appear to be synergistic. Since craniofacial and dental development have not been completed until the adolescent period, it is not surprising that dental late effects are commonly found in survivors of childhood cancer. Chronic problems involving target tissues lead to impairment of growth and development of hard and soft tissues, which may result in orofacial asymmetry, xerostomia, dental caries, trismus and a variety of dental abnormalities. Generally, the nature and degree of these complications vary widely and depend on several factors including the type and location of malignancy, the age of the patient, total dosage and timing of chemotherapeutic agents, and the initial oral health status and the level of dental care before, during and after therapy.

Late oro-dental effects of childhood neoplasia and treatment (Figure 10.9)

The majority of those children for whom oncology treatment results in a stable remission can expect to follow a healthy life. Recurrence of the original malignancy may occur although the likelihood of this becomes increasingly remote as time passes. Consequently, successfully treated paediatric oncology patients are never 'discharged', their health being regularly monitored throughout their life.

With the exception of those children treated with radiotherapy to the oro-facial region, the majority of children are no more prone to dental and periodontal disease than the well child, and often exhibit excellent oral health. However, long-term oro-dental effects of radiotherapy can influence dental management.

Growth disturbances

Following head and neck radiotherapy, facial growth can be impaired and alterations to developing teeth can occur. Children younger than 5 years of age are affected more

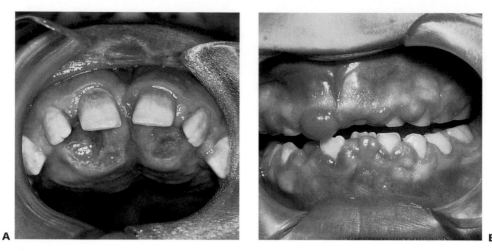

Figure 10.9 A Severe renal osteodystrophy in a child in end-stage renal failure. There has been gross expansion of the maxilla in an attempt to produce red blood cells because of failure of erythropoiesis. This is similar to events in β-thalassaemia. **B** Gingival overgrowth due to ciclosporin A treatment after kidney transplantation. The teeth are also hypoplastic and small because of renal disease in infancy.

severely than older patients. An altered craniofacial growth pattern with diminished mandibular growth, is often associated with a field of irradiation that includes a portion of ascending ramus and the entire condyle of the mandible. Dental effects may include:

- Incomplete calcification.
- Enamel hypoplasia.
- Arrested or altered root development, and premature closure of the root apices can complicate permanent tooth development.
- Microdontia and agenesis of teeth are also common.

The exact nature and extent of damage depends on the stage of dental development and the timing and dosage of irradiation. The lack of specificity of cytotoxic agents in terms of differentiating neoplastic cells from metabolically active normal cells, such as ameloblasts and odontoblasts, can result in abnormalities of dental development. Microdontia, enlarged pulp chambers, shortening, thinning and blunting of the root apex and delayed tooth eruption have been frequently reported in children receiving chemotherapy. Enamel opacities, hypocalcification and a high rate of dental caries have also been reported in several studies, however, it remains unclear whether these findings are due to direct alteration of enamel formation or maturation or to alterations in the oral environment (saliva and flora), diet and home care often observed among young patients on chemotherapy.

Xerostomia
Cranial irradiation can also irreversibly damage the acini cells of the major salivary glands and xerostomia can occur in children. This condition is often transient due to the lower dosage of radiation used and greater regenerative capacity of the exocrine

cells in children. Generally, there is a lower incidence of radiation-induced dental caries in children compared with adults. Regular nightly fluoride mouth rinsing is required to prevent enamel demineralization during this critical period.

Other less common effects
Epidermal and mucosal changes include skin hyperpigmentation, cutaneous telangiectasia, subcutaneous tissue atrophy and permanent thinning or loss of hair. Disturbances of intellectual, endocrine and germ cell development have also been reported following cranial irradiation. However, the mean age of dental maturation in children following cranial irradiation is within the normal range.

Since most craniofacial tumours are treated by combined chemotherapy and head and neck irradiation, it is difficult to know the exact effect of each treatment. In general, late oro-dental effects are more severe in patients who receive a higher-dosage treatment either with chemotherapy or radiotherapy. Dental aberrations are more severe and extensive in patients younger than 6 years of age due to the immature development of the permanent teeth. Total body irradiation in bone marrow transplantation appears to increase the risk of disturbance to dental development.

Complications associated with bone marrow transplantation
Almost all children undergoing bone marrow transplantation develop the typical oral mucosal changes of ulceration, keratinization and erythema. All tend to maximal about 4–14 days post transplantation. Mucosal atrophy is also frequently associated with ulceration between 1 and 3 weeks after bone marrow transplantation. During this period oral pain is often severe with many patients requiring narcotic analgesia. The use of keratinocyte growth factor (palifermin) has been demonstrated to reduce this complication in adults undergoing autologous transplantation and paediatric studies of this promising treatment are in progress.

As mentioned previously, oral infection with *Candida albicans*, herpes simplex, cytomegalovirus and varicella zoster are the major infective agents seen in children undergoing bone marrow transplantation, if inadequate prophylaxis is given. These conditions can be life-threatening if not treated aggressively at diagnosis.

Oral manifestations of defective haemostasis are common but seldom serious and include mucosal bleeding or crusting of the lips and gingival oozing.

Graft versus host disease (GVHD)
This condition occurs when transplanted T cells recognize the host tissues as foreign. GVHD is a major problem following bone marrow transplantation with clinical manifestations in up to half of patients. The acute form of GVHD tends to occur within weeks of bone marrow transplantation, with signs of fever, rash, diarrhoea and abnormal liver function leading to jaundice. Chronic GVHD may follow some months later and is characterized by lichenoid or scleroderma-like changes of the skin, keratogingivitis, abnormal liver function, pulmonary insufficiency and intestinal problems. Oral manifestations of GVHD vary with the severity of the conditions but often include:
- Mild oral mucosal erythema.
- Painful desquamative gingivitis.
- Angular cheilitis.
- Loss of lingual papillae.

- Lichenoid patches of the buccal mucosa.
- Striae on the buccal mucosa.
- Xerostomia.

Management of chronic GVHD requires a multidisciplinary approach. Long-term systemic immunosuppression with prednisone and other agents is often needed. Topical treatments such as dexamethasone mouthwashes can be effective. Careful attention to oral health with close communication with the treating medical team is needed to give the best outcomes.

Nephrology

Renal disorders
Renal diseases are classified as acute, chronic, acquired or congenital conditions.

Acute renal failure
- Results in a sudden onset of impaired renal function and perfusion.
- Can occur subsequent to septicaemia, dehydration, severe burns and blood loss, glomerulonephritis, pyelonephritis, tumour lysis and ureteric obstruction.

Chronic renal disease
The most common chronic conditions affecting the kidneys are:
- Ureteric reflux causing reflux nephropathy or hypoplasia.
- Obstructive uropathy.
- Glomerulosclerosis.
- Medullary cystic disease.
- Systemic lupus erythematosus.
- Cystinosis.

End-stage renal failure
- Leads to a progressive drop in glomerular filtration rate that results in hypertension, fluid retention and build-up of metabolites that are not excreted normally.
- Medical management is directed toward prevention of fluid and electrolyte imbalance, restriction of proteinuria, correction of hypoalbuminaemia, hypocalcaemia, hyperphosphataemia and control of anaemia and hypertension.
- In children with severe renal failure, drug treatment is often inadequate and artificial filtration by either peritoneal dialysis or haemodialysis becomes necessary.

Acquired conditions
- Urinary tract infections, usually from coliform bacteria from the intestinal tract and cystitis (bladder infection).
- Acute glomerulonephritis usually accompanies β-haemolytic streptococcal infections and often resolves with antibiotic therapy in most children. However, 3–4% may develop post-infection chronic renal failure and subsequently need dialysis.

Medical complications can be overcome with successful renal transplantation, which is now the preferred treatment of choice for children with end-stage renal failure.

Despite the restricted availability of donor organs, renal transplantation has a high success rate. Complications associated with immunosuppression due to ciclosporin (Sandimmun) and prednisone (Predsone) therapy to prevent organ rejection need to be considered in dental management. The most common oral manifestations following renal transplant are gingival hyperplasia (Figure 10.10B) and opportunistic infection from commensal oral flora.

Dental implications

Impaired renal function can result in several oral manifestations including:

- Uraemic stomatitis.
- Oral ulceration.
- Intrinsic and extrinsic tooth staining.
- Excessive supragingival calculus.
- Enamel hypoplasia and hypocalcification.
- Delayed dental development.

Uraemic stomatitis may develop when the serum urea level is greater than 300 mg/mL. It occurs as ulcerated or non-ulcerative forms involving the tongue and buccal mucosa predominantly. Both forms have a tendency to bleed and are susceptible to secondary infection by oral commensal organisms.

Renal osteodystrophy (Figure 10.9A)

Lytic lesions of the mandible or maxilla, known as Brown's tumours, can also occur in severe renal failure due to secondary hyperparathyroidism. Histologically, these lesions are similar to giant cell tumours and usually resolve following correction of hypocalcaemia and hyperphosphataemia with vitamin D metabolites. Hypocalcaemia occurs

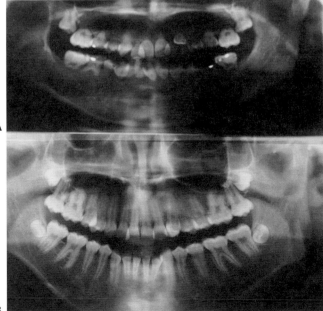

A

B

Figure 10.10 Effects of radiation to the head and neck. A set of identical twins, the first of which (**A**) had acute lymphoblastic leukaemia diagnosed at 18 months. She relapsed during the first remission and received a bone marrow transplant and total body irradiation (TBI). The comparison with her sister (**B**) at 15 years of age is dramatic. There is agenesis of some permanent teeth, arrested root development of the incisors and first permanent molars, and microdontia.

due to increased phosphate retention and decreased calcium absorption. Active calcium absorption from the gut depends on the presence of the active metabolite, 25-hydroxy-cholecalciferol (vitamin D_3). However, vitamin D metabolism is impaired due to failure of the hydroxylation of 25-hydroxy-cholecalciferol to 1,25-dihydroxy-cholecalciferol in the diseased kidney. In an attempt to raise serum calcium there is a secondary hyperparathyroidism and calcium is removed from bone stores giving rise to the characteristic radiographic appearance of a renal osteodystrophy.

Dental management

The observed dental changes depend on the time of onset of renal disease. Those teeth calcifying during renal failure will exhibit chronological hypoplasia or hypomineralization of the enamel and dentine. Developing teeth are often stained green or brown due to the incorporation of blood products such as unconjugated bilirubin or haemosiderin respectively. Caries is often minimal in these children, possibly due to urea metabolites in the saliva, but supragingival calculus formation is markedly increased, even when oral hygiene is adequate.

- Consultation with a renal physician or nephrologist is often required before these children can receive routine dental treatment.
- Children with acute renal conditions should have elective dental treatment postponed until restoration of their renal function.
- Emergency or palliative care is only indicated following pre-treatment screening for elevated bleeding time or APTT.
- Extraction of pulpally involved primary teeth is the preferred treatment option due to the risk of chronic bacteraemia following pulpotomy or pulpectomy.
- Symptomatic patients with proteinuria or on long-term steroid therapy are best managed in the hospital environment where blood pressure and fluid balance can be monitored before treatment. Fluids and electrolytes in such children can be adjusted by the nephrologist and steroid supplementation can be given prior to general anaesthesia or a major dental procedure.

Dialysis

Children receiving dialysis often exhibit somatic growth retardation, and are pale and anaemic on presentation. They also have a bleeding tendency due to increased capillary fragility and thrombocytopenia. In addition, children on haemodialysis receive anticoagulation with intravenous heparin, and can experience other complications such as infection of the port site and increased risk of hepatitis. In children receiving peritoneal dialysis, complications can occur with catheter placement including peritonitis and exit-site infections. However, peritoneal dialysis is easier to manage in children, requiring less time for the fluid exchange, less restriction of food and fluid intake, and fewer haemodynamic problems compared with haemodialysis.

- Children on haemodialysis and anticoagulant therapy can be successfully managed with pretreatment DDAVP and antibiotic prophylaxis to prevent infection of the access device.
- Any dental treatment, especially extractions, should be performed the day after dialysis when the heparin is no longer active (heparin half-life is 4 hours but residual effects can occur for 24 hours).

- Sockets should be packed with a haemostatic agent and sutured well. Platelet transfusions are to be avoided if possible.
- Children on continuous ambulatory peritoneal dialysis can be managed more conservatively.

Drug interactions

Drug interactions can occur in children with end-stage renal failure who are managed with long-term antihypertensives and steroids. Medications that are metabolized in the kidney or nephrotoxic should be avoided in children with renal insufficiency. These include:

- Ceralotin (cephalothin).
- Paracetamol (acetaminophen).
- Non-steroidal anti-inflammatory agents.
- Tetracycline.

Dentists should also be aware that renal excretion of drugs is also impaired and their half-life may be extended. However, if children are adequately haemodialysed it may be necessary to increase dosage of drugs to obtain the necessary pharmacological effect. Adjustment of a drug dosage as well as timing of intake should be made in consultation with the child's nephrologist.

Renal transplantation

A pretransplant dental assessment is essential to reduce the risk of oral complications following organ transplant and immunosuppression. The presence of dental caries and oral infections will necessitate delay in transplantation until all potential foci of infection are eliminated. Comprehensive dental treatment and institution of a rigorous preventive programme are recommended prior to transplant to reduce the risk of subsequent oral diseases. Antibiotic prophylaxis as per the protocol for prevention of infective endocarditis is essential prior to invasive surgical procedures.

Gastroenterology

Hepatic and biliary disorders

Biliary atresia

In this condition there is congenital obliteration or hypoplasia of the bile ducts resulting in biliary cirrhosis and portal hypertension. In severe cases, transplantation is necessary.

α_1-Antitrypsin deficiency

- Deficiency in hepatic secretion of α_1-globulin.
- Leads to progressive hepatomegaly and cirrhosis.
- Treated by liver transplantation.

Liver function tests

- Full blood count and coagulation profile should be routinely tested.
- Alanine aminotransferase (ALT): 7–47 U/L.
- Alkaline phosphatase: 60–391 U/L.

- γ-Glutamyl transpeptidase: 5–43 U/L.
- Total bilirubin.
- Albumin (a decrease may reflect impaired protein synthesis).

Dental implications
- Coagulation problems are of major concern due to the reduction in production of vitamin-K-dependent clotting factors (II, VII, IX, X).
- Patients are immunocompromised. Children are usually mildly anaemic due to destruction of red blood cells. High levels of circulating red-blood-cell degradation products may become incorporated in developing enamel. High levels of unconjugated bilirubin will cause green developmental staining of enamel.

Dental management
- Consultation with paediatric gastroenterologist and haematologist.
- Aggressive management of caries with extraction of suspect teeth, especially prior to transplantation.
- Coagulopathies are usually managed with fresh frozen plasma to replace deficient clotting factors.
- Antibiotic prophylaxis required.

Hepatitis A (infectious hepatitis)
Transmission period is very short (3 weeks). The important point to note is that there is no carrier state. If a patient is hepatitis-A positive treatment should be delayed for at least 4 weeks.

Hepatitis B (serum hepatitis)
Interpretation of hepatitis B test results
- If the HBsAg test is positive the blood is automatically tested for the 'e' antigen. If 'e' is negative, the patient is a chronic healthy carrier.
- If the 'e' antigen is positive the patient is a chronic active carrier.

Chronic healthy carrier (HBsAg +ve, e −ve)
- The degree of infectivity of these patients, although significant, is thought to be less than that of chronic active carriers. The liver function test for this patient should be normal.

Chronic active carrier (HBsAg +ve, e +ve)
- The chronic active carrier has active viral replication and is very infective. These patients have active liver disease, and their liver function may be abnormal.
- It is important to liaise directly with the patient's doctor in the first instance when planning dental treatment and to do so again at regular intervals while the patient is under the care of the paediatric dental unit.

Liver function tests
These are useful in chronic active carriers. Liver function tests should be considered in chronic healthy carriers (HBsAg +ve, e −ve), if recently diagnosed or just recently become negative for HBsAg, and in patients who have just recovered from hepatitis A.

Hepatitis C (non-A, non-B hepatitis)

The hepatitis C virus (HCV) is the cause of what was previously termed non-A, non-B hepatitis. Patients with antibodies to HCV are chronic carriers and are potentially infectious. They are usually asymptomatic although their liver enzymes may be intermittently abnormal. Transmission of HCV is primarily by blood or blood products; however, the virus can be detected, by polymerase chain reaction (PCR), in the saliva of chronic carriers.

Liver transplantation

Children with end-stage liver disease and doubtful prognosis are candidates for liver transplantation. Unfortunately, there is an acute shortage of organs for transplantation and many children succumb to their illness before a donor organ is found. Complete oral and radiographic evaluation is essential prior to transplantation. Any potential foci of oral infection, including exfoliating primary teeth should be eliminated before transplantation can proceed. Teeth with large carious lesions, even if not pulpally involved, should be extracted.

Blood transfusion with packed red cells or partial exchange transfusion with coagulation factors is often required. Prophylactic antibiotic therapy before surgical procedures should be instituted. The main management problem with children undergoing liver transplantation is that of immunodeficiency.

Immunosuppressive therapy includes various corticosteroids and ciclosporin. Ciclosporin is both nephrotoxic and hepatotoxic and can cause hypertension. However, most children are more easily treated post transplantation due to the cure of their original disease. This is especially true of children with end-stage hepatic failure.

Clinical Hint

Gingival overgrowth and candidiasis can result from ciclosporin and nifedipine therapy. Meticulous oral hygiene should be instituted and gingivectomy considered to assist development of the permanent teeth following transplantation.

Oesophageal disorders

Neuromuscular control of the lower oesophageal sphincter is inadequate in some children resulting in chronic gastro-oesophageal reflux disease (GORD). The exact pathophysiology of GORD is unknown, although gastric motor abnormalities characterized by delayed gastric emptying have been observed in some children. Regurgitation is not always clinically obvious or symptomatic and 24-hour oesophageal pH monitoring may be necessary to demonstrate significant GORD. Symptomatic children are given oral metoclopramide hydrochloride (Maxolon) to prevent reflux whereas in children with concurrent oesophagitis, a histamine H_2 antagonist such as cimetidine is helpful. Surgical treatment is required if medical therapy fails.

Increasingly, paediatric dentists may be the first professionals to observe the chronic effects of undiagnosed GORD on the primary dentition, namely severe dental erosion of the canine and molar teeth. If a diagnosis of GORD is suspected, prompt referral to a gastroenterologist is recommended for endoscopy and a pH monitor. Comprehensive dental treatment with stainless steel crowns is usually required to restore the lost vertical dimension.

Inflammatory bowel disease (see Chapter 8)

Commonly, 'chronic inflammatory bowel disease' refers to ulcerative colitis and Crohn disease that may represent ends of a spectrum of tissue reaction to a common agent. Establishing an aetiological agent is difficult. Both conditions present as a chronic inflammatory process of the gastrointestinal tract with acute exacerbations. Of particular interest to the dentist, is the association with oro-facial granulomatosis that sometimes precede the onset of ulcerative colitis by 1–2 years.

Oral changes reported in some children include linear ulceration or fissuring of the buccal and labial mucosa, diffuse swelling of the lips, angular cheilitis and diffusely swollen erythematous gingivae. These lesions may improve with sulfasalazine (Salazopyrin) therapy but usually reappear on the buccal mucosa periodically.

Endocrinology

Diabetes mellitus

Type 1 or insulin-dependent diabetes mellitus is the most common form of diabetes in children. Approximately 2 in 1000 children between the ages of 5 and 18 years have the disease. The development of type 1 diabetes is the result of viral or toxic insults to the pancreatic islets in the child genetically predisposed to developing the disorder. An autoimmune mechanism has also been suggested in the destruction of the insulin-producing β cells. The goal of treatment is to control blood glucose to a normal level and thereby reduce the potential complication of hyperglycaemia and ketoacidosis. This generally involves administration of an intermediate-acting insulin. Pancreatic transplantation is now a potential cure for juvenile diabetes and is currently under critical investigation.

Relatives of patients with diabetes are 2.5 times more likely to develop the disease than the population at large. Presenting symptoms include:

- Polydipsia.
- Polyuria.
- Weight loss with polyphagia.
- Enuresis.
- Recurrent infections and candidiasis.
- Glucosuria may also be present.
- Ketoacidosis and coma may be seen in poorly controlled or undiagnosed cases.

A diagnosis of diabetes is made when fasting blood glucose levels above 18 mmol/L are recorded, in conjunction with an abnormal oral glucose tolerance test and glucosuria with or without ketonuria.

Dental implications

- Periodontal disease is the most consistent oral finding in children with poorly controlled diabetes. These children exhibit increased alveolar bone resorption and inflammatory gingival changes. This may mimic the clinical manifestation of chronic generalized juvenile periodontitis.
- Xerostomia and recurrent intraoral abscesses may also be present in severe cases.
- Enamel hypocalcification and hypoplasia along with reduced salivary flow can predispose these patients to an increased risk of early childhood caries.

- Altered oral flora changes can occur with an increase in *Candida albicans*, haemolytic streptococci and staphylococci.

Dental management
- Children with well-controlled diabetes can receive dental treatment in the usual way, except when a general anaesthetic is required. For routine dental appointments, the child should eat a normal meal prior to the dental procedure although a glucose source should always be available to treat the sudden onset of hypoglycaemia.
- Fasting before a general anaesthetic requires careful monitoring and adjustment of blood sugar levels during the fasting period since hypoglycaemia related to general anaesthesia can be fatal.
- Post-surgical healing can be delayed, particularly in poorly controlled cases and oral sepsis can be an additional risk in the delicate control of a diabetic child.
- All children treated under general anaesthesia should be admitted to the paediatric hospital and their care supervised by the paediatric endocrine team. It is standard practice to start a dextrose and insulin infusion to avoid complications during the fasting period to facilitate adjustment of blood sugar levels.
- Prophylactic antibiotic therapy is recommended prior to surgical procedures.

Pituitary disorders
Hypopituitarism
Hypopituitary dwarfism, resulting from anterior pituitary insufficiency is either idiopathic or secondary to pituitary or hypothalamic disease (craniopharyngioma, infections, granulomatous disease and trauma). Although other pituitary hormones may be deficient, usually there is an isolated deficiency in growth hormone (GH). Treatment consists of supplemental GH that stimulates the differentiation of epiphyseal growth plate precursor cells and induces clonal expansion of cartilage cells. Hypopituitarism has effects on adrenal gland activity that may lead to hypothyroidism and increase the risk of hypopituitary coma. This may be precipitated by any stressful event including trauma, surgery, general anaesthesia or infection.

Early detection and therapeutic management are essential to minimize the growth disturbance. Although treatment will prevent loss of stature proportional to age, it cannot make up for any deficiency present at diagnosis.

Dental implications
- Hypopituitarism can decrease linear facial measurements (particularly in the posterior facial height) and linear cranial base measurements.
- Children often present with an open bite accompanied by the typical immature hypopituitary facies.
- Somatic skeletal development is consistently more retarded than craniofacial development, although tooth eruption and root formation can be delayed or incomplete.
- Early orthodontic assessment is required to monitor oro-facial growth and development.

Hyperpituitarism

Gigantism or acromegaly results from primary hypersecretion of pituitary hormones and pituitary hyperplasia is usually associated with pituitary neoplasm, which are extremely rare in children. Hypersecretion of hormones, however, may be a secondary finding in conditions such as hypogonadism, hypoadrenalism and hypothyroidism due to a decreased hormonal negative feedback.

Severity of the craniofacial manifestations of hyperpituitarism is dependent on the time of onset and the duration of the hypersecretion. In children with open epiphyses, hypersecretion of growth hormone results in generalized overgrowth of skeletal and soft tissues with marked increase in height and size.

Gigantism, although rare, is usually associated with an eosinophilic adenoma but can be also associated with a hypothalamic tumour. In adolescents with closed epiphyses, hypersecretion leads to acromegaly which consists chiefly of enlargement of the distal parts of the body (fingers and toes) with little, if any, increase in overall height.

Dental implications

- Precocious and accelerated development of the craniofacial skeleton.
- Prognathism.
- Accelerated dental development and eruption.
- Enlarged crenated tongue, and coarse facial features.
- Radiographically, there is a marked thickening of the cranium and cortical bone of the mandible.
- Osseous structures exhibit overdevelopment with poor maturation and bone quality (osteoporosis) and hypercementosis of tooth roots is common.

Dental management

Dental management of patients with pituitary disorders focuses mainly on the management of the associated craniofacial malformations. Treatment needs to be planned carefully and coordinated in a multidisciplinary setting. No contraindications exist for comprehensive dental healthcare.

Thyroid disorders

Hypothyroidism

Hypothyroidism may be either a congenital (cretinism) or an acquired disorder (juvenile myxoedema or Hashimoto's thyroiditis). Thyroid hormone deficiency is most often secondary to a primary disease of the thyroid and less commonly associated with hypothalamic and/or pituitary insufficiency. Cretinism is rare in those countries where prenatal testing is performed. It can be attributed to aplasia, hypoplasia or maldescent of the gland, familial inborn metabolic errors, maternal intrauterine teratogens, iodide deficiency and idiopathic causes. Juvenile myxoedema can stem from a multitude of causes including thyroidectomy, thyroid irradiation, autoimmune diseases, infection or medication.

General hypothyroid changes include somatic growth retardation, diminished physical activity, decreased circulation, poor muscle tone, speech disorders, delayed mental development, and craniofacial manifestation. These changes are obviously dependent on the age of onset of the disease, the degree of thyroid hormone production lag, and the timing of diagnosis and treatment.

Treatment focuses on supplementing the deficient hormone with a synthetic derivative (levothyroxine sodium) or animal thyroprotein. In most developed countries, abnormal thyroid function is screened soon after birth by measurement of thyroid hormone levels (T3 and T4) and early management instituted immediately following initial diagnosis.

Dental implications
- Decreased vertical facial growth.
- Decreased cranial base length and flexure, maxillary protrusion, and open bite with typical immature facial patterns.
- Delayed eruption of teeth and increased spacing between both primary and permanent teeth.
- Developmental anomalies such as enamel hypoplasia have been reported.

Hyperthyroidism
Although of undetermined aetiology, hyperthyroidism (thyrotoxicosis) has an association with immunological deficiencies, infectious diseases, and hereditary disorders and childhood neoplasm. The most common associations are Graves' disease, toxic multinodular goitre, toxic adenoma and subacute thyroiditis. Thyrotoxicosis is more common in females and is most likely to appear between 12 and 14 years of age. It is usually associated with a goitre and has a cyclic clinical course.

Changes associated with hypothyroidism can mimic a state of hyperactivity of the sympathetic nervous system and typical clinical manifestations include nervousness, emotional instability, heat intolerance, loss of weight despite increased appetite, insomnia, marked perspiration, changes in skin, hair and nails, and gastrointestinal disturbances. In addition, ocular abnormalities such as eyelid lag, exophthalmos and widening of the palpebral fissures are demonstrated with various cardiovascular abnormalities.

Dental implications
- Include accelerated growth and development of the craniofacial complex and skeleton.
- Precocious eruption of teeth.
- Periodontal and periapical destruction.
- Osteoporosis.
- Typical oro-facial changes are increased vertical facial height with anterior open bite and mild mandibular prognathism.

Dental management
The principal concern in children with thyroid disorders is the increased risks associated with general anaesthesia. The hypothyroid patient is at risk of developing congestive cardiac failure that may be precipitated by general anaesthesia. Anaemia, if present, further increases the hazards, as does cardiomegaly that may result in sudden hypertension during the anaesthetic induction. The potential adverse cardiac effects of hyperthyroidism also increase the risks associated with general anaesthesia, particularly in children with chronic cardiac rhythm disturbances. The untreated patient is also at risk from oral infection or surgical procedures as thyroid crisis may be precipitated.

Oral infections seem to have an injurious effect on the thyroid gland, either directly or through toxic substances and may aggravate hyperthyroidism or exacerbate symptoms associated with hyperfunction. Oral infections should be treated aggressively in conjunction with the help of the child's endocrinologist. Antithyroid drugs may produce parotitis and agranulocytosis, which predispose the patient to bleeding episodes, ulceronecrotic lesions and chronic oral infections.

The general management of such patients is analogous to that of patients with hypertensive disease. Dental appointments should be kept to a short duration and treatment as simple as possible. Preventive treatment is preferable to operative procedures, where possible.

Parathyroid disorders
Hypoparathyroidism
This condition usually results from structural or functional deficiencies in the parathyroid glands occurring during early childhood, parathyroidectomy occurring during thyroidectomy, irradiation of the gland, neoplasm or autoimmune disease.

Treatment focuses on maintaining normal serum calcium by medication, diet supplementation, and vitamin D therapy. Changes in hypoparathyroidism include prolonged hypocalcaemia with a resultant hyperphosphataemia, neuromuscular excitability and tetany. Cardiovascular dysfunction, idiopathic epilepsy, ectodermal defects and craniofacial manifestations can also occur with permanent physical and mental retardation occurring if diagnosis and treatment are delayed.

Dental implications
- Circumoral paraesthesia and spasm of the facial muscles has been reported in severe hypocalcaemia.
- Hypoplasias of enamel.
- Hypodontia and root anomalies are common clinical findings.
- Tooth eruption can be markedly delayed or arrested.
- Increased risk of acute and chronic oral candidiasis has also been reported.

Pseudohypoparathyroidism (PHP)
This condition is also known as Albright's hereditary osteodystrophy. Inheritance of PHP is classically an X-linked dominant disease in which there are adequate parathyroid hormone levels but inadequate response to the hormone in bone and kidney. In general, males are more severely affected than females although females are more commonly encountered.

Dental implications
- Round full facies with short neck.
- Delayed or incomplete eruption of teeth.
- Enamel hypoplasia.
- Short tooth roots.

Hyperparathyroidism
Excessive production of parathyroid hormone may result from a primary defect in the gland (adenoma hyperplasia, hypertrophy) or secondarily as a compensatory phenomenon, usually correcting hypocalcaemic states due to rickets or from chronic renal

disease. Primary disease results in hypercalcaemia and hypercalcinuria producing muscle weakness, gastrointestinal disturbances, polyuria, kidney stones, soft-tissue calcification, osseous malformation (osteoporosis and osteomalacia) and pain. Whitlock (1970) summarized these changes as 'stones, bones, abdominal groans and psychic moans'. In infants and young children there may be failure to thrive, poor feeding and muscular hypotonia leading to mental retardation, convulsions and blindness.

Bony lesions are called brown tumours because they contain areas of haemorrhage, containing an abundance of multinucleated giant cells, fibroblasts and haemosiderin. Generalized osteoporosis with cortical resorption is the most common bone lesion and radiographic signs include multiple rarefactions, loss of typical trabeculation, ground-glass appearance and metastatic calcifications.

Dental implications
- Increasing tooth mobility.
- Severe malocclusion and drifting of teeth with no apparent pathological periodontal pocketing have been reported.
- Radiographic changes with metastatic soft-tissue calcifications, periapical radiolucencies, root resorption, loss of lamina dura, and generalized loss of radiodensity.

Dental management
Generally, routine dental treatment involves no treatment modifications provided there are no associated medical complications present. Manifestations of Addison's disease (adrenal insufficiency) may accompany hypoparathyroidism and thus the child may be at risk from stressful procedures such as oral surgery and general anaesthesia.

Hyperparathyroidism may be associated with cardiac arrhythmias that increase the risk of cardiac arrest during general anaesthesia. Risk of pathological fracture in advanced cases of disease should be a consideration during oral surgical procedures. Splinting of mobile teeth is a useful adjunct to prevent further drifting following stabilization of the dentition.

Adrenal gland disorders
Adrenal glands are composed of two endocrine systems termed the cortical and medullary systems. The adrenal cortex is concerned with the production of three major classes of steroid hormones: glucocorticoids, mineralocorticoids, and sex hormones. Glucocorticoids (cortisol) have an important role in carbohydrate, fat, and protein metabolism, assist in the maintenance of normal blood pressure, and protect the body against stresses of various types. Mineralocorticoids (aldosterone) help maintain salt and water balance through their action on the kidney. Adrenal sex hormones help complement the actions of the gonadal steroids in the development of sexual characteristics and reproductive capability.

Adrenal insufficiency
The major problems associated with adrenal hypofunction are the result of glucocorticoid and mineralocorticoid deficiency. Primary adrenal insufficiency (Addison's disease) is a chronic condition characterized by:
- Anorexia.
- Weight loss, vomiting.

- Salt craving.
- Nausea.
- Weakness.
- Skin hyperpigmentation.

There are low blood cortisol levels and an acute adrenal crisis can be precipitated by a relatively minor stress. Management is with immediate steroid supplementation. Secondary adrenal insufficiency is caused by prolonged administration of steroids resulting in the suppression of endogenous cortisol. Children do not usually present with obvious clinical signs unless stressed and an adrenal crisis can occur without warning.

Congenital adrenal hyperplasia

Congenital adrenal hyperplasia (CAH) arises when there is enzymatic (21-hydroxylase) deficiency in the biosynthetic pathway between cholesterol and cortisol. Clinical manifestations include failure to thrive, vomiting and dehydration associated with excessive loss of sodium in the urine (salt-wasting form) and hyperkalaemia. Management includes restoring electrolyte balance with mineralocorticoid replacement therapy.

Adrenocortical hyperfunction

Cushing's syndrome refers to the clinical condition characterized by manifestations of adrenocortical hyperfunction such as 'moon facies', truncal obesity, hirsutism and poor wound healing. It maybe iatrogenic or secondary to treatment of inflammatory or immune diseases with high-dose glucocorticoids. Management is bilateral adrenalectomy or pituitary surgery.

Dental management

It is important to confirm the diagnosis with the endocrinologist before commencement of dental treatment. An assessment of the potential for adrenal suppression can be made from the duration and dosage of previous treatment. Supplemental steroids should be given following medical consultation and proportional to the degree of adrenal suppression and the perceived stress of the dental procedure. In general, doubling or tripling the daily dose is appropriate before the procedure and a rapid taper to original dosage over 3 days is recommended. Use of conscious sedation or general anaesthesia and prophylactic antibiotic treatment is recommended for invasive surgical procedures.

Neurology

Febrile convulsion

This is a term used to describe a child under 5 years of age who has a seizure in response to a febrile illness. It usually occurs with body temperatures over 38°C and when no other cause can be determined. Recurrent, non-febrile seizures are termed as epilepsy.

Epilepsy

Epilepsy is the most common disorder in paediatric neurology and the predominant aetiologies are birth injury and congenital abnormalities.

Convulsions can be classified as:

- Generalized, either tonic–clonic (grand mal) or absence (petit mal).
- Focal (partial), either simple or complex.

Lennox–Gastaut syndrome is an intractable form of severe epilepsy with clinical features of head-dropping attacks, atypical petit mal and brief tonic–clonic seizure usually at night.

Modern treatment is usually restricted to the use of one anticonvulsant medication and slowly increasing the dose to achieve therapeutic blood levels and minimizing side effects. About 70% of children do very well, with only minimal problems, even if treatment is long term. However, drowsiness, ataxia, excessive salivation, hyperactivity and aggressive behaviour are common complications of anticonvulsant therapy. Gradual reduction of multiple medications has a beneficial effect in terms of increased alertness, and a reduced number of seizures. Phenytoin sodium (Dilantin) is still probably the most effective drug for grand mal seizures but the cosmetic side effects such as hirsutism and gingival hypertrophy have reduced its use in favour of carbamazepine (Tegretol).

Dental implications
The major oro-dental concerns with epileptic children are gingival enlargement (Figure 10.11) and the precipitation of a seizure in the dental surgery.

Dental management
Management of gingival hypertrophy (Figure 10.9B) is dependent on oral hygiene and dental development at diagnosis. In the permanent dentition, full mouth gingivectomy may be required, but gingival overgrowth will recur if oral hygiene is not optimal. Maintenance of adequate oral hygiene may be especially difficult in children with additional intellectual disability and is highly dependent on the motivation and skill of the parents and caregivers. Battery-operated plaque removers with small circular heads are beneficial in the maintenance of good oral hygiene in the more intractable cases. The use of daily chlorhexidine-containing gels is effective in reducing the inflammatory component of the gingival overgrowth. It is important to always keep the interests of

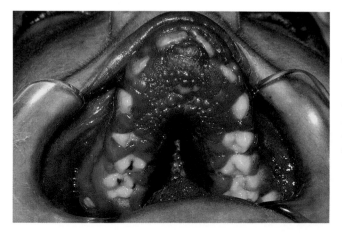

Figure 10.11 Severe phenytoin gingival enlargement in a child with cerebral palsy. The hypertonicity of the oral musculature has caused the protrusion of the anterior teeth and the orthopaedic compression of the maxilla.

the child in mind, particularly with regard to aggressive surgical treatment that may not benefit the child in the long term.

The general goal of dental management is the avoidance of a seizure. It is important to know the type of epilepsy and any precipitating factors, medications and dosage, compliance and degree of seizure control before commencing treatment. In addition, drug interactions with anticonvulsants are common and their half-life and blood levels can be increased substantially. Consultation with the child's neurologist is essential before commencement of treatment.

The following management protocol is recommended for prevention and control of seizures in the dental surgery:

- Reduce stress to the child by behavioural management and conscious sedation techniques.
- Reduce direct overhead lighting, particularly for the photosensitive form of epilepsy.
- Avoid seizure-promoting medications such as CNS stimulants and local anaesthetics containing adrenaline (epinephrine).
- Emergency drugs such as oxygen, intravenous or rectal diazepam (Valium) and intravenous phenobarbital sodium should be readily available.
- Pre-arranged transfer to a paediatric hospital, in case required.

General anaesthesia is preferable in children with poor seizure control as the abnormal neural activity is completely ablated during the procedure. Dental trauma is an obvious consequence in the child with frequent, poorly controlled seizures. Removable appliances are contraindicated in an epileptic child due to potential airway obstruction.

Cerebral palsy

The cerebral palsies are a heterogeneous group of static encephalopathies that have in common a disorder of posture and movement. The motor disability is permanent and the clinical manifestations are variable. Cerebral palsy can be simply classified into:

- Spastic (hemiplegia, paraplegia and quadriplegia).
- Dyskinetic (choreo-athetoid and dystonic).
- Ataxia.
- Mixed.

Adverse prenatal and perinatal events that affect the brain account for the known causes of cerebral palsy, although most causes are unknown.

The cognitive ability of a child with cerebral palsy cannot be quickly determined. Time is required with these children to assess their physical and mental abilities. Many patients with cerebral palsy have no cognitive impairment at all and may use a form of verbal communication that requires an electronic aid and operator patience. It is often not necessary to change voice tone or level of language when addressing these children.

Maxillary protrusion and generalized anterior tooth spacing are common sequelae due to abnormal oro-facial neuromuscular tone. Tongue thrust, dribbling, mouth breathing, and peri-oral sensitivity are also common clinical presentations. Dental caries and periodontal disease may be severe due to neglect and following surgery to reposition the major saliva gland ducts to reduce drooling.

Dental management

Reflex limb extension patterns may be triggered during dental visits if care is not taken. These contractions may occur during transfer of the patient from wheelchair to the dental chair. Discuss the transfer with the parent or caregivers before offering assistance. The reflex may also be stimulated if the child's head is loose or unsupported. Ensure that the child is stabilized in the chair with blankets and pillows or restrained with a belt or webbing. If a reflex pattern occurs where the limbs are in extension:

- Raise the chair.
- Stabilize the head in the midline.
- Bring the arms forwards.
- Reassure the child.

Gag, cough, bite and swallowing reflexes may be impaired or abnormal in children with cerebral palsy. If the gag reflex is more exaggerated, treat the patient in a more upright position with the neck in slight flexion and the knees bent upwards, if possible. Mouth props may be used, however, for those patients with impaired swallowing, there is an increased risk of aspiration. Hand-held props and a floss ligature help to reduce this possibility. Rubber dam is especially useful in these cases as well.

If the patient's bite reflex to oral stimulation is still present, introduce instruments from the side rather than the front. To allow dental examination, apply gentle pressure with the forefinger on the anterior border of ascending ramus and in the retromolar triangle. This reduces the risk of a bitten finger. Nitrous oxide sedation may help to reduce involuntary movements during dental treatment.

Hydrocephalus

Most cases of hydrocephalus result from obstruction to cerebrospinal fluid (CSF) flow, either within the cerebral ventricles or in the subarachnoid space. As the ventricles enlarge due to the accumulation of CSF, intracranial pressure increases resulting in serious neurological impairment if not decompressed. The postnatal causes of hydrocephalus are varied including bacterial infection, haemorrhage and neoplastic obstruction, but prenatal causes are often undiagnosable. Treatment by insertion of a shunt is usually appropriate in infants with severe hydrocephalus. Many children with hydrocephalus have other developmental deficits such as learning disabilities or paraplegia.

Children with hydrocephalus undergoing dental treatment require antibiotic prophylaxis if they have shunts that directly empty into the major blood vessels (ventriculo-atrial) to prevent septicaemia and shunt infection. It is generally considered that children with ventriculoperitoneal and spinoperitoneal shunts do not require prophylactic antibiotic cover, unless specified by the neurologist.

Spina bifida

In this condition there is a herniation (meningomyelocele) of the spinal cord, nerve roots and meninges through a wide deficiency in the laminae and spinous process of one or more vertebrae, usually at the sacral or lumbosacral levels. The exposed cord is dysplastic and almost always non-functional often resulting in paraplegia. Early operative closure is performed where possible to prevent infection and subsequent orthopaedic and urological management are necessary. Rehabilitation is best provided by coordinated multidisciplinary clinics.

Children with spina bifida have a higher prevalence of latex allergy (gloves, rubber dam) compared with the general paediatric population. The use of vinyl gloves is recommended. Many children are confined to a wheelchair and spinal comfort should be optimized in a similar way as for children with cerebral palsy. Otherwise, routine dental management can be undertaken in the clinic setting.

Muscular dystrophies

A muscular dystrophy is a progressive, genetically determined, primary degenerative myopathy. The clinical features include increasing muscle weakness, poor muscle tone, abnormal movements, skin changes and progressive joint and skeletal deformity. Duchenne's muscular dystrophy and dystrophia myotonica are the two most common forms and current treatment is to slow the effects of disuse atrophy. Ambulation is usually not possible after 12 years of age.

Oral manifestations include craniofacial deformity with protrusive spaced anterior teeth due to poor oro-facial tone and associated mouth breathing, tongue thrust and open bite. Poor plaque control, gingivitis and anterior tooth trauma are common oral findings. Dental management strategies are similar to those used in children with cerebral palsy, using head and body supports and mouth props. Sedation and general anaesthesia are often necessary to manage children with muscular dystrophy due to their inability to tolerate routine procedures in the dental chair.

Respiratory disease

Asthma

Australia has one of the highest rates of childhood asthma in the world with 1 in 5 children and 1 in 7 adolescents affected. It is a respiratory condition characterized by increased responsiveness of the airways to a wide variety of stimuli, leading to widespread narrowing of the airways resulting in symptoms of dyspnea, wheezing, and coughing. Precipitating factors include emotional stress, exercise, cold air, viral respiratory infections, air pollution, and aspirin. The condition is reversible, either spontaneously or as a result of bronchodilator therapy. Currently there is an emphasis on prophylactic medications to prevent episodes rather than simply treating acute attacks.

Bronchodilators include β_2-adrenergic drugs such as salbutamol sulphate (Ventolin) and theophylline (Nuelin). Preventive agents include disodium cromoglicate (Intal) and oral corticosteroids such as prednisone and inhaled corticosteroids such as beclometasone dipropionate (Beclovent) and salmeterol xinafoate (Seretide).

Dental implications

- The major concern to the paediatric dentist is the exacerbation of an acute attack in the dental surgery.
- Avoid any known precipitating factors prior to dental treatment and ensure that the child has the appropriate medication (inhaler) for emergency use if an asthmatic attack occurs during dental treatment.
- Some bronchodilator and corticosteroid medications may cause extrinsic staining of the teeth due to changes in oral flora and may also predispose to oral candidiasis.
- Children on high-dose corticosteroids (>1600 µg/day) may be immunocompromised and may also require additional supplemental corticosteroids on the day of dental treatment due to adrenal suppression.

- Children are often mouth breathers causing gingivitis and swelling of anterior gingival tissues.

Dental management
- Regular dental prophylaxis may be necessary if extrinsic staining is present.
- Advise parents to brush their child's teeth following administration of medication or use an aqueous mouth rinse if oral hygiene is not possible, particularly during the night to reduce the risk of dental erosion.
- Children who have been admitted to hospital with frequent episodic asthma within the past 12 months or those managed with high-dose oral corticosteroids are not suitable for day surgery and should be admitted preoperatively to be adequately prepared by the paediatric respiratory team.
- Avoidance of adrenaline-containing local anaesthetic solutions is recommended due to their potential adrenergic effects if injected intravenously.
- There are no known contraindications to the use of nitrous oxide or sedative doses of diazepam (Valium) or hydroxyzine pamoate (Vistaril) for asthmatic children.

Cystic fibrosis
This multisystem disorder is an autosomal recessive condition affecting all mucus-secreting exocrine glands of the body, especially the respiratory and gastrointestinal systems. The heterozygote frequency is estimated to be 1 in 25 in the Caucasian population. Cystic fibrosis is characterized by chronic respiratory obstruction and infection, intestinal malabsorption and growth retardation. Sexual development is often delayed. Although the disease is currently incurable, aggressive symptomatic treatment has improved survival and quality of life in recent years. The major cause of death is respiratory failure from recurrent chest infections.

Children were previously treated with broad-spectrum tetracyclines and often exhibited classic intrinsic staining and enamel hypoplasia of the permanent dentition. However, in Australia this practice stopped in the early 1970s and the incidence of enamel anomalies has decreased dramatically in recent years. Increased and altered rates of salivary flow seem not to predispose to dental caries, possibly due to long-term use of antibiotics.

Dental management
- Dental management should be based on optimal prevention including strict oral hygiene and diet control. Routine dental treatment can be undertaken provided pulmonary involvement is stable and well controlled with medication.
- Local anaesthetics with vasoconstrictors are not contraindicated.
- Long appointments should be avoided. However, the use of conscious sedation or general anaesthesia must be carefully discussed with the respiratory paediatrician and only used when routine pain management is not possible.
- Physiotherapy and prophylactic antibiotic treatment is required both preoperatively and postoperatively in cases of severe pulmonary involvement.
- Although, life expectancy has increased with current medical therapies, there should be a rational and pragmatic approach to treatment planning and expectations.

Tuberculosis

Tuberculosis is an infectious disease caused by *Mycobacterium tuberculosis* that involves granulomatous inflammation and caseating necrosis in the lung tissues. The most common presentation in children is malaise, anorexia, and weight loss, fever and cough with signs of cervical lymphadenitis. Children are managed with long-term antibiotic treatment specific to the infectious organism. Chemoprophylaxis is given to other family members and contacts to prevent spread of the disease. The bacille Calmette Guérin (BCG) vaccine is used routinely in communities with a high prevalence of tuberculosis.

Dental treatment should not be performed until the diagnosis and causative agent have been identified and only then following consultation with the respiratory physician.

Other children with special needs

Children with special needs require dental appointments that are tailored to make best use of their abilities. The clinician who understands how to accommodate a child's disability will provide the secure environment required to successfully treat these children.

Attention deficit hyperactivity disorder (ADHD)

Attention deficit hyperactivity disorder (ADHD) is a common developmental disorder affecting about 3–5% of the population. Boys are affected much more commonly than girls. It is characterized by developmentally inappropriate degrees of impulsivity, inattention and often hyperactivity. The symptoms are noted from early childhood, usually well before school entry and are present in all settings.

The term ADHD is currently used to describe a range of children with varying functional difficulties, but who share the feature of poorly sustained attention. Some are extremely impulsive, some aggressive, others quiet and restless. Many have low self-esteem. Comorbidities include developmental language disorders, anxiety, oppositional-defiant behaviours, fine motor and coordination difficulties and specific learning disabilities. Virtually all children with ADHD have deficits in short-term auditory memory.

Assessment

The assessment of a child for the diagnosis of ADHD requires a number of essential components. These include:

- Detailed developmental history.
- Physical, neurological and neurodevelopmental examination.
- Detailed standardized behaviour rating scale data, e.g. Conners Parent and Teacher Rating Scale (Goyette et al 1978) rating scale, from at least two sources, usually school and home.

Management

Management of the child with ADHD involves three broad approaches:

- Behavioural.
- Educational.
- Pharmacological.

Many other approaches are commonly applied to these children, including dietary modification, 'natural' or complementary therapies of diverse types, and behavioural optometry. There is little evidence to support the broad use of any of these interventions, though some individuals report benefits.

Psychostimulant medication is the principal pharmacological therapy for ADHD. The two stimulants most commonly prescribed are methylphenidate (Ritalin) and dexametamine.

- Significant clinical improvements in approximately 75% of correctly diagnosed children.
- Onset of behavioural effect is usually noticeable within 30–60 minutes of ingestion.

Other medications sometimes used in ADHD include the antihypertensive drug clonidine, antidepressants (selective serotonin re-uptake inhibitors, reversible monoamine oxidase inhibitors, and tricyclics) and occasionally neuroleptics.

Dental implications

The visit to a dentist is likely to raise anxiety levels in any child and indeed their parents. In a child with ADHD this anxiety may manifest in overexcited behaviour. Many parents worry about the effect of their child's behaviour on others. They have become accustomed to failure having taken their 'difficult' child to dentists only to be told that it is not possible to provide treatment/care. This may result in either an excessively protective/embarrassed parent with constant apologies on behalf of the child or else an overly firm parent exerting inappropriate, heavy-handed disciplinary actions throughout the encounter. In either situation the child's behaviour is likely to be reactive towards the parent thus precluding the establishment of a successful relationship with the dental practitioner.

Successful management of these children may be facilitated in ADHD using similar strategies to those employed in other disabilities. In general the chance of success is raised if the dental practitioner takes control of the situation early. By creating an atmosphere of confidence the parental anxiety is often alleviated allowing the child and the dentist to establish a relationship in a more relaxed environment. Likewise a gentle but firm approach will convey to the child a confidence and a structure to the situation within which it is easier for them to conform.

It is useful for the dental practitioner to have an understanding of the current management strategies being employed by the family at home and in school. For example if a child is used to raising their hand prior to speaking it is useful for the dentist to employ the same strategy. Clear instructions should be given to the child maintaining eye contact throughout and taking care not to over burden the short-term memory. Such instructions need to be given at a time when the child is not distracted by other activities in the dental surgery.

The use of the tell-show-do method of behaviour direction has been shown to have value in the management of children with ADHD. Praise and encouragement have an important role in the management of these children and good behaviour should be reinforced and rewarded.

Management strategies

- The current medication scheme should be discussed with both the parents and the prescribing practitioner. It is often helpful to either change the dose or the timing of medication to optimize the action at the time of the dental visit. There is also some suggestion that morning appointments may be more successful, however this may be related to the timing of medication rather than anything else.

- A preventive approach is essential.
- It is again important to realize that many of these children are already struggling to master other life skills.
- Tooth brushing and controlling diet both require concentration, motivation and understanding all of which can be problematic for the child with ADHD. Tooth-brushing charts for the child to take home and mark off daily are more likely to be successful than verbal instructions to brush daily.
- Repetition is important in building up self-confidence in the child.
- Multiple short visits have a higher chance of success than few, prolonged visits.
- However it is important to realize that oral health is only one of many priorities for the family of a child with ADHD, and the multiple demands made of the parents need to be weighed against the need for dental care.

Developmental disabilities and intellectual disabilities

Developmental disabilities are described as differences in neurological-based functions that have their onset before birth, or during childhood, and are associated with long-term difficulties. People with intellectual disability have an IQ of less than 70, deficits in adaptive functioning and an onset before 18 years of age.

The term developmental disability includes all people with an intellectual disability, however, not all people with a developmental disability have an intellectual disability. People with cerebral palsy and autism have a developmental disability, but not all of them will be intellectually disabled.

As in many cases of treating medically compromised children, the first appointment is often one in which to familiarize both the dentist with the child's condition and the child with the dental environment. Find out the patient's likes, dislikes and behaviour patterns. Offer verbal support and allow time to develop a rapport with the child.

Take a thorough medical history. Developmental delay is a broad term covering children with a range of medical conditions and syndromes. It is essential that obscure syndromes be researched before performing treatment. Photocopy relevant information for the child's file.

Support of the parent or caregivers is extremely important in reinforcing and administering preventive advice, oral hygiene practices and diet modification. Consultation with the school or institution may be required to modify diet.

Children with intellectual disabilities have a higher incidence of:

- Tooth wear.
- Poor plaque control.
- Malocclusion.
- Self-inflicted traumatic injuries and tooth grinding.

Management of permanent toothwear in the patients with an intellectual disability

Study models should be taken at the earliest signs of tooth wear to establish the rate of toothwear over time. The causes of the toothwear should be established and if possible eliminated. Gastro-oesophageal reflux is common in people with developmental disabilities and must be addressed by appropriate referral to gastroenterology. The incidence of tooth grinding is also higher in this population and should be addressed where possible by appropriate means.

Only treat the toothwear restoratively if there is:

- Uncontrolled toothwear over time.
- Loss of vitality or risk of loss of vitality.
- Aesthetic issues.
- Functional issues.

The restorative treatment of choice is overlaying of worn teeth using an indirect composite resin material with minimal tooth preparation. Two treatment sessions using sedation will be required for many patients with developmental disabilities to adequately take impressions and maintain isolation for cementation procedures.

Management of poor plaque control

All patients with intellectual disabilities require assistance to maintain adequate oral hygiene to prevent gingivitis. Carers should be trained in techniques to deliver oral care in a safe and effective manner. However, some patients may be tactile defensive and require referral to a speech pathologist for an oral desensitization programme. These programmes include vibration and extra-oral massage to treat tactile-defensive behaviour.

Malocclusion

There is a higher incidence of hypotonicity and hypertonicity of oral musculature in people with intellectual disabilities. These patients may also have unusual oral habits such as tongue thrusting which creates malocclusions. Many patients with intellectual disabilities will be able to manage conventional orthodontics with an appropriate level of support. However, for those patients with challenging behaviours, conventional orthodontics may not be possible. An orthodontist to consider interceptive orthodontic measures that may reduce the degree of malocclusion should see all children with intellectual disabilities who are developing a malocclusion in the mixed dentition stage.

Tooth grinding

Many parents and caregivers seek dental consultation because of tooth grinding and the worry or associated dental damage. It can be quite annoying for families, teachers and caregivers, and consideration should be given to whether or not the behaviour has other implications such as attention seeking in changed family circumstances. Tooth grinding is either physiological or pathological.

Physiological tooth grinding

- Often occurs during times of concentration or at night during sleep, although it may occur at any time.
- Begins early during the development of the primary dentition usually once the primary first molars erupt.
- Usually diminishes once the primary teeth have exfoliated.
- No treatment is usually required other than parental reassurance.
- If wear is excessive threatening pulp exposure, then extraction or restoration will be required.

- Unusual to reflect any generalized systemic condition and dental anthropologists regard this grinding as a phenomenon of 'tooth sharpening' termed thegosis.

Pathological tooth grinding
- The amount of wear exceeds that which is felt to occur normally. Children may lose up to half the crown length in upper anterior teeth. Extensive enamel loss with wear facets and exposed dentine is unusual in posterior teeth.
- Often seen in children with underlying neurological disorders or medical problems such as Down's syndrome, cerebral palsy or head injury.
- An increase in grinding intensity in these children may reflect other pathology such as otitis, salivary gland infection or generalized pain elsewhere in the body.

Management of tooth grinding
- If there has been extensive loss of tooth structure in the primary dentition, it will be essential to monitor any changes in the first permanent molars. Treatment may involve the placement of stainless steel crowns on the second primary molars. This will not only protect the permanent teeth but preserves the vertical dimension of occlusion and tends to decrease grinding.
- Tooth grinding that is associated with self-mutilation of the soft tissues is extremely difficult to manage and some strategies are discussed in Chapter 8.
- It must be noted that when, in the most severe cases, extractions of permanent teeth are contemplated, eventually, all teeth will probably be lost. For those cases of intractable grinding and self-mutilation, the removal of only a few (anterior) teeth invariably leads to removal of all teeth in the arch.

Vision impairment
- Allow the child to make full use of their tactile sense and their sense of smell when familiarising them to the dental environment and dental procedures.
- Offer verbal and physical reassurance to the child once a rapport has been established. They cannot see your smile.
- Paint a picture in the mind of your patients by describing the treatment and the environment throughout the procedure. A startle reflex may occur if patients are not warned before different instruments are introduced into the mouth without warning.
- Many visually impaired people are photophobic. It is important to ask parents and children about light sensitivity. Safety glasses should preferably be tinted.

Hearing impairment
- Investigate how the child communicates.
- A common fault is to talk loudly rather than slowly. If the patient lip-reads, face the child and speak clearly and slowly.
- It is useful to learn basic sign language. It should be noted that even within the English-speaking world, there are different signing languages in different countries.
- Make it easy for patients to maintain visual contact because these children may be startled if they are touched without visual contact.

- Deaf children may be very sensitive to vibration, so introduce high-speed and low-speed drills carefully.
- If a hearing aid is worn the volume may need adjustment. Try to avoid blocking the ears and the hearing aid with the forearms when operating, as this will create feedback.

Oro-motor dysfunction in patients with developmental disabilities

Children with cerebral palsy and global developmental delay often present with poor oral functions including:
- Hypertonicity.
- Hypotonicity.
- Dysphagia – difficulty in swallowing.
- Dysphasia – difficulty in speaking.
- Sialorrhoea – difficulty in swallowing resulting in drooling.

Drooling
The parents will often present with their primary concern being excessive drooling. The paediatric dentist has a significant role in the management of sialorrhoea. The options for the management of drooling are:
- Eliminate aggravating factors (dental caries, malocclusions).
- Referral to a multidisciplinary team for oro-motor function therapy.
- Medications.
- Surgery.

Surgical management
- Re-routing the submandibular duct to the posterior tonsillar pillar.
- 70% cases described as good to excellent.

Risks and side effects
- Ranula formation.
- Loss of the gland.
- Increased caries risk.
- Aspiration of saliva due to dysphagia.

Pharmacological agents
- Benzatropine (Cogentin).
- Trihexyphenidyl hydrochloride (benzhexol hydrochloride; Artane).
- Scopolamine transdermal patches.
- Glycopyrrolate.
- Botulinum toxin A (Botox).
Side effects of medications are:
- Xerostomia.
- Dental caries.

- Urinary retention.
- Flushing.
- Drying of all mucous membranes.
- Trihexyphenidyl can cause behavioural changes.

Oro-motor function therapy

Oro-motor function therapy is carried out by multidisciplinary teams that may include speech pathologists, occupational therapists, physiotherapists and dentists. The focus of oro-motor function therapy is to develop the oral skills required to manage saliva control. This multifaceted approach may include a number of elements such as:

- Behaviour modification.
- Proprioceptive neuromuscular facilitation.
- Postural adaptations.
- Oral screens and dental appliances designed to stimulate oral musculature.

Dental appliances

These are individually designed to produce the desired movement of the tongue, lips or jaw (Figure 10.12). Common goals include:

- Establishment of correct tongue position.
- Stimulation of lip closure.
- Stimulation of tongue elevation, lateralization.
- Stimulation of jaw stabilization.
- Reduction in mouthing behaviour.

Autistic spectrum disorder

Autistic spectrum disorder (ASD) is defined as a severe developmental disorder characterized by the classic triad of:

Figure 10.12 A dental appliance with a movable bead in palate for use in oro-motor function therapy.

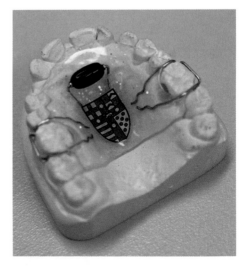

- Impaired communication.
- Impaired socialization.
- Repetitive and restricted patterns of behaviour.

ASD is genetic in origin, however, there are still aspects of the aetiology that are not fully understood. It is also a biological disorder with a number of associations. Approximately 70% of affected individuals have moderate or severe learning difficulties, some have raised serotonin levels and there may be other co-morbidities such as fragile X syndrome, Rett's syndrome, phenylketonuria and epilepsy.

The dental management of autistic children can be a huge challenge for the paediatric dentist mainly because of the child's behaviour and their impaired communication. Problems associated with the dental treatment of a child with ASD include:

- Impaired communication – there is limited speech and understanding and communication aids such as Makaton and Pictorial Exchange Communication System (PECS) may need to be used.
- Behaviour may be erratic and unpredictable, and some children have ADHD-type traits.
- Lack of eye contact, absence of 'theory of mind' and sense of humour.
- Drug history – many are cariogenic and some cause dry mouth.
- Trauma due to the association with epilepsy.
- Late diagnosis of the condition and therefore access to early care is delayed.
- Processing sensory information – many children are hyposensitive or hypersensitive to smells, sights and sounds and touch.
- Problems with treatments, dietary restrictions, avoidance of fluoride and amalgam, use of confectionary for the reinforcement of good behaviour as part of a behavioural approach.
- Child may be idiosyncratic about food.
- Anxiety – both child and parent will be anxious about the visit.

Clinical management

Although prevention is the key element to managing any child with special needs, this is especially true for the child in the autistic spectrum. Local anaesthesia and inhalation sedation is limited to the higher-functioning children with autism where communication is not severely compromised.

General anaesthesia is the most frequently used approach – especially for those children who are young and present with extensive disease. Such treatment should obviously be definitive and comprehensive including preventive as well as curative elements.

Important tips for management

- Establishing the behaviour of tooth brushing as early as possible is extremely important for these children, not only for oral health but also because it is the most successful way of initiating a dental examination.
- Use behavioural approaches such as applied behavioural analysis to establish patterns of behaviour around tooth brushing.
- Remember that it may not be the brushing that the child dislikes – it may be the paste. Explore other flavours.

- Some echolalic children are able to copy words and expressions, if this applies you can then teach the parents to encourage the child to say 'ahhhh' which will help three people – the parent to brush, you the dentist to examine the teeth visually, and lastly the child's medical doctor to examine the throat! Then try the sound 'eeeeeee' – thus displaying the upper anterior gingival margins, which are sometimes quite difficult to access.
- Actively looking for evidence of trauma should be routinely done because of the association with epilepsy.
- Make contact with the families as soon as possible through the local child health networks and development teams.
- Familiarize yourself with the different communication aids that the child may be using. Photographs or images can be put together in the form of a storyline so that the child is prepared for the dental visit. This helps to reduce any build-up of anxiety by making events more predictable for the child.
- Frequent visits to the dental setting will give you opportunities to learn about the child and give preventive support.
- Send out a pre-appointment questionnaire style letter and an information leaflet.
- Maximize your communication, e.g. put yourself in a position where the child can see you so that you get their attention using the child's usual name at the beginning of the sentence. Your language must be simple with the minimum of social language and you must speak slowly. It is also important to limit any background noises in the surgery.
- Dietary counselling must be specific to each individual child. If dietary reinforcers are being used, encourage the use of low-sugar safe snacks and consider the use of sugar-free confectionery.
- Extraordinary children require extraordinary dentists. Paediatric dentists who care for a large number of these children need to be attracted by differences, need to be flexible and need to be prepared for the challenge.

Genetics and dysmorphology

Diagnosis

Although generally uncommon, many children with genetic abnormalities will present to the paediatric dentist with specific dental anomalies associated with their condition or medical problems that complicate their dental management. Never assume that all conditions will have been diagnosed before they present, as many children are often diagnosed as having significant genetic disease quite late in childhood, either because the disease has late manifestations or because features have simply been missed. When taking a history it is always useful to draw a simple three-generation family pedigree (Figure 10.13).

Many disorders do not follow mendelian inheritance patterns, but are clearly of 'familial' or hereditary nature. Many important and common conditions fall into this group; they are often not single entities but heterogeneous and are seen as the end result of multiple gene effects against a variable environmental background (multifactorial or polygenic), e.g. cleft lip and palate.

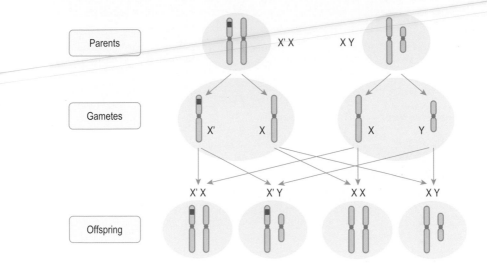

Figure 10.13 Calculation of risk in an X-linked recessive disorder: 50% of the boys are affected and 50% of the girls will be carriers.

One in 170 live-born births has a major chromosomal abnormality. Chromosomal abnormalities, particularly those involving imbalance of the autosomes usually result in developmental delay and dysmorphic features, and often include multi-system anomalies. These include numerical abnormalities (trisomy 21 or Down's syndrome) and structural abnormalities such as segmental deletions (cri-du-chat syndrome), duplications and translocations. Sex chromosome numerical abnormalities are better tolerated than autosomal abnormalities and include examples such as Turner's syndrome in females and Klinefelter's syndrome in males. Many other genetic disorders are caused by mutations *within* genes, which cannot be detected by chromosome analysis, but may be able to be confirmed by targeted gene testing after a syndrome is recognized (see Table 10.1).

The first step in making a diagnosis is the recognition that the child is dysmorphic or unusual looking. It is the pattern of dysmorphism rather than a single feature that aids diagnosis. Accurate diagnosis is the key to prognosis, management and sometimes the underlying genetic cause of the disorder. It also helps the parents as it removes the anxiety of uncertain aetiology and prognosis.

The diagnostic procedure involves history, clinical examination and laboratory investigations. Based on the above information, children can be divided into three basic groups, those with:
- Fetal environmental syndromes.
- Developmental defects.
- Genetic syndromes.

If a spot diagnosis cannot be made, refer to the index in books on dysmorphology or a syndrome electronic data bank (POSSUM; www.possum.net.au) and search for a possible diagnosis by the list of expressed features. Laboratory investigations include radiographic survey, chromosomal analysis, biochemical screening of urine or blood

Table 10.1 Classification of genetic abnormalities

	Defect	Examples
Chromosomal structure	Aneuploidies (abnormal number of chromosomes)	Down's syndrome, trisomy 21 Klinefelter's syndrome (XXY) Turner's syndrome (45,X)
	Chromosomal deletions, duplications and translocations	18q- (deletion of part of long arm of chromosome 18)
Single gene defects	Autosomal dominant	Cleidocranial dysplasia Osteogenesis imperfecta
	Autosomal recessive	Cystic fibrosis
	X-linked	Haemophilia Ectodermal dysplasia
Polygenic disorders	Multiple minor gene abnormalities interacting with environmental influences	Cleft palate Diabetes mellitus Spina bifida Schizophrenia

Adapted from Jones KL. Smith's recognizable patterns of human malformation, 5th ed. WB Saunders, Philadelphia, 1997.

or cultured fibroblasts for specific enzymatic or protein deficiencies if a metabolic disorder is suspected. Referral to a genetics clinic is often required to further elaborate a diagnosis and to assist with specialized genetic testing and genetic counselling.

It is not the intention of this section to detail those anomalies with a major cranio-facial or orofacial manifestation, of which dental clinicians should be aware. The reader is directed to texts and online sources that more comprehensively cover these conditions (see References and further reading).

Terms used in morphogenesis
Sequence
A pattern of multiple anomalies arising from a single structural defect or event, and previously termed anomalad. Usually originate early in development with single problems that create secondary anomalies and manifest with multiple defects at birth or later. These sequences may be divided into three basic groups.
1. Malformation sequence
   - Poor formation of tissue.
   - May be single or multiple but are primary structural abnormalities.
   - Poor prognosis for normal growth in the areas affected.
   - Recurrence rate of 1–5%.
   - Example: cleft palate.
   Malformations may present as:
   - Accessory tissue (e.g. polydactyly, periauricular skin tags).
   - Hamartomas (e.g. haemangioma/lymphangioma).
   - Incomplete morphogenesis:
     - agenesis (e.g. salivary gland agenesis)
     - hypoplasia (e.g. enamel hypoplasia in amelogenesis imperfecta)

- incomplete septation (e.g. ventral septal defect (VSD))
- incomplete migration of ectomesenchyme (e.g. Di George association).
  - Failure of cell death (apoptosis) (e.g. spina bifida, cleft palate, syndactyly).
2. Deformation sequence
   - Unusual forces acting on normal tissues, usually from abnormal intrauterine pressures.
   - Good prognosis for normal growth and a low risk of recurrence.
   - Examples are:
     - talipes
     - micrognathia
     - torticollis.
3. Disruption sequence
   - Destruction or breakdown of normal tissue, which may result from vascular, infective or physical causes.
   - Low risk of recurrence, poor prognosis for normal growth in affected areas.
   - Examples:
     - deafness from congenital rubella
     - bizarre facial clefting from amniotic bands
     - hemifacial microsomia (from stapedial artery haemorrhage).

Syndrome
- A recognizable pattern of malformation.
- Multiple defects of related pathogenesis, arising directly from a single cause (genetic or acquired).

Association
- Non-random occurrence of several morphologic defects not identified as a syndrome or sequence.
- Low risk of recurrence.
- Example: VATER association (**V** vertebral anomalies and VSD, **A** anal atresia, **T-E** tracheoesophageal fistula with oesophageal atresia, **R** radial and renal dysplasia).

Risk of recurrence in genetic disorders
Autosomal dominant
There is a 50% risk to each offspring of a single affected parent. Many dominant conditions have variable expression and so the manifestations may be increased or reduced compared to the parent. New dominant genetic conditions can also occur.

Autosomal recessive
Carriers do not express the trait. If both parents are carriers, the risk of the child being affected (homozygous; the trait will be expressed) is 25%, the risk of being a carrier is 50%, and the chance of neither being a carrier or affected is 25%. If one parent is a carrier there is a 50% chance of the child being a carrier.

X-linked (sex-linked)
- 50% risk of transmission from female carriers to sons (who would then be affected) or daughters (who would then be a carrier).

- No male-to-male transmission from affected fathers to sons, but all daughters will be carriers.

The terms 'X-linked recessive' and 'X-linked dominant' are used to describe sex-linked conditions with an altered frequency of phenotypic expression. Males usually have only one X chromosome; males with an X-linked abnormality are described as hemizygous for the trait, and will be affected. Females usually have two X-chromosomes; female carriers of an X-linked trait are heterozygous. In X-linked recessive disorders, female carriers can be unaffected, or affected (manifesting carrier) but the latter are usually much less severely affected than males. Rarely, females are homozygous for an X-linked trait, so will be affected as severely as a hemizygous male. 'X-linked dominant' traits manifest in females and males, but males are often more severely affected.

The degree of phenotypic expression in heterozygous females is determined by the pattern of X inactivation (Lyonization: see Chapter 9) in each tissue. For example, female carriers of haemophilia A will show a measurable (but subclinical) reduction in factor VIII; and those that carry X-linked hypohidrotic ectodermal dysplasia may also show some phenotypic variation in the dentition such as microdontia and oligodontia, but not to the same extent as in hemizygous males. The increased frequency of affected females with some 'X-linked dominant' conditions, such as incontinentia pigmenti or focal dermal hypoplasia (Goltz–Gorlin syndrome) may be explained by male lethality for these mutations in hemizygous males.

Prenatal tests for genetic abnormalities
Ultrasound
Ultrasound has become a routine investigation for most pregnancies. It is non-invasive to the mother and the fetus and there are many anomalies that may be diagnosed by this technique. Common ultrasound techniques include the first trimester nuchal translucency measurement (a screening examination for Down's syndrome risk) and the mid-trimester fetal morphology scan.

Amniocentesis
This is the sampling of cells from amniotic fluid at around 15–18 weeks. A number of tests can be performed including:
- Karyotyping.
- Sex determination.
- DNA diagnosis.
- Enzyme assays.

Chorionic villus sampling
This test is performed earlier than amniocentesis, at around 10–12 weeks. Similar tests are performed to those done with amniocentesis although it has the advantage of earlier diagnosis.

Population screenings
- Mid-trimester maternal alpha fetoprotein levels for neural tube defects.
- Mid-trimester maternal serum 'triple test' for Down's syndrome risk.
- First trimester maternal serum screening (combined with NT scan) for Down's syndrome risk.

Postnatal tests
Cytogenetics
For any baby with dysmorphic features or multiple abnormalities.

DNA analysis
For specific disorders; direct mutation detection or linkage analysis.

Neonatal screening tests
A range of newborn screening tests is undertaken in each country, but the tests offered vary significantly between centres. Commonly performed tests include those for:
- Phenylketonuria.
- Cystic fibrosis.
- Congenital hypothyroidism.
- Galactosaemia.
- Thalassaemia.
- Sickle cell disease.
- Aminoacidopathies.
- Organic acidaemias.
- Fatty acid oxidation defects.

Genetic counselling
Genetic counselling is the process of providing diagnostic assessment, information and support to families or individuals who have, or are at increased risk for, birth defects, chromosomal abnormalities or a variety of inherited conditions. Genetic counselling specialists include clinical geneticists and genetic counsellors. Genetic counselling involves medical assessment and investigation, interpretation of information about the disorder, analysis of inheritance patterns and risks of recurrence, and review of available management options with the family. Genetic counsellors also provide supportive counselling to families, and refer individuals and families to genetic support groups or other community or state support services.

Dental management
The aim of dental management should be to be a part of a team approach in the care of the child. The overall aim is to reduce the handicapping consequences of the condition. Restorative and surgical management of the specific dental disability (e.g. enamel hypoplasia or hypodontia) should be addressed with a long-term comprehensive management plan. This must involve several dental disciplines such as orthodontics, periodontics, oral surgery and restorative dentistry working together to coordinate a treatment plan. Overall success in management is measured by the total rehabilitation of the child and family.

References and further reading

Endocarditis
See Appendix E.

Haematology
Johnson WT, Leary JM 1988 Management of dental patients with bleeding disorders: review and update. Oral Surgery, Oral Medicine, and Oral Pathology 66:297–303

Morimoto Y, Yoshioka A, Sugimoto M et al 2005 Haemostatic management of intraoral bleeding in patients with von Willebrand disease. Oral Diseases 11:243–248

Piot B, Sigaud-Fiks M, Huet P et al 2002 Management of dental extractions in patients with bleeding disorders. Oral Surgery, Oral Medicine, Oral Pathology, Oral Radiology, and Endodontics 93:247–250

Warrier AI, Lusher JM 1983 DDAVP: a useful alternative to blood components in moderate hemophilia A and von Willebrand's disease. Journal of Paediatrics 102:228

Immunodeficiency
Flaitz CM, Hicks MJ 1999 Oral candidiasis in children with immune suppression: clinical appearance and therapeutic considerations. ASDC Journal of Dentistry for Children 66:161–166

Moyer IN, Kobayashi RH, Cannon ML 1983 Dental treatment of children with severe combine immunodeficiency. Pediatric Dentistry 5:79

Porter SR, Scully C 1994 Orofacial manifestations in the primary immunodeficiency disorders. Oral Surgery, Oral Medicine, and Oral Pathology 78:4–13

Acquired immunodeficiency syndrome
Eldridge K, Gallagher JE 2000 Dental caries prevalence and dental health behaviour in HIV infected children. International Journal of Paediatric Dentistry 10:19–26

Hicks MJ, Flaitz CM, Carter AB 2000 Dental caries in HIV-infected children: a longitudinal study. Pediatric Dentistry 22:359–364

Ramos-Gomez FJ, Flaitz C, Catapano P 1999 Classification, diagnostic criteria, and treatment recommendations for orofacial manifestations in HIV-infected pediatric patients. Collaborative Workgroup on Oral Manifestations of Pediatric HIV Infection. Journal of Clinical Pediatric Dentistry 23:85–96

Oncology
American Academy of Pediatric Dentistry Clinical Affairs Committee; American Academy of Pediatric Dentistry Council on Clinical Affairs 2005–2006 Guideline on dental management of pediatric patients receiving chemotherapy, hematopoietic cell transplantation, and/or radiation. Pediatric Dentistry 27(7 Reference Manual):170–175

da Fonseca MA 2004 Dental care of the pediatric cancer patient. Pediatric Dentistry 26:53–57

Dahllöf G, Barr M, Bolme P et al 1988 Disturbances in dental development after total body irradiation in bone marrow transplant recipients. Oral Surgery, Oral Medicine, and Oral Pathology 65:41–44

Ferretti GA 1990 Chlorhexidine prophylaxis for chemotherapy and radiotherapy induced stomatitis: a randomized double-blind trial. Oral Surgery, Oral Medicine, and Oral Pathology 69:331–338

Reid H, Zietz H, Jaffe N 1995 Late effects of cancer treatment in children. Pediatric Dentistry 17:273–284

Nephrology
Lucas VS, Roberts GJ 2005 Oro-dental health in children with chronic renal failure and after renal transplantation: a clinical review. Pediatric Nephrology 20:1388–1394

Gastroenterology
Dodds AP, King D Gastroesophageal reflux and dental erosion: case report. Pediatric Dentistry 19:409–12

Little JW, Rhodus NL 1992 Dental treatment of the liver transplant patient. Oral Surgery 73:419–426

Seow WK, Shepherd RW, Thong YH 1991 Oral changes associated with end-stage liver disease and liver transplantation: implications for dental management. Journal of Dentistry for Children 58:474

Wondimu B, Németh A, Modéer T 2001 Oral health in liver transplant children administered cyclosporin A or tacrolimus. International Journal of Paediatric Dentistry 11:424–429

Endrocrinology

Dahms WT 1991 An update in diabetes mellitus. Pediatric Dentistry 13:79

Lalla E, Cheng B, Lal S 2007 Diabetes-related parameters and periodontal conditions in children. Journal of Periodontal Reseach 42:345–349

Twetman S, Petersson GH, Bratthall D 2005 Caries risk assessment as a predictor of metabolic control in young type 1 diabetics. Diabetic Medicine 22:312–315

Whitlock RI 1970 The jaw: lesions associated with hyperparathyroidism. Transactions of the International Conference on Oral Surgery 322–329

Neurology

Nelson LP, Ureles SD, Holmes G 1991 An update in paediatric seizure disorders. Pediatric Dentistry 13:128

Respiratory disease

Zhu JF, Humberto HA et al 1996 Dental management of children with asthma. Pediatric Dentistry 18:363–370

Developmental and behavioural paediatrics

Chew LC, King NM, O'Donnell D 2006 Autism: the aetiology, management and implications for treatment modalities from the dental perspective. Dental Update 33:70–80

Goyette CH, Conners CK, Ulrich RF 1978 Normative data on revised Conners Parent and Teacher Rating Scales. Journal of Abnormal Child Psychology 6:221–236

Klein U, Nowak AJ 1998 Autistic disorder: a review for the paediatric dentist. Pediatric Dentistry 20:312–317

Levine MD, Carey WB 1983 Developmental-behavioral Paediatrics. WB Saunders, Philadelphia

Monroy PG, da Fonseca MA 2006 The use of botulinum toxin-a in the treatment of severe bruxism in a patient with autism: a case report. Special Care Dentistry 26:37–39

Pilebro C, Bäckman B 2005 Teaching oral hygiene to children with autism. International Journal of Paediatric Dentistry 15:1–9

Genetics and dysmorphology

Gorlin RJ, Cohen MM, Levin LS 1996 Syndromes of the head and neck, 4th edn. Oxford University Press, Oxford

Jones, KL 1997 Smith's recognizable patterns of human malformation. 5th edn. WB Saunders, Philadelphia

Online Mendelian Inheritance in Man. Available at: www.ncbi.nlm.nih.gov/sites/entrez?db=OMIM

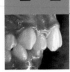

11 Orthodontic diagnosis and treatment in the mixed dentition

Contributors

John Fricker, Om P Kharbanda, Julia Dando

Introduction

The primary aim of orthodontic assessment in a growing child is to differentiate between a developing normal occlusion and a potential malocclusion. It is essential to have a sound understanding of facial growth and dental development, and the ability to recognize the rate and direction of facial and dental growth versus the general physical maturation of the child. Many cases of apparent malocclusion in the mixed dentition are actually part of the normal process of dental development. Incisor irregularities, spacing and apparent ectopic eruption of teeth may present early in the mixed dentition yet self-correct with growth and development.

Correction of dental arch irregularities, occlusal and jaw relation abnormalities and elimination of functional interferences, may be classified as preventive or interceptive. The term 'preventive' applies to the elimination of factors that may lead to malocclusion in an otherwise normally developing dentition. 'Interceptive' implies that corrective measures may be necessary to intercept a potential irregularity from progressing into a more severe malocclusion. Neither the appliances used nor the treatment itself should interfere with the often rapid changes in eruption of permanent teeth and the dynamic nature of occlusal adjustment. It is important to understand that even when such procedures are carried out, a majority of these children will go on to require some further treatment in the permanent dentition.

Orthodontic assessment

An orthodontic assessment in common with other specialties must include a good history, a thorough clinical examination and any relevant investigations. The information gathered leads to a diagnosis, which in turn allows treatment planning. This topic is covered in detail in Chapter 1. Additional points relevant to aid orthodontic diagnosis, however, will now be discussed.

The child should be assessed for both skeletal and dental problems.

Skeletal classification
This describes the relationship between the maxilla and mandible relative to the cranial base.

Skeletal Class I – the maxilla and mandible are in a normal relationship (orthognathic).

Skeletal Class II – the mandible appears small relative to the maxilla (retrognathic). This could be due to:

- Small mandible.
- Large maxilla.
- Combination of both.

Skeletal Class III – the mandible appears larger than the maxilla (prognathic). This could be due to:

- Large mandible.
- Small maxilla.
- Combination of both.

Dental relationships

Dental relationships are recorded with the teeth in occlusion. It describes the antero-posterior relationship of the upper and lower molars according to Angle's classification and the anteroposterior incisor relationship according to the British Standards Institute classification (1983). Angle's classification of malocclusion is based on the relationship of the upper and lower first permanent molars.

Molar relationship

- Class I implies a normal anteroposterior relationship with the mesial cusp of the upper first permanent molar occluding with the fossa of the lower first permanent molar.
- Class II molar relationship implies disto-occlusion of the lower first permanent molar with the upper first permanent molar and is a reflection of a retrognathic skeletal pattern with increased overjet.
- Class III molar relationship implies a mesially positioned lower first permanent molar and is a reflection of a prognathic mandible and anterior crossbite.

Incisor relationship

- Class II Division 1 (proclined upper incisors).
- Class II Division 2 (retroclined upper incisors).
- Class III (anterior crossbite).

Complicating factors in any malocclusion

These include:

Intra-arch problems

- Crowding.
- Dentoalveolar disproportion (discrepancy between tooth and jaw size).
- Space loss (premature loss of primary teeth, delayed eruption of permanent teeth).
- Local tooth displacement.
- Spacing.
- Physiological.
- Dentoalveolar disproportion.
- Missing teeth (congenital absence, traumatic loss).
- Supernumerary teeth.
- Eruption of teeth.
- Ectopic teeth.
- Impactions.
- Transpositions.
- Retained deciduous teeth.

Inter-arch problems:
- Increased overjet.
- Increased overbite.
- Open bites.
- Anterior (most common).
- Lateral.
- Crossbites.
- Anterior.
- Posterior (unilateral/bilateral).
- Tooth size discrepancies (Bolton's ratio).

Other factors
- Habits.
- Digit sucking.
- Pacifiers.
- Mouth-breathing.
- Abnormal swallowing.
- Trauma.

Orthodontic examination

Extra-oral
The physical status of the child should be included here, and if relevant, height and weight should be recorded on a standard growth chart. It is essential to determine if the face of the child is also growing normally. The face is examined with the child sitting upright. This is important because the mandibular rest position will change if lying back.

Frontal view
- Shape of face – long and thin/normal/short and square.
- Symmetry – initial assessment from the front. Looking at the child from above and behind will confirm asymmetry. It is important to look at the position of the chin at rest and in occlusion. A deviation would suggest a functional shift is occurring rather than a true asymmetry.
- Facial proportions – from the front the face can be divided vertically into thirds. The height of the midface (supraorbital ridge to base of nose) should therefore equal that of the lower face (base of nose to chin) However, it may be increased or decreased (Figure 11.1).

Lateral view
- Profile – convex/straight/concave.
- Skeletal pattern – Class I, II, III.
- Nose – small/normal/prominent.
- Chin – recessive/normal/prominent.
- Nasolabial angle – acute/normal/obtuse. If the angle is obtuse, orthodontic treatment involving the extraction of permanent teeth will have a detrimental effect on the profile.

- Lip position – competent (closed), incompetent (apart).
- Lower lip – normal/everted.
- Labiomental sulcus – normal/deep.
- FMPA – imagine a line connecting the ear to the eye (Frankfort horizontal) and construct an angle with the lower border of the mandible. This angle (FMPA) will help to assess growth direction.

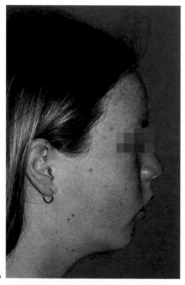

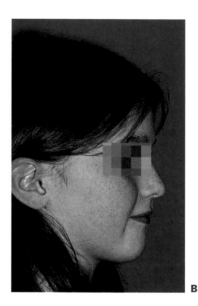

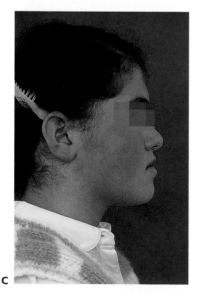

Figure 11.1 Evaluation of facial profile. **A** Child with retrognathic chin and convex face suggestive of skeletal Class II pattern. **B** Normally growing chin – Class I pattern. **C** Prominent chin with concave profile, suggestive of Class III skeletal pattern.

- Extreme types are vertical growers (with an angle >32°) and horizontal growers (with an angle of <20°). Growth direction is an important consideration in treatment planning (Figure 11.2).

Intra-oral

A record should be made of:
- Tooth quality and any existing restorations or active caries.
- Level of oral hygiene.
- Condition of the soft tissues.

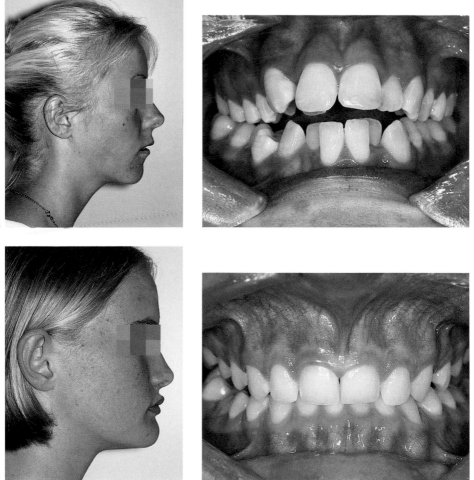

Figure 11.2 A, B Vertical grower with a long thin face, high FMPA. **B** Tendency for anterior open bite. Note the increase in lower face height. **C, D** Horizontal grower with square face and low FMPA. **D** Tendency for deep bite. Note the decrease in lower face height.

- Gingival condition.
- Abnormal frenal attachments.
- Tongue position.
- Erupted teeth.
- Assessment of crowding/spacing in both arches.
- Overjet, overbite, canine and molar relationships.
- Anterior or posterior crossbites and any associated functional shift into occlusion.
- Centrelines.
- In relation to each other (upper to lower).
- In relation to the facial midline (upper to face and lower to face).

Investigations

These are determined by the findings at examination.

- Panoramic radiograph – will give an overall picture of the developing dentition and jaws. It is the standard radiograph used in orthodontic assessment. Additional films may be needed to allow a more detailed analysis of suspected pathology.
- Bitewings.
- Periapical films.
- Lateral cephalogram – this is useful to assess skeletal discrepancy when treatment is to be started. Tracing of the film and subsequent cephalometric analysis will aid diagnosis and treatment planning. This film can also be used as a baseline to monitor future growth.
- Posteroanterior (PA) cephalogram – for transverse discrepancies or asymmetry.
- Anterior occlusal films – only for location of impacted canines, supernumeraries, or ectopic teeth.
- Study models are essential baseline records that are also used in treatment planning and space analyses.
- Any other relevant tests (i.e. pulp sensibility testing).

Evaluation of crowding

In the permanent dentition it is easy to assess the amount of crowding by taking measurements directly from a study model. Treatment will depend on the severity of the problem and may involve arch lengthening or extractions. In the mixed dentition, however, a prediction of future crowding is necessary.

Mixed dentition analysis

The purpose of a mixed dentition analysis is to determine the space available in the dental arch for the permanent successors to erupt. To complete this analysis it is necessary to first record the arch length and the mesiodistal widths of the mandibular permanent incisors.

Measurement of arch length

The conventional way to determine arch length is to measure directly from a set of study casts. Soft wire can be adapted from the mesial of the first permanent molar to follow the arch form around to the mesial of the contralateral first molar. The wire should be shaped to the ideal arch form and not follow any teeth out of alignment. Once the arch length has been determined, it is then necessary to estimate the space required for the permanent successors. Mesiodistal dimensions of erupted teeth can be obtained directly from a study cast. Unerupted teeth can be measured by one of two methods:

- Using periapical radiographs with allowances for magnification (Modified Hixon–Oldfather method).
- Using tooth size prediction formulas (Tanaka & Johnston 1974).

Both methods are based on the high correlation between the sizes of the permanent mandibular incisors and the combined sizes of premolars and permanent canines. Thus, it is possible to forecast the amount of space required for the unerupted teeth and to plan interceptive and or preventive space management requirements (see Figure 11.4 below).

The difference in values between arch length and tooth size will indicate the amount of crowding or spacing present.

Summary

At the end of diagnosis a clinician should have gathered the following information:

- Growth pattern – normal, Class I, Class II, Class III.
- Growth trend – horizontal, vertical.
- Sequence and stage of eruption of teeth.
- The dental arch relations – crossbites.
- Number of teeth missing or supernumeraries.
- Tongue of digit habits.
- Overjet and overbite.
- Amount of crowding and spacing.
- Is the child likely to grow normally or would he or she benefit from orthodontic intervention?

Crowding and space management in the mixed dentition

Space management can minimize the development of crowding in the permanent dentition. It essentially involves:

- Space maintenance following the premature loss of primary molars.
- Utilization of the leeway space by placement of holding arches.

Space maintenance

The best space maintenance treatment is the preservation of the primary molars until natural exfoliation. Although dental health education and improved caries prevention have lowered the number of children who develop malocclusion because of premature loss of primary teeth, it is still one of the most common controllable causes of malocclusion.

When a primary second molar is lost prematurely due to caries or to the ectopic eruption of the first permanent molar, the first permanent molar will drift mesially. This is most pronounced in the maxilla with a more rapid shift of the molar and causing a Class II malocclusion. The earlier the loss of the second primary molar and the less the root development of the permanent molar, the greater will be the amount of bodily mesial shift of the permanent molar.

Factors to consider for placement of space maintainers

Placement of a space maintainer requires care of the appliance and oral hygiene maintenance. A child with poor oral hygiene and high caries risk is not the ideal case for such therapy. Before a decision is made to provide a space maintainer it is often essential to critically evaluate its merits, the need, and the benefit it would provide to the development of normal occlusion.

Anterior teeth

- Loss of one or more primary incisors results in negligible space loss if canines and molars are present.
- If the eruption of a permanent incisor is delayed, space loss may occur because of migration of adjacent teeth.

Posterior teeth

- Whenever a primary second molar is lost prematurely, whether before or after the eruption of the first permanent molar, there will be some loss of arch length caused by the mesial drift of the permanent molar (Figure 11.3).
- Space maintenance is critical in children who have a normal arch length and loose a primary molar. Any loss of space in these children will result in crowding of the permanent teeth.
- Where space has already been lost it is necessary to regain space and then fit a space maintainer.

Types of space maintainer
Removable

- Removable space maintainers have the shortcomings of all removable appliances.

Figure 11.3 An ankylosed lower second primary molar in infraocclusion. The tooth is subgingival and grossly carious. Uprighting of the first permanent molar is required initially, followed by surgical removal, and placement of a space maintainer.

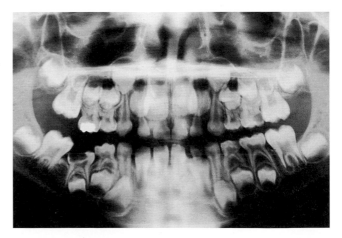

- They may be worn at the whim of the patient.
- May be broken.
- Easily lost when removed by the patient.

A removable space maintainer that is only worn at night is often sufficient to hold space and prevent the mesial drift of permanent molars. Night-only wearing of the appliance also reduces the risk of loss or breakage by the patient. The appliance should be washed and inserted immediately before going to bed, then removed, washed and placed in a safe place when not worn. Hawley's appliance is a typical example.

Fixed space maintainers (Figure 11.4)

- Fixed appliances have the advantage that they are worn continuously and do not require patient cooperation in wearing them.
- It should be noted that the placement of a fixed appliance in a child at high risk of caries may compromise those teeth which are banded, or even adjacent teeth.
- Band and loop appliance is typically used in cases of unilateral loss.
- Nance appliance or lingual arch can be used if the loss is bilateral.
- Distal shoe appliances can be used if the first permanent molar is not yet erupted, but are not widely used because of risks of infection.

Utilization of the leeway space

- The combined mesiodistal width of the deciduous molars is greater than that of the premolars. This residual space can be used to relieve mild crowding (1–2 mm) elsewhere in the arch.
- A transpalatal arch is used in the maxilla.
- A lingual arch is used in the mandible.

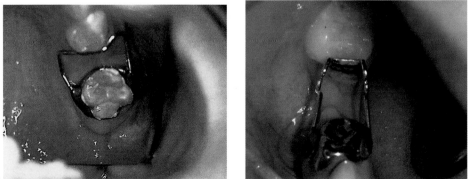

A   B

Figure 11.4 A A band and loop space maintainer. The placement of a space maintainer must not compromise the permanent tooth. Bands should be cemented with a luting glass ionomer as a protection against caries and the appliance reviewed regularly. As the premolar erupts, the appliance is removed when there is interference with normal emergence. **B** A distal shoe space maintainer is placed following early loss of the second primary molar prior to the eruption of the first permanent molar. It prevents mesial migration of the permanent tooth.

Regaining space (Figure 11.5)

Within an arch, space may need to be regained when migration of permanent teeth has already occurred following the loss of adjacent deciduous teeth. Furthermore, space maintenance would then be needed until the permanent successor erupted. In the maxilla, this would intercept a developing Class II dental relationship secondary to mesial migration and rotation of the first molar. In the mandible it could prevent a mild dental Class III relationship by uprighting tipped lower molars. In individuals with a developing skeletal discrepancy, the dental correction would have no effect on the underlying skeletal problem.

In general tooth movement is slower in cases with severe horizontal growth pattern (low FMPA). Conversely it is rapid in vertical growers, and space loss can occur very quickly. Early fitting of a space maintainer will prevent space loss. If space is to be regained it is essential that the mechanics should not extrude the teeth at all.

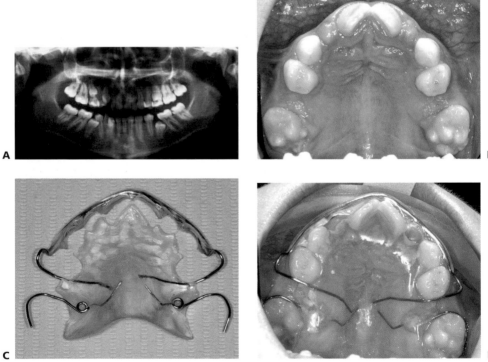

Figure 11.5 A The failure to place a space maintainer following bilateral extraction of primary second molars has resulted in forward movement of the first permanent molars thereby reducing the available space for the second premolars. **B–D** The ACCO appliance is used for uprighting maxillary permanent molars to regain space. To maximize anchorage, acrylic is flowed over the labial arch wire and this limits the proclination of incisors as the molars are distalized.

Radiographs and study models are essential aids in assessing space needs. It is important to note whether teeth have moved bodily or have tipped into the space. Tipping can be easier to resolve than bodily tooth movement. Radiographic examination should also locate the permanent second molars and establish space available for distalization of the first permanent molars.

Appliances used to regain space
- Uprighting mechanics:
  - Sectional fixed appliance.
  - Removable appliances – ACCO appliance (Figure 11.5).
  - Full arch fixed appliances.
- Distalizing appliances:
  - Distalizing springs or screws.
  - Open coil springs.
  - K loop.
  - Extra-oral headgear.
- Lip bumpers – to upright and distalize lower molars.

Permanent molars can be uprighted to regain space for the eruption of premolars by using removable appliances. These are most successful where there is a dental and skeletal Class I pattern with normal vertical proportions.

Timed extraction of teeth to resolve intra-arch crowding

The total amount of arch length deficiency is the key to planning of timed extractions. For this to be beneficial a cephalometric analysis should show the child to be growing within a normal pattern and that all the permanent teeth are present radiographically and in the normal order of eruption.

Extraction of deciduous canines
- Premature loss of a primary canine as the permanent lateral incisor erupts will result in a midline shift to the same side. Extraction of the contralateral deciduous canine will help prevent a shift occurring.
- In cases with crowding, the loss of primary canines should be managed by placement of a fixed lingual arch to support the incisors and prevent lingual tipping as the midlines correct themselves.
- As the permanent canines erupt it may be necessary to reduce the mesial of the primary first molars and then, as the first premolars erupt, reduce the mesial of the second primary molar.

Serial extraction
Where there is an arch deficiency of >4 mm, serial extraction may be considered. The purpose of this treatment is to encourage the early eruption of the first premolars ahead of the permanent canines. The premolars are then removed, allowing room for

the canines to erupt spontaneously. Serial extraction is usually limited to the upper arch. Serial extractions in the lower arch usually result in lingual collapse of the lower anterior segment.

Contraindications
Serial extraction should not be performed in the following circumstances:
- Class I malocclusions where the lack of space is slight and the teeth show only mild crowding.
- Where there is a skeletal discrepancy in the dental arches.
- When there is a deep overbite or an open bite, these should be treated before undertaking serial extraction.
- When there are permanent teeth congenitally absent from the dental arch.

Treatment stages in serial extraction
- First, the primary canines are removed to allow spontaneous alignment of the permanent incisors.
- The primary first molars are removed to allow the eruption of the first premolars.
- Once the first premolars are erupted, they are removed and a space maintainer is issued to allow the permanent canines to erupt.
- Further orthodontic treatment is usually required to align teeth achieve correct root angulation and incisor torque.

Thus serial extraction is a planned procedure which demands a minimum of 5 years' supervision by the dentist of the developing occlusion. Without such a commitment, the objectives will not be fully achieved and at times the child may well be left with a more severe malocclusion.

Spacing

Spaces in the deciduous dentition are normal and there is an increased chance of good alignment in the permanent dentition. During the early mixed dentition stage, physiological spacing is common in the anterior region with the incisors appearing splayed. As the permanent canines erupt this will resolve spontaneously and early treatment should not be contemplated.

Dentoalveolar disproportion and tooth size discrepancies can also lead to spacing. Definitive treatment is carried out in the permanent dentition when space closure or tooth build-ups should be considered.

Management of missing teeth

Spaces in the deciduous dentition are normal and there is an increased chance of good alignment in the permanent dentition. During the early mixed dentition stage, physiological spacing is common in the anterior region with the incisors appearing splayed. As the permanent canines erupt this will resolve spontaneously and early treatment should not be contemplated.

Dentoalveolar disproportion and tooth size discrepancies can also lead to spacing. Definitive treatment is carried out in the permanent dentition when space closure or tooth build-ups should be considered.

Hypodontia is the term used to describe the congenital absence of one or more teeth. These teeth have not developed from the initiation stage of tooth development (see Chapter 9).

Diagnosis

An understanding of the normal sequence and average age of eruption of permanent teeth will alert the practitioner to the possibility of congenital absence. Any delay in the normal eruption time of permanent teeth or exfoliation of primary teeth should be investigated radiographically. The orthopantomogram (OPG) film will provide the best view for investigation of premolars and molars but is often unclear in the incisor region because of the narrow focal trough. It may be necessary to supplement this with either periapical films or, in the maxilla, an anterior occlusal film.

For most children a radiographic survey at age 7 years will demonstrate the presence or absence of all permanent teeth except for third molars. It should be noted, however, that there is a large variation especially in the second premolar region. Third molars are generally not radiographically visible before the age of 9 years. A radiograph will show the tooth follicle before calcification begins, and there is a range in development time between the presentation of the follicle and calcification commencing, especially for second premolars.

Management

Where a permanent tooth is diagnosed as congenitally absent, there are two choices in management:
- Retain the space after loss of the primary tooth and insert a prosthetic replacement.
- Orthodontics to close the space.

The preferred treatment choice will depend on the severity of the condition (number of absent teeth), location of the missing teeth and the underlying skeletal pattern.

Class I patterns

The jaw relationship is normal. If the missing tooth is located in the posterior segments, space closure is often the treatment of choice. Occlusal relationships, however, will dictate the decision. On the other hand if one or more incisors are missing it is more appropriate to consider space opening and prosthetic replacement.

Class II patterns

This malocclusion is characterized by a smaller mandible with an increased overjet. The preferred option for missing teeth in the maxilla, is to close space and reduce the overjet at the same time. The permanent canines can replace lateral incisors, but size, shape and colour must be considered. Restorative techniques using resin veneers and acid-etch can be used to reshape the canines as lateral incisors, restoring the anatomy of the substituted teeth and providing a balanced smile.

Class III patterns

The maxilla is proportionally smaller than the mandible and there can be a dental crossbite either anteriorly or posteriorly. If teeth are missing in the lower arch, and the skeletal problem can be camouflaged with orthodontics only, it may be advantageous to close space. Conversely if teeth are missing in the maxilla, space opening and tooth replacement is the preferred option to avoid further constriction of the arch.

Tooth loss due to trauma

Traumatic loss of a maxillary incisor can be treated orthodontically within the same guidelines as those for congenital absence of teeth.

Orthodontic aspects of supernumerary teeth

Development and aetiology

Supernumerary teeth may be found in any part of the dental arch; however, the most frequent sites are in the regions of the maxillary midline and the third molars. Because the supernumerary teeth develop late, they are not often found in the primary dentition and when they do develop with the primary teeth they usually erupt. Tubercular and inverted supernumerary teeth are most often unerupted, and they commonly delay or inhibit the eruption of the central incisors. Supernumerary teeth in the region of the lateral incisors, either in the primary or permanent dentition, usually erupt into the arch.

Orthodontic effects

Delay or failure of eruption

The failure of a permanent tooth to erupt leads to malocclusion as adjacent teeth shift into the area that should be occupied by the permanent tooth. Moreover, the supernumerary tooth can be a cause of ectopic eruption of other teeth, producing a malocclusion. Supernumeraries can result in:

- Displacement of permanent teeth.
- Rotations.
- Diastemas.
- Development of dentigerous cysts.
- Resorption of roots of adjoining teeth.

Treatment planning

- Even though supernumerary teeth may not produce a malocclusion, they should be removed as soon as possible after detection to avoid future problems.
- A supernumerary primary incisor may be retained if there is sufficient room for it. The tooth should be extracted when the permanent lateral incisor is ready to erupt.
- If there is an extra permanent lateral present with the primary supernumerary, it may be removed at the same time. Usually, the more distal of the two teeth is the supernumerary tooth.
- Identification of a supernumerary tooth that is similar in form and size to the adjacent tooth can be made by comparing the teeth with those on the opposite side of the dental arch. The tooth that more closely resembles the size and shape the normal lateral incisor should be retained.

Extraction of over-retained primary teeth (Figure 11.6)

The earlier that one can recognize and remove over-retained primary teeth that may be causing ectopic eruption of a succedaneous tooth, the better the chance that a permanent tooth will erupt in a satisfactory position. The greatest damage that may result from over-retained primary teeth comes in the wake of ankylosed primary molars (Figure 11.3).

Diagnosis

The ankylosed primary molar may not be recognized in the very early stage. The condition can readily be diagnosed a short time later because the vertical level of the occlusal surface of the ankylosed tooth becomes noticeably lower than the level of adjacent teeth, and as time progresses this difference in vertical level becomes more extreme.

Because ankylosed teeth seem to be submerging, they have been called 'submerged' teeth, but the term cannot be applied accurately to ankylosed teeth. The continued vertical eruption of the uninvolved adjacent teeth and the vertical growth of the alveolar process and periodontium creates the illusion that the ankylosed tooth is submerging.

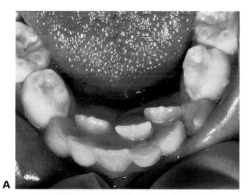

A

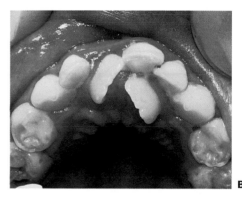

B

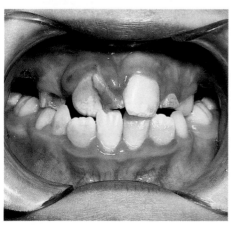

C

Figure 11.6 A, B Common presentations of anterior crowding. It is important to inform parents and children of where teeth will erupt. Lower permanent incisors form lingually to the primary teeth and in patients with tooth to base bone discrepancy, they will erupt behind the primaries. It is often wise to facilitate removal of such teeth, as in **B** and **C**, to avoid the development of a crossbite.

Management

- Ankylosed primary molars may be retained as long as they are maintaining arch length (i.e. preventing mesial shifting of the first permanent molars) or as long as they do not prevent the eruption of the succedaneous teeth.
- If there is evidence of root resorption these teeth will eventually be lost normally and there is no indication for early removal.
- The union between the cementum and dentine of the tooth and the bone of the alveolar process is physically strong and removal may require a surgical procedure, depending on how far the tooth has been submerged.
- A space-maintaining appliance must be used if the primary tooth is removed before the imminent eruption of the succedaneous tooth.

An over-retained tooth often accounts for the ectopic eruption, or impaction, of the succedaneous tooth. Because the ankylosed tooth is ultimately unable to withstand the mesial shifting of the first molar and the loss of arch length, extraction of an ankylosed primary tooth is an effective means of interceptive-preventive orthodontics.

Ectopic eruption of permanent canines

The incidence of impacted canines in the maxilla is 2% and the majority lie in a palatal position. The anomaly can be associated with small or absent lateral incisors. In about 12% of cases with impacted canines, the lateral incisor root will undergo some resorption.

The normal age of eruption is 11 ± 2 years and the crown should certainly be palpable in the labial sulcus at 9–10 years of age. If the canine is not palpable further investigation is indicated. Radiographs are taken at right angles to each other and the technique of parallax used to localize its position.

Interceptive extraction of the deciduous canines can improve the position of the permanent teeth and the maximum improvement will be seen within 12 months (Ericson & Kurol 1988) The success of this approach is reduced, however, if the arch is already crowded (Power & Short 1993).

Ectopic eruption of first permanent molars (Figure 11.7)

This can be an indication of an inadequate arch length, and a radiographic survey is required to confirm the presence of premolar teeth. The permanent teeth may resorb the distal margins of the second primary molars; this is more common in the maxilla.

Management

- Where there is impaction of the permanent molar against the distal of the second primary molar, slicing or discing of the distal surface of the primary molar will allow the spontaneous eruption of the permanent molar.
- Placement of orthodontic separators or brass ligature wire is usually difficult and uncomfortable, and has mixed success.

- Where the resorption of the primary molar is advanced, the loss of this tooth is indicated and space-regaining mechanics should be considered once the permanent molar has erupted.
- Parents should be warned that further orthodontic treatment is usually required because of arch length deficiencies.

Extraction of first permanent molars (Figures 11.8, 11.9)

Gross caries involving the first permanent molars poses a difficult dilemma in treatment planning. The early presentation of the patient is essential in obtaining favourable results. The basic questions about whether these teeth should be removed or restored are:

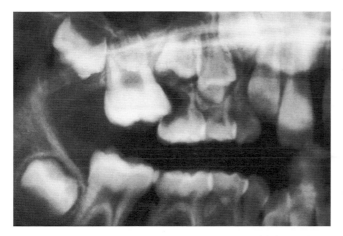

Figure 11.7 Ectopic eruption of the first permanent molars, causing resorption of the primary teeth. In this position, it is unlikely that the first permanent molars will erupt and space loss has already occurred. The primary molars were extracted and a space-regaining appliance constructed.

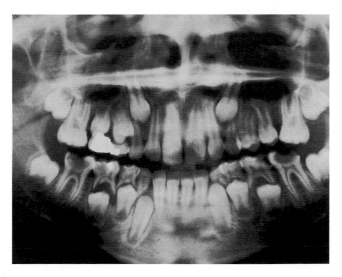

Figure 11.8 Gross caries affecting the lower first permanent molars. Both teeth are non-vital and should be removed. This is a perfect time for extraction as the second molars will migrate mesially. The upper molars should be retained with a night-time removable appliance to prevent overeruption.

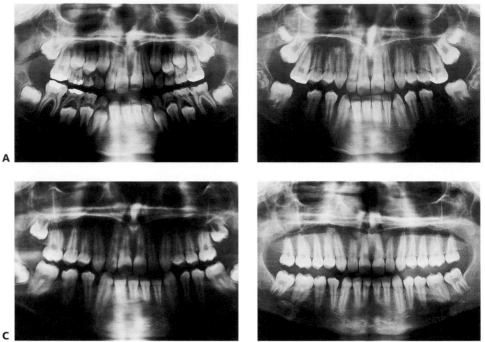

Figure 11.9A–D Serial panoramic radiographs showing mesial migration of the second and third permanent molars following timed extraction of carious first permanent molars.

- What is the long-term prognosis for the tooth?
- What is the status of the pulp?
- Are the root apices fully formed?
- Are the third molars present?

General considerations

- The decision to extract is often best made in conjunction with an orthodontist.
- If the tooth is not restorable no matter what the occlusion, then it should be removed. Even if successful root canal treatment can be completed, the status of the crown is most important. Commonly, these teeth have extensive loss of tooth structure with only an enamel shell remaining.
- Non-vital immature teeth have a poor prognosis. Root canal treatment is usually not indicated in these teeth, especially as they would need an apexification procedure.
- If the upper molars are retained, a removable appliance such as a Hawley should be used to prevent overeruption of these teeth before the eruption of the lower second molars.
- The ideal time for lower first permanent molar extraction is before alveolar eruption of the second molar. These teeth will migrate mesially and assume the position of the first molar.

- If three molars are grossly carious and require removal it is probably better to keep the extractions symmetrical and extract all four teeth.
- The presence of absence of third molars may influence a decision to extract the first molars, but ultimately it will be the long-term prognosis of the first molars that determines the final treatment plan

Timing of extractions

Although the timing of extractions will be determined in individual cases, some general rules should be followed if possible.

Class I (with no crowding)
- Extract teeth that are not restorable.

Class I (crowding) or Class II
- Extract lower first permanent molars as early as practicable.
- Retain upper first permanent molars until the second molars begin to erupt.
- Extraction of the upper first permanent molars should coincide with ongoing treatment for crowding.

Class III
- Extract teeth that are not restorable.

Basic requirements of orthodontic appliances

- Permit control of the amount, distribution, duration and direction of the force they exert.
- Be atraumatic to the oral tissues and not be adversely affected by oral secretions.
- Allow teeth and soft oral tissues to function normally.
- Allow wearer to maintain oral hygiene.
- Exert sufficient force or offer sufficient anchorage resistance to induce histological bone changes necessary for desired orthodontic tooth movement.
- Respond to the control of the operator.
- Allow movement of individual teeth or of groups of teeth in desirable directions.

Safety measures in appliance treatment

Appliances should be regularly examined. Loose molar bands can result in caries due to failure of the cement lute, or cause trauma to the soft tissues because of excessive movement from biting forces. Archwires should be carefully fitted with the distal ends either cut as they leave the molar tube, or turned in. Failure to do this will result in irritation of the buccal mucosa. Broken cribs or springs on removable appliances may need chairside modification or repair in the laboratory.

Removable appliances

Although removable orthodontic appliances cannot produce all types of tooth movement (Figure 11.10), they possess several advantages. They are laboratory fabricated

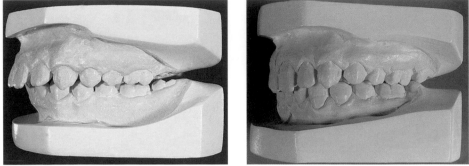

A   B

Figure 11.10A,B Study models of a child with mild proclination of the upper anterior teeth and a tendency for a Class II molar relationship. Following treatment with a simple Hawley appliance, the molar relationship has improved and the upper incisors are now normally inclined. The overjet and overbite are reduced to within normal limits.

and hence require less chair time, are easily removed by the child/patient for oral hygiene and are often low cost. The conventional removable appliance is the Hawley appliance.

Design
Removable appliances should include:
- Acrylic base plate or body.
- Retentive components.
- Adams' cribs.
- C clasps.
- Ball retainers.
- Passive labial bow.
- Active components/tooth-moving components
- Springs.
- Screws.
- Biteplanes.

Other design considerations
- For successful tooth/teeth movement to occur, the active components of the appliance should produce force in the desired direction whereas anchorage is derived from the acrylic plate that remains stationary.
- The acrylic plate should fit well against the palatal mucosa and must occupy the interdental spaces. The plate should be of even thickness, for strength and to house the retentive components and springs.
- The anchorage of the appliance is derived from palatal tissues, and from the teeth through the clasps.
- The posterior border of the maxillary appliance should be placed anterior to the junction of the hard and soft palate. It should be thin and gently merge with the palatal mucosa.

- The lower appliance should have smooth borders with sufficient relief to accommodate the functioning of the lingual frenum.

Springs

Spring design (finger, Z or retractors) should ensure adequate springiness and range of action while retaining strength.

For lingual/palatal movement: Labial bow/long labial bow
For labial movement: Z spring or T spring
For mesial movement: Finger spring
For distal movement: Finger spring
For canine retraction: Canine retractor – labial/palatal

- The active arm of the spring should be in surface contact with the tooth to be moved.
- The point (area) of force application should be close to the cervical margin/gingival margin to minimize tipping.
- To increase the range of action, helices are incorporated into the spring design.
- Activate slowly, close to the gingival margins, without causing trauma to the oral tissues.
- There should be no hindrance/obstacle in the path of movement of teeth.

Labial bow

An active labial bow produces both horizontal and vertical force vectors resulting in palatal/lingual tooth movement. It is used for retraction of proclined incisors. Since the labial bow causes tipping of the crown, simultaneous labial root tipping occurs.

   Prerequisites for activating a labial bow are:

- Bite opening – this should be achieved prior to incisor retraction.
- Ensure sufficient space is available.
- The activation should be gradual and gentle.
- Ensure sufficient relief of acrylic is provided palatal to the incisors before activation.

Anterior biteplanes

- The acrylic behind the upper incisors is thickened. In occlusion, there is contact of the lower incisors with the acrylic, with open bites in the buccal segments.
- In a growing child with a mild Class II tendency, bite opening may result in forward posturing of the mandible.
- Bite opening is a combination of supra-eruption of the mandibular molars and intrusion/stabilization of the vertical position of the mandibular incisors. Hence a child with a normal or horizontal growth pattern is the most suitable case for bite opening.
- Children with vertical facial growth (that is, with a high FMPA) are not suitable cases for treatment with biteplanes. The biteplane will cause an open bite tendency to worsen, and have a detrimental effect on the profile.
- An active labial bow can be used to retract incisors after adequate bite opening, thus reducing an overjet.
- Biteplanes are also used to relieve interferences in the buccal segments, which may be hindering tooth movement.

Posterior biteplanes
- The acrylic is extended to include coverage of the occlusal surfaces of the posterior teeth.
- Allows rapid correction of an anterior crossbite.
- Unlock the molars for maxillary expansion.

Treatment of anterior crossbites

Up to 10% of children present with crossbites. Three types of anterior crossbite may present in the mixed dentition.

Ectopic incisors
An incisor may erupt ectopically either palatally in the maxilla or labially in the mandible to a crossbite relationship in centric occlusion. This may occur in a child with a balanced skeletal relationship. Early treatment is only necessary if there is a deviation on opening and or closing or if there is a traumatic occlusion or periodontal concern. Otherwise treatment can be delayed until the full permanent dentition erupts.

Skeletal Class III malocclusion
An anterior crossbite may be associated with a skeletal Class III discrepancy such that, although the incisors are positioned correctly within the alveolar ridges, they are in negative overjet on closing into centric occlusion with no deviation of mandibular closure.

Pseudo Class III malocclusion
This pattern occurs where there is an habitual mandibular closure pattern such that the mandible goes into a protrusive bite and thus crossbite of incisors avoiding traumatic occlusion with lingual position of one or more maxillary incisors. Thus anterior shift of the mandible can affect the growth of both the maxilla and the mandible with undesirable muscle adaptation.

Management
Tongue blade
If there is only one permanent incisor in crossbite without an excessive overbite, a tongue blade, or paddle pop stick may be used to correct this. The stick is placed lingual to the upper tooth in crossbite and the patient instructed to close firmly against the stick while it is held in position against the chin. The child should hold it there while biting against it and another person should count to 50 out loud as in one apple, two apples etc, so as to bring up to approximately a minute. Repeat this six times per day with an interval of at least half an hour. Correction is often complete within a few days.

Incline planes
Where there is a functional shift of the mandible into an anterior crossbite, an acrylic inclined plane can be fitted to the lower incisors to restrict the forward posturing and place pressure on the palatal of the maxillary incisors to push them labially. Alternatively a composite build-up of the lower incisors will mimic the action of an incline

plane. (It is preferable to choose a shade of composite resin that is easily distinguished from normal tooth structure to facilitate safe removal).

Treatment is usually complete within a few weeks. This appliance works best where there is a slight increase in overbite, which helps to retain the incisors in positive overjet once the appliance is removed.

Removable appliances (Figure 11.11)

- These appliances should only be used to correct crossbites of dental origin.
- A modified Hawley appliance can be used in the maxilla to correct one or two teeth in crossbite.
- Ensure there is adequate space to move the teeth into the desired position and movement will occur rapidly.
- Occlusal surfaces of both the primary and permanent molars should be covered to open the bite and allow free labial movement of the teeth in crossbite.
- Adams' clasps are placed on the first permanent molars.
- If the primary molars are present, ball-ended clasps can be fabricated to engage the interproximal areas of these teeth.

Where a single tooth is in crossbite, a Z-spring placed palatally to the malposed tooth can be used, or if both central incisors are in crossbite, two springs can be used to provide sweep arms on the palatal surface. Initially, the appliance should be fitted and checked for comfort with the springs passive. The springs are then activated 1–2 mm at a time. The patient is reviewed after 4 weeks to reactivate the springs as required and to check the retention of the appliance.

As with all removable appliances the success of treatment is reliant on cooperation and compliance. If these qualities can be encouraged and the patient takes responsibility for the wearing of the appliance, treatment will progress satisfactorily. Occasionally the crossbite may also be due to a labially placed lower incisor. This must also be corrected, but is dependent on available space. If this is not available definitive treatment may need to be delayed.

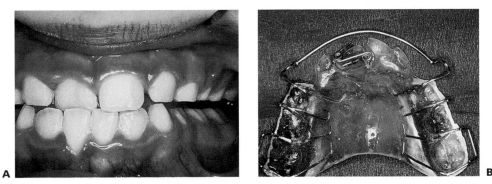

Figure 11.11 A Anterior dental crossbite involving the tooth 11. **B** Hawley appliance was used to correct the malocclusion with Adams' cribs on the first permanent molars, ball retainers between the primary molars, posterior bite planes and a labial bow. A Z-spring is activated approximately 2 mm to procline the incisor. The crossbite was corrected within 4 weeks and was self-retaining due to the amount of overbite.

Figure 11.12 Correction of an anterior crossbite with a fixed appliance.

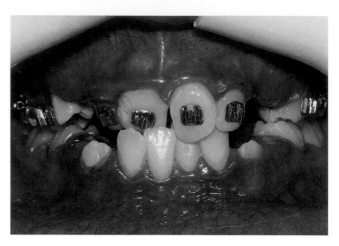

Fixed appliances (Figure 11.12)

- Fixed appliances can be used when two or more incisors are in crossbite.
- Brackets are bonded to the incisors with bands cemented to the first permanent molars.
- A labial 0.016″ arch wire is used with vertical loop stops mesial to the molar tubes. These loops are expanded to procline the incisors, and the round wire permits labial tilting of the incisors to correct the crossbite.
- Where the incisor crossbite is a combination of palatal inclination of maxillary incisors and labial inclination of the lower incisors, fixed appliances can be used in both upper and lower arches on the incisors and first permanent molars.
- Class III elastics (from maxillary molars to mandibular canines) can be used. The elastics need to be worn 24 hours per day, except for tooth brushing, and replaced every 3–4 days. This appliance will provide rapid correction of the crossbite within 6 months.

Treatment of posterior crossbites

A posterior crossbite is an abnormal, buccolingual relationship of a tooth or teeth when the two dental arches are brought into centric occlusion. There are two types of posterior crossbite:

- Dento-alveolar

Insufficient arch length or prolonged retention of deciduous teeth can deflect teeth during eruption and produce a crossbite. Prolonged digit sucking can also cause palatal tilting of teeth and narrowing of the maxillary arch.

- Skeletal

A skeletal crossbite is related to size discrepancy between the maxilla and mandible. This could be a narrow maxilla, a wide mandible, or a combination of both.

It is possible that both dental and skeletal causes may contribute to crossbites of variable severity.

Management
- In children with a normally growing mandible, posterior crossbites should be treated as early as possible to allow normal growth and development of the dental arches and temporomandibular joints. When planning treatment it is important to determine whether the crossbite is unilateral or bilateral.
- The majority of crossbites are bilateral but often present as unilateral when the teeth are in full intercuspal position. In these cases the dental midlines will not be coincident on closing and there will be a deviation of the mandible towards one side at the end on closing.
- When the teeth are closed with the dental midlines coincident, the posterior segments will be in an edge-to-edge, buccolingual position, reflecting the overall constriction of the maxillary dental arch, and bilateral maxillary expansion is indicated.

Cross-elastics
- When only a single molar is in crossbite, this can often be corrected with a bonded attachment, button or hook, to the palatal of the maxillary and buccal of the lower molar.
- An elastic is stretched between these teeth; it is worn 24 hours per day and changed every time it breaks (which is often).
- Crossbites will normally correct within 3–4 months with continuous wearing of the elastic. The major change will be reflected in the position of the maxillary molar because of the cancellous nature of the maxillary alveolar bone as against the denser bone around the mandibular molar.

Removable appliances (Figure 11.13)
- Lateral maxillary expansion can be achieved with a parallel expansion screw that is housed in the upper acrylic plate.
- To ensure delivery of sufficient force on the teeth and palate the appliance should have excellent tissue contact and anchorage with clasps on teeth.

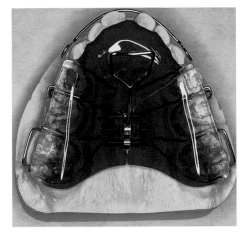

Figure 11.13 Maxillary appliance with a midpalatal expansion screw.

- Provide acrylic relief palatal to anterior teeth.
- The labial bow should be passive. When expansion occurs the bow becomes activated.
- The majority of the expansion appliances have a pitch of 1 mm. A full turn is achieved with four turns of the key.
- The conventional expansion schedule is one-quarter turn every second or third day. Some clinicians prefer one turn per week.
- An expansion appliance with posterior occlusal coverage work faster as they disclude the buccal occlusion.

It is extremely difficult to achieve unilateral expansion. A jackscrew offset in the palate will move one or two teeth, but there will usually also be some expansion on the contralateral side. Always expand beyond the correction of the crossbite and retain, because relapse potential is high. It is important to remember that correction is dental only, as the major component of tooth movement is tipping.

Fixed appliances (Figures 11.14, 11.15)
Slow maxillary expansion – quad helix/nickel titanium expanders

- A quad helix is attached to molar bands which are then cemented to the first permanent molars.
- The activation of this appliance is controlled by the dentist.
- Reactivation is carried out at alternate visits. It can be done intra-orally using triple-beak pliers, or by removal of the appliance which is then expanded by hand.
- The expansion should continue until the molars are overcorrected, then retained with the same appliance for a further 3 months. The crossbite is usually corrected within 4–6 months.
- The quadhelix can be used simultaneously with full bonded appliance treatment.
- Nickel titanium expanders require less adjustment than conventional stainless steel quad helix appliances.
- They cause a pre-determined amount of expansion.

Figure 11.14 A quad helix appliance is used to correct posterior crossbites in the mixed dentition. These appliances are simple to construct, are well tolerated by the patient and are efficient. They have the advantage that they are fixed and will also act as retainers once the malocclusion is corrected.

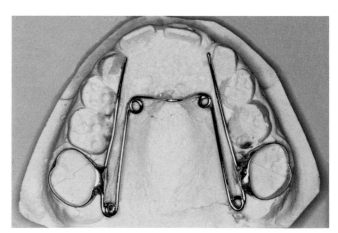

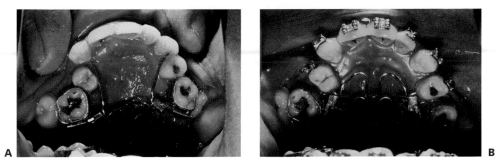

Figure 11.15A,B Maxillary expansion using a nickel–titanium (NiTi) expander. This appliance also achieves molar derotation.

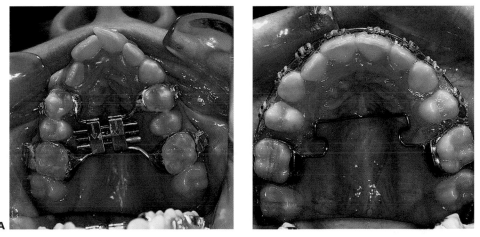

Figure 11.16 **A** Rapid maxillary expansion appliance. **B** Following expansion, a rigid retainer (e.g. transpalatal arch) should be used during the fixed appliance treatment phase to limit relapse.

- Cooling the expander allows it to be constricted and inserted into lingual tubes on the maxillary molars.
- As it warms to body temperature it becomes springy and exerts continuous force on the teeth thereby causing arch expansion.
- The expanding forces also cause simultaneous derotation of the molars.

Rapid expansion – Hyrax screw (Figure 11.16)
- Rapid maxillary expansion (RME) is indicated for severe cases of bilateral crossbite in which correction requires skeletal expansion. It involves the splitting of the midpalatal suture producing an orthopaedic increase in maxillary width. This can easily occur in a growing child, preferably before the age of 9 years. The split is evident on an occlusal radiograph, being widest at the incisors.

- The appliance uses a midpalatal screw (Hyrax) soldered to bands on the first permanent molars and the primary molars or premolars. In contrast with the removable appliance, the screw is activated a quarter turn twice each day and the patient should be monitored once a week.
- As the expansion proceeds, a diastema will show between the central incisors. This will close as the overstretched supragingival transseptal fibres relapse. The parents and patients should be warned of this. As with any expansion technique, the crossbite should be overcorrected and retained in this position for at least 3 months with the same appliance.

Habits: digit sucking

One of the most common oral activities of the infant and young child is thumb and finger sucking. Sucking habits are perfectly normal in infancy. The infant will suck on any object brought into contact with the lips. This reflex behaviour may last for several years. It is an adaptive reflex common to mammals.

Because it is a normal activity, thumb and finger sucking may be ignored in infancy. Thumb or finger sucking that is discontinued by age 2–3 years produces no permanent malformation of the jaws or displacement of the teeth. Continued beyond the time that the permanent incisor teeth erupt, it is almost always a factor in producing malocclusion in the anterior portion of the mouth.

The majority of older children who continue thumbsucking, have what is termed an 'empty' habit. It is just something they have always done. These children are usually receptive to reasons why they should stop and many actually want to give up. A minority, however, (especially if the habit has restarted) may have underlying social or psychological problems and these should be investigated.

Malocclusion from digit sucking
- Proclination and protrusion of the upper incisor teeth.
- The lower incisors may or may not be displaced lingually by the abnormal sucking habit.
- Posterior crossbite due to overactivity of buccinator compressing the maxilla.
- Anterior open bite.
- Tendency for the tongue to perpetuate open bite with anterior tongue thrust. Proclined maxillary incisors and an anterior open bite favour the forward positioning of the tongue.

Control of digit sucking (Figure 11.17)
Chemical means
Chemical therapy employs either hot-tasting, bitter-flavoured preparations or distasteful agents that are applied to the fingers or thumbs. Such things as cayenne pepper, quinine and asafoetida have been used to make the thumb or fingers so distasteful that the child will keep them out of his or her mouth. These preparations are effective with a limited number of children, and only when the habit is not firmly entrenched.

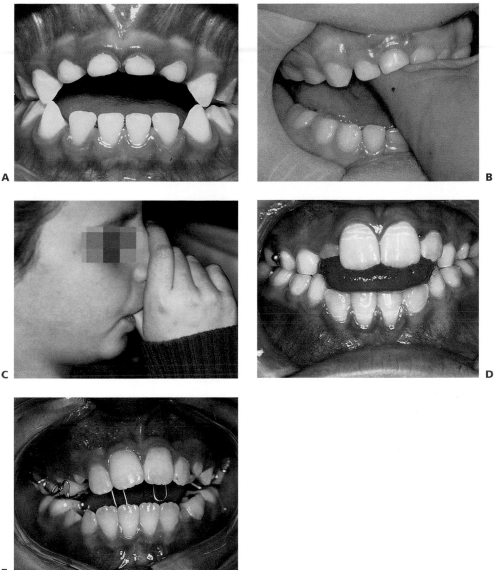

Figure 11.17 A An anterior open bite in the primary dentition caused by a dummy-sucking habit. Even a malocclusion of this size will improve once the habit has stopped and requires no active treatment. Note that the anterior teeth have been restored, due to early childhood caries associated with the dummy and a bottle at night. **B** Position of a thumb exerting orthopaedic as well as orthodontic forces. **C** Note the abnormal activity of the perioral musculature due to thumb sucking. **D** Resultant proclination of the upper anterior teeth, anterior open bite and abnormal tongue position in the mixed dentition. **E** Tongue guard appliance incorporating a mid-palatal screw expander.

Mechanical means
- A simple device for controlling thumb or finger sucking is the application of adhesive tape to the thumb or finger. In many instances this changes the character of the finger sufficiently to call the child's attention to the fact that it is being placed in the mouth.
- A Hawley appliance with a palatal bar may be fitted as a habit reminder. This is important because in many instances thumb- and finger-sucking habits are at the subconscious level of the individual's attention. Even though there may be some desire on the part of the child to discontinue the act, they may find it difficult to do so unless made aware of when they are sucking the thumb or finger.
- A fixed appliance consisting of bands on the first molars and an anterior tongue crib will ensure compliance, as the child cannot remove it.
- Often the child will respond to simple encouragement and explanation of the effect of digit sucking on the teeth. The child's own desire to break the habit means they react positively to such encouragement.
- The critical time for the elimination of digit sucking is as the permanent incisors erupt. This generally coincides with entry into school, where peer pressure can be a powerful inducement to discontinue the habit.
- Psychological assessment is often beneficial in older children.

Correction of developing Class II skeletal malocclusions

Developing Class II skeletal malocclusions may benefit by the use of functional appliances. Functional appliances are those that alter the abnormal functioning of orofacial musculature thereby bringing about normalization of growth and occlusion (Figure 11.18).
- By using functional appliances, there is an expectation of changes in the facial skeleton by growth modification.
- The simplest functional appliance is the anterior biteplane which can reposition the mandible more anteriorly in a growing child.
- Appliances can be fixed or removable.
- Functional appliances can be classified as tooth borne (active or passive) and tissue borne depending upon the structures from which they derive anchorage. All functional appliances are tooth borne except the Frankel appliance which is tissue borne.
- Functional appliances help posture the mandible forward. The degree/amount of vertical and sagittal repositioning may cause variable tissue (muscle) responses.
- Those appliances that displace the mandible within the freeway space are intended to stimulate muscle activity and are called myodynamic appliances.
- Others can cause extreme/severe displacement of the mandible and rely on passive muscle tension, and are called myotonic appliances.

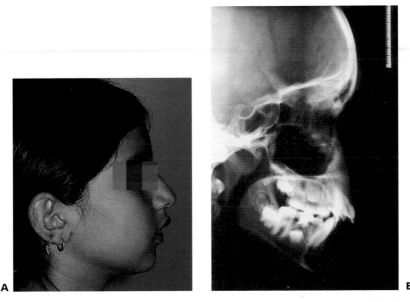

Figure 11.18 A An ideal case for treatment using a functional appliance: a child with a normal maxilla, a small mandible and a normal growth pattern. **B** Lateral cephalogram showing proclination of the upper incisors.

Indications and case selection for functional appliances
- A growing child preferably during or prior to peak pubertal growth spurt.
- Retrognathic small mandible.
- Large overjet (>5 mm).
- Horizontal or normal growth trends.
- Normal or low incisor mandibular plane angle.
- Maxillary incisors not placed forward but can be proclined.
- No or minimal crowding in the upper and lower anterior teeth.
- A willing and cooperative child.

Effects of functional appliances
- Regulate the function of the oral/perioral musculature such as abnormal swallowing and thereby restrains normal development.
- Mandible is postured forward.
- Remodelling of the glenoid fossa takes place.
- Maxillary growth can be restrained.
- Retraction of maxillary anterior teeth.
- Supra-eruption of lower posterior teeth.
- Mesial movement of lower buccal teeth and restraint or distalization of upper buccal teeth.
- Increase in lower posterior face height.

- Reduction in overjet.
- Bite opening.
- Proclination of the lower anterior teeth.
- Increase in arch width.
- Improvement in facial profile.

Evolution of functional appliances

The activator or the monoblock was the first functional appliance. It was mainly propagated and researched in Europe (1910, 1940). This appliance was extensively used in clinical practice. Research showed that it brought about a correction of malocclusion mainly by dentoalveolar changes with minimal alterations in the underlying skeletal structures.

Balters in 1950 felt that abnormal posturing of the tongue and perioral musculature were responsible for Class II malocclusion. He introduced the 'bionator' appliance (Figure 11.19), which has an extended labial bow to keep the peri-oral musculature away from the maxilla thereby allowing transverse maxillary growth to occur. The coffin spring in the palate is expected to normalize tongue posture. A number of other modifications were made to existing designs with the aim to make the appliance more acceptable to wear.

There are certain inherent problems with the functional appliance:

- Requires the child's cooperation.
- The bulk of the appliance.
- Speech problems.
- Cannot correct individual tooth malpositions.
- The majority of the above-mentioned limitations have been overcome with the introduction of the twin block appliance.

Clark's twin block appliance (Figure 11.20)

The twin block appliance is a two-piece functional appliance. The upper and lower blocks are made in acrylic and meet each other in the premolar region at an angle of about 70°. This is sufficient to maintain mandibular forward posturing. A child can

Figure 11.19 The bionator appliance.

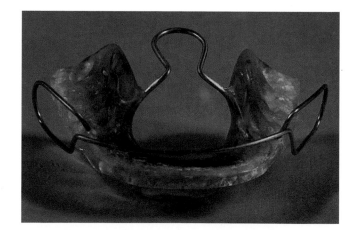

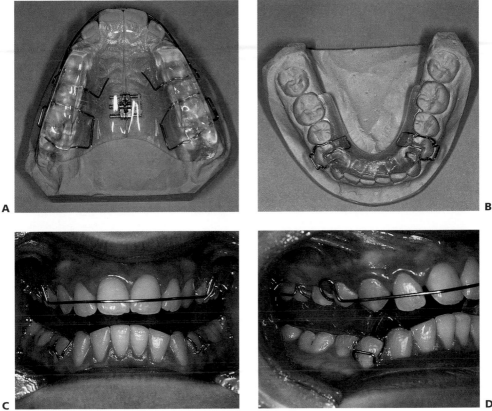

Figure 11.20A–D Clark's twin block appliance.

speak, eat and live with the appliance in place. Being the only full-time functional appliance it is expected to bring about rapid skeletal, dental and neuromuscular adaptations.

The upper twin block can house an expansion screw as well as springs for individual minor tooth/teeth movement. Hence while mandibular repositioning is in progress, simultaneous expansion of the maxilla and alignment of minor tooth malpositions can take place thereby eliminating the need for pre-functional phase treatment, resulting in an overall shorter treatment time.

The twin block appliance offer flexibility of use with fixed appliances that may be required for finishing and detailing in the second phase of occlusal settlement. Hence, the total treatment time could be even shorter.

Treatment sequence (Figures 11.21, 11.22)
1. Case selection and treatment planning.
   - Prepare complete records.
   - Phase out need for any major pre-functional orthodontic treatment or the possibility of simultaneous tooth movement with active phase.

- Record bite – advance mandible to edge-to-edge position for bite registration.
2. Active phase.
  - Appliance issue and follow-up.
  - Acrylic trimming for selective eruption of teeth for bite opening and sagittal molar correction.

Figure 11.21A–C Guides for trimming of molar blocks in the twin block appliance that allow eruption of the molars into a Class I relationship.

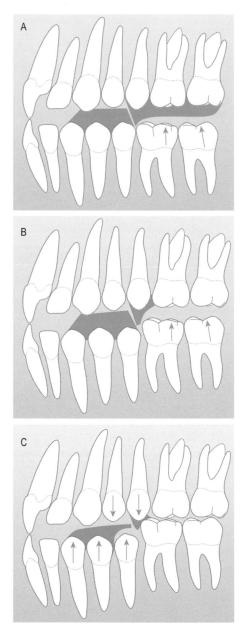

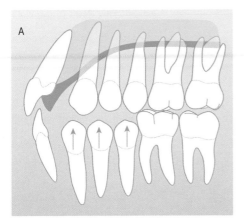

Figure 11.22 A, B The modified biteplate that maintains mandibular repositioning and allows settling of the buccal segments.

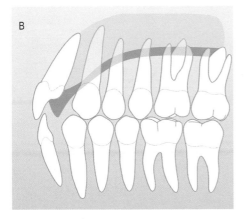

3. Support phase.
   - The modified acrylic biteplate holds the mandible forward.
4. Finishing and detailing with fixed appliances.

Instructions for patients wearing Clark's twin block appliance

- The appliance should be worn 24 hours per day except for cleaning and sport including swimming.
- The key to success is eating with the appliance as this enhances the adaptation of the muscles and ligaments of the temporomandibular joints as the mandible is protrusion.
- The usual length of treatment is 12 months, and this is usually followed by a second phase of treatment to detail the interdigitation of the upper and lower teeth.

References and further reading

Crowding
Becker A, Kurnei-R'em RM 1992 The effects of infra occlusion: Part I. Tilting of the adjacent teeth and local space loss. American Journal of Orthodontics and Dentofacial Orthopedics 102:256–264

Bolton WA 1962 The clinical application of a tooth-size analysis. American Journal of Orthodontics 48:504–529

Irwin RD, Herold JS, Richardson A 1995 Mixed dentition analysis: a review of methods and their accuracy. Internation Journal of Paediatric Dentistry 5:137–142

Moorres CFA, Chadha JM 1965 Available space for the incisors during dental development: a growth study based on physiological age. Angle Orthodontist 35:12–22

Papandreas SG, Buschang PH 1993 Physiologic drift of the mandibular dentition following first premolar extractions. Angle Orthodontist 63:127–134

Staley RN, Kerber PE 1980 A revision of the Hixon and Oldfather mixed dentition prediction method. American Journal of Orthodontics 78:296–302

Tanaka MM, Johnston LE 1974 The prediction of the size of unerupted canines and premolars in a contemporary orthodontic population. Journal of the American Dental Association 88:798–801

Space management

Brennan MM, Gianelly AA 2000 The use of the lingual arch in the mixed dentition to resolve incisor crowding. American Journal of Orthodontics and Dentofacial Orthopedics 117:81–85

Wright GW, Kennedy DB 1978 Space control in the primary and mixed dentitions. Dental Clinics of North America 22:579–601

Timed extraction

Dale J 1994 Interceptive guidance of occlusion, with emphasis on diagnosis. In: Graber TM, Vanarsdall RL, eds. Orthodontics, current principles and techniques, 2nd edn. Mosby, Philadelphia

Gianelly AA 1994 Crowding: timing of treatment. Angle Orthodontist 64:415–418

Jacobs S 1987 A reassessment of serial extraction. Australian Orthodontic Journal 10:90–96

Jacobs SG 1992 Reducing the incidence of palatally impacted maxillary canines by extraction of deciduous canines. A useful preventive/interceptive orthodontic procedure. Australian Dental Journal 37:6–11

Little RM 1987 The effects of eruption guidance and serial extraction on the developing dentition. Pediatric Dentistry 9:65–70

Mackie IC, Blinkhorn AS, Davies PHJ 1989 The extraction of permanent molars during the mixed-dentition period – a guide to treatment planning. Journal of Paediatric Dentistry 5:85–92

Ectopic eruption

Brearley LJ, McKibben DH 1973 Ankylosis of primary molar teeth. I. Prevalence and characteristics. Journal of Dentistry for Children 40:54–63

Ericson S, Kurol J 1988 Early treatment of palatally impacted maxillary canines by extraction of the primary canines. European Journal of Orthodontics 10:283–295

Jacobs SJ 2000 Radiographic localization of unerupted teeth: further findings about the vertical tube shift method and other localization techniques. American Journal of Orthodontics and Dentofacial Orthopedics 118:439–447

Power SM, Short MBE 1993 An investigation into the response of palatally displaced maxillary canines to the removal of deciduous canines and an assessment of factors contributing to favourable eruption. British Journal of Orthodontics 20:215–223

Proffit WR, Vig KWL 1981 Primary failure of eruption. American Journal of Orthodontics 80:173–190

Southall PJ, Graveley JF 1989 Vertical parallax radiography to localize an object in the anterior part of the maxilla. British Journal of Orthodontics 16:79–83

Maxillary expansion

Bishara SE, Staley RN 1987 Maxillary expansion: clinical implications. American Journal of Orthodontics and Dentofacial Orthopedics 91:3–14

Fricker JP 2000 Early intervention: the mixed dentition. Annals of the Royal Australasian College of Dental Surgery 15:124–126

Glineur R, Boucher C, Balon-Perin A 2006 Interceptive treatments (ages 6–10) of transverse deformities: posterior crossbite. L'Orthodontie Française 77:249–252

Kennedy DB, Osepchook M 2000 Unilateral posterior crossbite with mandibular shift: a review. Journal of the Canadian Dental Association 17:569–573

Thilander B, Wahlund S, Lennartsson B 1984 The effect of early interceptive treatment in children with posterior cross-bite. European Journal of Orthodontics 6:25–34

Digit sucking

Larsen E 1987 The effect of dummy sucking on the occlusion: a review. European Journal of Orthodontics 8:127–130

Mitchell EA, Taylor BJ, Ford RP et al 1993 Dummies and the sudden infant death syndrome. Archives of Disease in Children 68:501–504

Oulis CJ, Vadiakas GP, Ekonomides J et al 1994 The effect of hypertrophic adenoids and tonsils on the development of posterior crossbite and oral habits. Journal of Clinical Pediatric Dentistry 18:197–201

Functional appliances

Bishara SE, Ziaja RR 1989 Functional appliances: a review. American Journal of Orthodontics and Dentofacial Orthopedics 95:250–258

Clark WJ 1988 The twinblock technique. American Journal of Orthodontics and Dentofacial Orthopedics 93:1–18

Twelftree CC 1998 Functional appliances. In: Fricker JP, ed. Orthodontics and dentofacial orthopaedics. Tidbinbilla, Canberra

12 Management of cleft lip and palate

Contributors

Nigel M King, Julie Reid, Roger K Hall

Introduction

Cleft lip and cleft palate are fusion disorders that affect the midfacial skeleton. The aetiology, although often unknown, may be genetic, teratogenic or inherited. Clefting may occur in isolation or as a feature of around 300 different syndromes (Shah & Wong 1980). Cleft palate, with or without cleft lip, is one of the more common congenital malformations in humans.

Although many factors have been associated with this condition, from a practical preventive aspect the aetiology remains undetermined. The incidence varies worldwide between 0.8 and 2.7 cases per 1000 live births and is affected by region, gender, ethnicity and maternal characteristics. Racial differences are apparent with native Americans having the highest incidence (followed by Maoris, Chinese, Anglo Saxons) and African Americans the lowest (Vanderas 1987). The offspring of patients with a cleft lip have an increased risk of 1 in 20 of having a clefting condition. If other siblings or close relatives also have clefts, then the frequency is 1 in 6 (Bixler 1981).

More recent Scandinavian studies have claimed to show a rise in incidence of the cleft condition. The authors have proposed several contributory factors such as decreased neonatal mortality, the use of some medications during pregnancy (i.e. retinoic acids) and an increase in intermarriage and childbirth in people with the cleft conditions.

Clefting disorders are now increasingly diagnosed prenatally at the routine first trimester ultrasound screen (at 18–20 weeks); 80–100% of mothers-to-be in all developed countries have an antenatal ultrasound screen and this is becoming universal. The identification or suspicion of a cleft at this examination may be followed by three-dimensional magnetic resonance imaging (MRI) examination at 22–26 weeks in major hospitals, for confirmation and additional information. The diagnostic accuracy is not greatly different between ultrasonography (80%) and MRI (88%) for complete clefts of lip and palate. Partial lip clefts present the greatest difficulty in ultrasound diagnosis with only 26% accuracy, and isolated palate clefts are only rarely diagnosed by ultrasound, depending on the fetal position and an open mouth (yawning) at the time of examination. Where suspected however, an MRI will be done because of the high frequency of syndromes and other anomalies associated with isolated cleft palate.

The incidence of delivered babies with clefts is decreasing in some countries where mothers are making the choice of having a medical termination of the pregnancy following diagnosis of a cleft. Even where termination is not acceptable, prenatal screening provides knowledge of the impending birth of a baby with a cleft, which allows both the family to prepare for this event and forward medical planning for the delivery and subsequent special neonatal care. In Victoria, Australia, for the year 2003–2004, pregnancy outcome figures for cleft lip and palate show that 3% were stillborn or neonatal deaths and 20% of pregnancies were terminated (7% <20 weeks and 13% >20 weeks). For cleft lip, terminations were 8% with 2% stillbirths; for isolated cleft palate, terminations were 9% and neonatal deaths 4%, reflecting the greater difficulty in ultrasound diagnosis for these groups and perhaps also maternal perception that these were less serious defects, more easily repaired.

Often in the past, many children born with cleft lip and palate conditions received inadequate care as a result of diagnostic errors, failure of recognition of the full spectrum of problems, and the use of inappropriate or ill-timed procedures. Although cleft lip and palate is a single anomaly, its consequences affect numerous systems and functions that include facial growth, the dentition, speech and language, hearing and genetics. The inevitable social and psychological impact on the child, their parents and the family, must also be considered. To avoid these problems, specialists, throughout the world, have elected to form multidisciplinary teams to manage children with cleft lip and palate. Consequently, the team is exposed to a sufficient number of patients each year to maintain clinical expertise, and is thus well prepared to provide care for new cases. The specialities of the team usually include plastic surgery, maxillofacial or craniofacial surgery, dentistry (paediatric dental, orthodontic and oral surgical care, etc.), ENT surgery, audiology, speech pathology, psychology, nursing and social services. In some cases, genetics, ophthalmology and neurosurgery are also involved.

To better understand the characteristics of the various types of clefts of the lip and palate and the implications it is proposed to first review the resulting anatomy. The management and thus the roles of various specialists will then be considered.

The anatomy of the facial skeleton in cleft lip and palate

Clefts of the lip and palate may be unilateral or bilateral, complete or incomplete. The presentation of clefting conditions can be categorized into the following groups.

Clefts of the lip and alveolus (primary palate)

These may vary from an incomplete cleft (forme fruste) to a minimal defect involving just the vermilion border, to a complete defect extending from the vermilion border to the floor of the nose with clefting of the alveolus. The primary palate forms anterior to the incisive foramen. The defect may also exist as a Simonart band which is a fine strip of soft tissue connecting both sides of the cleft.

The nasal alar cartilage on the side of the cleft is displaced and flattened to a greater or lesser degree, depending on the extent and width of the cleft. The tip of the nose tends to deviate to the non-cleft side.

The cleft may be unilateral or bilateral and the latter may be symmetrical or asymmetrical in extent. In bilateral clefts the median portion of the lip contains the philtrum and is attached to the columella and the premaxilla. In humans, except for a brief period in the early embryo, the 'premaxilla' does not exist as separate entity. The term is retained with reference to cleft lip and palate conditions, however, due to its descriptive convenience and homology with experimental animals. The term 'premaxilla,' therefore, refers to that portion of the maxilla anterior to the incisive foramen and mesial to the canine teeth. The columella appears deficient and the alar cartilages are flattened on both sides.

Unilateral cleft lip and palate

Varying degrees of clefting in the lip and palate can exist, in a wide range of combinations. In complete clefts, a direct communication exists between the oral and nasal cavities on the cleft side (Figure 12.1A). There can be substantial variation in the degree of palatal shelf separation.

Premaxillary segment and nasal septum

The premaxillary segment in the frontal view, tilts upward into the cleft. The cartilaginous nasal septum is also bent in the same direction. The nostril on the non-cleft side is constricted and may be functionally occluded. This constriction is due to a combination of deviation of the nasal septum and approximation of the alar base and columella. The alar of the cleft side is usually stretched and flattened.

The lip and columella

The anatomy of the orbicularis oris muscle is disrupted. The muscle fibres proceed horizontally from the corner of the mouth toward the midline and turn upward along the margins of the cleft. The muscle fibres terminate beneath the alar base in the

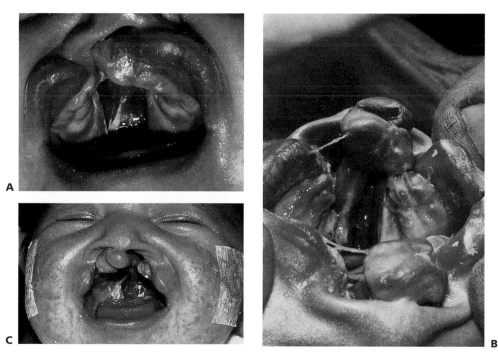

Figure 12.1 A Unilateral complete cleft lip and palate, showing the extent of the malformation in the palate. **B** Bilateral complete cleft lip and palate. The premaxillary segment is clearly visible as an extension of the nasal septum. The central incisors are contained within this process. **C** Anterior view of a child with a bilateral complete cleft of the lip and palate. The columella and philtrum are extremely short and there is a wide defect between the segments.

lateral segment and beneath the columella in the medial segment. Most fibres attach to the periosteum of the maxilla, but a few blend into the subepithelium. Where the cleft is less than two-thirds of the lip height, the muscle fibres above the level of the cleft remain intact. A protrusion of excess muscle may be seen and palpated on the lateral aspect of the cleft, due to heaping up of the disrupted fibres. The medial segment tends to be underdeveloped.

Vomer and palatal process

The palatal segment on the cleft side is often tilted medially and superiorly into the cleft. The vomer is deviated laterally at its line of attachment to the palatal process of the non-cleft side. This deviation may be so severe in some cases that the vomer assumes a nearly horizontal position at its inferior margin.

Bilateral cleft lip and palate

Clefting can be either symmetrical or asymmetrical. In the bilateral complete cleft lip and palate, both nasal chambers are in direct communication with the oral cavity. The palatal processes are divided into two equal parts and the turbinates are clearly visible within both nasal cavities. The nasal septum forms a midline structure that is firmly attached to the base of the skull but is fairly mobile anteriorly, where it supports the premaxilla and columella (Figure 12.1B).

Premaxilla

There is a malformation of the premaxilla characterized by its protrusion relative to the nasal septum. The columella is usually non-existent, with the lip attaching directly to the nasal tip. The basal bone of the premaxilla articulates with the cartilaginous nasal septum superiorly and the vomer posteriorly. In normal structure the alveolar process of the premaxilla is inferior to the basal component. However, in the bilateral cleft condition the alveolar component is anterior to the basal component, in horizontal arrangement. In these clefts, the premaxilla protrudes considerably forward of the facial profile and is attached to a stalk-like vomer and the nasal septum.

The lip and columella

The lip moiety in the medial segment contains only collagenous connective tissue. It is, therefore, grossly deficient in bulk and lacks the features normally produced by muscle (Figure 12.1C).

Although the columella would appear to be absent clinically, in anatomical terms it may be present in that the medial crura of the alar cartilages appear to occupy a normal position relative to the tip of the nose and the nasal septum. There is a deficiency of columellar skin, however, which complicates the re-establishment of normal anatomical relations during treatment.

The maxillary arch form generally appears normal at birth, but medial collapse of the maxillary segments occurs soon after. The medial aspects of the palatal processes are often tilted superiorly into the cleft.

Cleft palate

The cleft may involve only the soft palate, both soft and hard palates, but almost never the hard palate alone. Deficiency of mucosa and bone are the main features of clefts of the hard palate (Figure 12.2). The cleft may extend forward from the uvula to

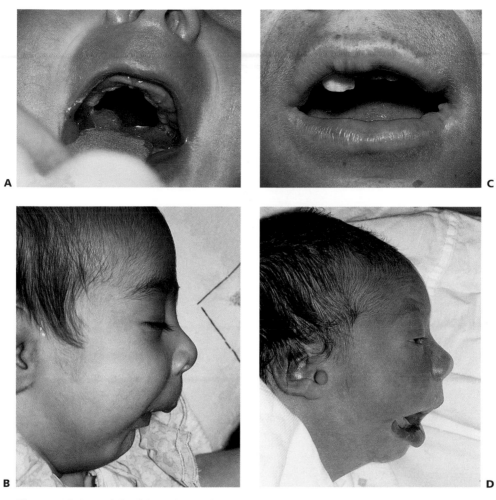

Figure 12.2 A Cleft of the palate with an intact lip and alveolus. This U-shaped cleft was associated with the Robin sequence and resulted from a failure of embryonic head rotation. This maintained the tongue in the oral cavity and the palatal shelves subsequently formed around the tongue, giving rise to the characteristic cleft shape. **B** Another manifestation of this condition is extreme micrognathia. The Robin sequence may also be associated with transverse clefts of the face. These transverse clefts may be rather subtle as demonstrated in **C**, or severe as in **D**. This latter patient has a first and second branchial arch deformity associated with Goldenhar's syndrome. Note the preauricular skin tag.

varying degrees, from a bifid uvula (Figure 12.3) to a 'V'-shaped cleft extending through the hard palate to the incisive foramen.

A 'U'-shaped cleft palate is seen in babies with Robin sequence (Figure 12.2). This is thought to be secondary to mandibular hypoplasia in the first trimester which causes the tongue to sit high in the mouth and prevent fusion of the palatal shelves.

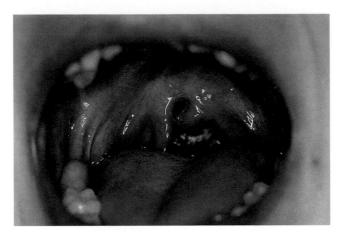

Figure 12.3 A bifid uvula associated with a submucous cleft palate. The fibres of tensor palati are not joined although the epithelium is intact. These children may present with nasal air escape due to a shortened palate a velopharyngeal incompetence. There is often a notch felt at the posterior border of the hard palate and a bluish median line extends to the uvula.

Submucous cleft palate

Clefting of the velum can be 'submucous' where the mucous membrane remains intact despite clefting of the underlying musculature. Submucous cleft palate occurs in around 1 in 1200 live births with only half of the cases having clinically significant symptoms. These clefts may present with:

- Bifid uvula (Figure 12.3).
- Zona pellucida (a very thin membranous portion of the soft palate).
- Abnormal insertion of velar musculature.
- Resultant palpable notch at the junction of the soft and hard palates.

Where there are no discernible anomalies on oral examination in the presence of a submucous cleft, the appropriate diagnoses is occult submucous cleft palate. In submucous cleft palate the levator musculature are aberrantly inserted onto the bony free edge of the hard palate rather than forming a muscular sling. Surgery is needed to restore the normal transverse position and function for speech and swallowing.

Current concepts of cleft management

The need for treatment

- Feeding difficulties usually due to lack of suction and in some cases lack of compression. Nasal regurgitation is often seen during feeding.
- Facial aesthetics.
- Speech and language delay.
- Speech problems associated with poor velopharyngeal closure and/or oro-nasal fistulae.
- Chronic middle-ear problems due to eustachian tube dysfunction.

- Malocclusion.
- Disruption of skeletal growth of the facial structures due to surgical intervention.

It is worth noting that general growth of the maxilla and the midface does not appear to be adversely affected in those cleft patients left untreated until physical maturity. However, the need for surgical interventional is dictated by functional and social pressures.

The cleft palate team

Treatment is generally undertaken in a coordinated interdisciplinary 'team' environment with a team leader. Cleft palate teams are located in the major paediatric hospitals throughout the world. A typical cleft palate team comprises:

- Plastic surgeons.
- Paediatric dentists.
- Orthodontists.
- Speech pathologists.
- Maxillofacial surgeons.
- Paediatricians.
- ENT surgeons.
- Nurses.
- Social workers.
- A team coordinator.

Other specialists, such as geneticists, periodontists, implantologists, and prosthodontists who are consulted as required in individual cases.

While there are many variations in techniques, sequencing and timing of treatment, there are, some commonly accepted aims and principles of treatment (Table 12.1). The appropriate specialists within a team aim to provide a rapid initial evaluation, often within hours of birth. Subsequent regular contact with family members through frequent review clinics ensures that social and psychological problems are identified and resolved early. Treatment plans can then be formulated and implemented in collaboration with fellow specialists. Regular follow-up appointments enable the accumulation of data on the outcome of clinical procedures, the psychological wellbeing of the patients, the effects of treatment on growth, postoperative function and appearance, which must then be used to help future patients under the care of that team.

Aims of cleft treatment

The ultimate goal is to attain normal form and function (especially speech and mastication) with the least possible damage to growth and development through surgical intervention.

Specific treatment objectives are:

- Provide a long mobile palate capable of completely closing off the oropharynx from the nasopharynx.
- Produce a full upper lip with a symmetrical cupid's bow and reconstruction of the columella and the alar architecture of the nose.
- Achieve an intact, well-aligned dental arch with a stable inter-arch occlusion.
- Provide a pleasing facial appearance.

Table 12.1 Protocols for total dental management of children with cleft lip and palate

Age	Paediatric dental	Orthodontic	General practitioner	Surgical
Birth	Initial contact and interview with parents Registration with Cleft Palate Scheme Arrange contact with parental support groups	Construction of presurgical orthopaedic appliance, if required		Initial assessment
3–5 months	Initial contact, if not at birth Introduce dental care plan Study models at time of lip repair			Primary surgical repair of lip
12 months	Review			Surgical repair of palate
2–6 years	12-monthly reviews for assessment of growth and development, caries and preventive advice		Initial visit – then 6 monthly for preventive advice, topical fluoride applications and fissure sealing	Possible revision of lip repair Pharyngoplasty if required Myringotomy and grommets by ENT
6–7 years	Fissure sealing of first permanent molars Composite resin restoration of hypoplastic teeth adjacent to cleft Preventive advice		Fissure sealing of first permanent molars Composite resin restoration of hypoplastic teeth adjacent cleft Preventive advice	Myringotomy and grommets by ENT as required
8–10 years	Case conference with surgical and orthodontic teams for bone grafting	Assessment for maxillary expansion prior to bone grafting Skeletal age assessments	6 monthly reviews Possible extractions of erupted supernumerary teeth Interim bridge or partial denture	Bone grafting at half to two-thirds root development of canine
11–12 years	Retention of palatal expansion		6-monthly reviews	
12–15 years	12-monthly review	Full fixed appliance treatment	Fissure sealing of bicuspids and second molars	Review and possible surgical revision if required
16–17 years	Restoration of teeth adjacent to the cleft Referral to general practitioner	Retention after orthodontic treatment	Restoration of teeth in the cleft region, including crowns, bridges, implants, dentures	Assessment of the need for orthognathic surgery

Adapted from Hall (1986).

Management of cleft lip and palate

When a baby is born with cleft lip and/or palate, the services of a team of specialists are needed from infancy until early adulthood. During that time, a number of primary and secondary surgical procedures need to be performed, each being preceded by a period of presurgical preparation of the child. Careful planning by the team members is essential to ensure that any proposed procedure is appropriate and that the timing of that procedure is in keeping with the overall development of the child. The management of children with cleft lip and palate can be considered on a chronological basis.

Cleft management in the neonatal period

Soon after birth, the parents need to be counselled about the intermediate and long-term implications of the cleft defect and the necessary surgery if this has not already been done following prenatally diagnosis.

Feeding

Efficient feeding is important for growth and development in infancy. A baby with a cleft of any kind may experience feeding difficulties. However, babies with cleft palate or combined cleft lip and palate usually have more problems than those with cleft lip. A cleft palate prevents the baby from sealing the oral cavity and generating the negative pressure necessary for efficient feeding. Babies with large clefts of the lip and palate may also have difficulty generating positive pressure (compression) which is also important for feeding. The early involvement of a feeding specialist from the cleft lip and palate team is essential to offer advice regarding appropriate feeding techniques. Breast-feeding is best for babies and should be encouraged. It is usually unsuccessful when there is a cleft palate therefore bottle feeding (especially using expressed breast milk) may be the most appropriate approach. Nasogastric tube feeding is inappropriate in most cases, although it may be required in those babies with other central disorders.

A simple and effective protocol is as follows:

- A compressible bottle with a cross-cut teat can be used to overcome the baby's lack of suction (and compression).
- Feeding in an upright posture to minimize nasal regurgitation.
- Restricting feeds to 30 minutes so the baby does not burn more energy than it consumes.
- The nipple of the feeding bottle should be positioned on the non-cleft side.
- Specialized feeding plates may be recommended in some centres especially for those infants with wide bilateral complete clefts.

Once the child is feeding well, and is progressively gaining weight, the child will be able to be able to cope with the primary surgery.

Presurgical orthopaedics (Figure 12.4)

The use of presurgical orthopaedics is controversial and varies between different centres. An impression of the maxillary arch is taken as early as 24 hours after birth.

Taking impressions in neonates and infants

When taking impressions in these young children, a fast-setting elastomeric material is superior to alginate. The authors successfully use a polyether bite-registration

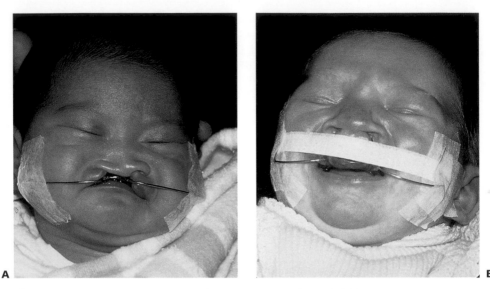

A   B

Figure 12.4 A Presurgical orthopaedic appliance. The plate is held by micropore tape to the cheeks. **B** Strapping aids in the positioning of the labial segments, especially in cases of bilateral complete clefts. Depending on the institution, these appliances are used in cases of bilateral cleft lip and those with very wide unilateral clefts as shown in **A**.

material for this purpose. Clinicians should be aware of the danger of alginate breaking on removal from undercut areas of the oronasal structures. For taking of impression:
- Place the child in a stabilized supine position.
- Extend the head with the feet elevated.
- Suction must be available.
- The impression should not be taken after a feed.
- Assistance should always be available.
  A passive acrylic appliance is constructed as in Figure 12.4 with the aim of:
- Normalizing oral function in regard to tongue posture.
- The presurgical orthopaedic appliance does not restore ability to generate negative intra-oral pressure but does provide a surface for the tongue to appose during feeding.
- Re-approximating grossly divergent maxillary segments to facilitate the primary repair.
  With bilateral cleft palates, the plates help prevent collapse of the buccal segments of the palate, if delayed closure of the hard palate is planned. These appliances need to be made by a specialist and fitted as soon as possible after birth to ensure their acceptance by the neonate.

Counselling and parent support

Careful counselling by an empathetic specialist is needed by the parents at this early stage (Young et al 2001). This is probably the first time that they have seen an unrepaired cleft of the lip or palate. It must be remembered, however, that parents have not had the benefit of a medical education and are usually unable to understand anatomical and medical terminology. They want to know about their child's problems and will certainly be confused and anxious. It is most important that they are attended by a team members who are both supportive and able to provide accurate information in a sympathetic manner, and in terms that can be understood by the parents. While this counselling must be done in a sympathetic manner, it must also be authoritative (King 1986). Parents will also often appreciate and benefit from the assistance available from members of a parent support group.

Timing of surgery

- Many surgical techniques have been described for the primary closure of cleft lip and palate. Unfortunately, there is still controversy regarding the precise timing of surgery and which is the most reliable technique that is consistent with ensuring optimal growth of the face and development of speech.
- **Lip repair** is generally undertaken at 10–12 weeks and almost certainly by 6 months of age, provided the infant is otherwise developing well.
- The timing of lip repair is less controversial than is palate repair and aims to restore the continuity of the orbicularis oris muscle of the lip, and with it, the appearance and notion of the upper lip (Figure 12.5). Recently introduced techniques that include the additional re-attachment of the muscles at the base of the nose have improved both the aesthetic result as well as the growth potential of the midface.
- **Palate repair** aims to reconstruct the abnormally inserted musculature of the soft palate to normalize movements of the soft palate and permit the development of normal speech. The extent and timing of palatal surgery is one of the major and continuing controversies in cleft management and relates to the perceived balance between the benefits of good speech development versus the deleterious effects on midfacial growth through surgical trauma and associated scarring.
- Depending on the institution, 'early' closure is carried out prior to the development of speech, between 6 and 18 months of age. It is likely to disturb the subsequent growth of the midface.

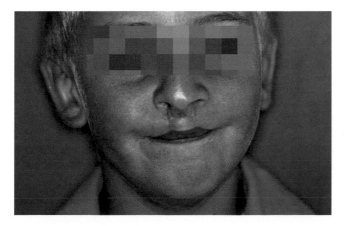

Figure 12.5 Surgical repair of a bilateral complete cleft lip with columella lengthening. The alar base is symmetrical although there is an accentuation of the cupid's bow and eversion of the vermillion border.

- 'Delayed' repair minimizes the growth disturbance but has a negative influence on speech development.
- Thus, a compromise is required which may be either:
  - to repair the palate late, but before speech patterns develop at approximately 2 years of age or,
  - to repair the soft palate only at the time of lip repair, leaving the hard palate open for later closure and using an acrylic plate in the meantime.

Cleft management in childhood

Speech and language problems

Children with clefts and other craniofacial malformations are at an increased risk of speech and language difficulties. Regular assessments are required to monitor the speech and language acquisition process, to assist in making surgical decisions and to provide therapy interventions.

During childhood, care needs to be exercised to ensure hearing is optimal for speech and language development. Otitis media is common in infants and children with cleft palate and some may have sensorineural loss as well. It is important to differentially diagnose any speech and language problems so that appropriate treatment can be arranged. The possible causes of communication problems in this group include:

- Developmental delay.
- Hearing problems.
- Oronasal fistulae.
- Dental malocclusion.
- Velopharyngeal incompetence (VPI).

Pharyngoplasty

Children with clefts are at increased risk of hypernasality and nasal air escape during speech. The speech pathologist's assessment of speech production is critical in the identification and management of this problem. This may involve simple clinical tests such as the mirror fogging test or more objective measures of velopharyngeal function during speech such as nasometry nasendoscopy or videofluoroscopy. These instrumental procedures assist the cleft palate team in planning surgery to improve velopharyngeal closure.

- If significant VPI is identified then surgery is usually needed. Velopharyngeal narrowing can be achieved using either a pharyngeal flap or sphincter pharyngoplasty. Alternatively, lengthening the palate by repositioning the velum using techniques such as intravelar veloplasty or a Furlow z-plasty may be indicated. Minor defects of the velopharyngeal sphincter can be improved with fat augmentation of the posterior pharyngeal wall and/or the soft palate. The assessment and surgical correction for VPI should ideally be performed before the age of 6 years. This is generally followed by a period of speech therapy based on several established principles. Although surgery (velopharyngeal narrowing and the closure of palatal fistulae) can be expected to improve structural obstacles which hinder the development of normal speech, postoperative speech therapy will still be needed to correct poor speech habits that have developed because of the structural malformation.

- Sometimes surgical correction of VPI is not possible. In this case a palatal obturator or a speech bulb may reduce the velopharyngeal space sufficiently for normal speech to develop.

General dental care
- Both preventive and therapeutic care is essential during childhood to minimize morbidity due to the loss of teeth.
- Oral hygiene instruction.
- Prophylactic measures to prevent the development of dental caries and periodontal disease.
- Restorative treatment to repair carious or malformed teeth.

Orthodontics
Isolated clefts of the lip and soft palate do not generally involve any dental deformity although in the latter case, growth retardation of the maxilla and consequent skeletal Class III jaw relation may occur as a result of postsurgical scarring. Where the hard palate is also involved, there is a greater likelihood of growth retardation and maxillary constriction in the buccal segments with an associated buccal crossbite.

Complete clefts of the lip and palate may require extensive orthodontic treatment, from shortly after birth in some cases, until physical maturity.

The first orthodontic referral is made routinely at 8 years of age, unless the child has been seen as a baby for presurgical orthopaedics. In such cases, the child can be reviewed with the paediatric dental appointments. In certain circumstances of incisor crossbite or other incisor relationship problems, it may be necessary to request an earlier orthodontic referral, at around 7 years of age, for correction of this problem; however, in most instances, the simple treatment involved comes within the province of normal paediatric dental care (i.e. palatal expansion). Orthodontic management in this instance can be divided into three stages.

Mixed dentition treatment (Figure 12.6)
Treatment may involve:
- Interceptive treatment such as minor tooth alignment to facilitate anterior alignment.
- Palatal expansion prior to alveolar bone grafting which may be a relatively short period of fixed appliance therapy to obtain optimal arch shape or to improve access for surgery. Expansion is commenced approximately 12 months prior to any alveolar bone grafting. Such grafting is usually undertaken when the cleft-side permanent canine tooth shows between half and two-thirds root development (Figure 12.7). The appliance is maintained for 4–6 months post-graft for stability, at which time it may be replaced with a passive retainer.
- Dentofacial orthopaedic appliances for children with grossly abnormal jaw development.

Secondary alveolar bone grafting (Figure 12.7)
Bone grafting should be timed to precede the eruption of the permanent canine tooth on the cleft side, which usually occurs at approximately 11 years of age. The aim of bone grafting is to:

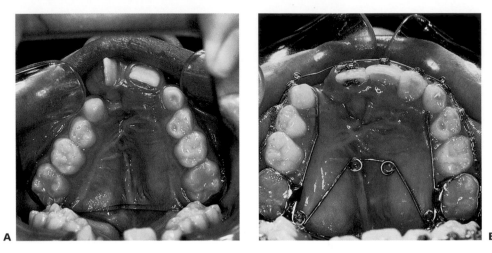

A   B

Figure 12.6 A One of the effects of early surgery and scarring is collapse of the palatal segments due to an inhibition of growth. Rotation of the central incisor adjacent the cleft can also be seen. **B** Palatal expansion with a quad helix appliance to correct the posterior crossbite and open space for the bone graft.

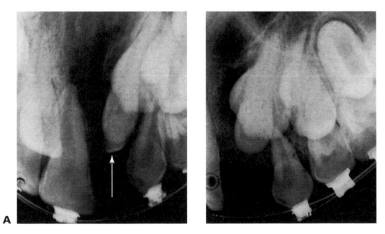

A

Figure 12.7 A Periapical radiograph of a cleft prior to bone grafting. The lateral incisor is present on the palatal aspect of the canine tooth. A small supernumerary tooth (arrowed) is also present, and was removed at the time of surgery. **B** The cleft has been filled with cancellous bone, harvested from the iliac crest. After 3 months there is already movement of the lateral and canine and both these teeth erupted through the graft to the mouth, where they were aligned orthodontically.

- Restore the bony contour of the alveolus.
- Stabilize the maxillary expansion.
- Provides a matrix through which teeth (especially the canine) may erupt.
- To allow to the teeth to have a healthy supporting periodontium.

Although some centres advocate bone grafting of the maxillary alveolar defect at the time of primary lip repair, the majority of teams do this as a secondary procedure, either 'early', before the eruption of the permanent lateral incisor or later, prior to eruption of the permanent canine tooth. The object here is to have these teeth erupting through and consolidating the bone graft.

Surgery
- Presurgical palatal expansion (if required) with fixed appliances such as a quad helix (Figure 12.6B).
- Preparation of recipient area is prepared by extraction of retained primary teeth several weeks prior to surgery.
- Bone harvest for the graft is usually autologous iliac crest cortico-cancellous bone, but may be obtained from the mandibular symphysis, tibia, rib, or calvarium.
- The procedure may include revision of lip and/or palate repair if necessary and will definitively close any remaining fistulae.

Clinical experience has shown that the timing of the operation, preoperative gingival health and careful tissue and graft handling during the surgical procedure are more important in determining the success of the operation than the anatomical source of the bone graft (Samman et al 1994).

Cleft management in adolescence and early adulthood

Orthodontics
Full permanent dentition correction
Once the full permanent dentition is established (excluding the third molars), final tooth alignment and interdigitation is undertaken. In the mixed dentition, only the minimum of active orthodontic treatment if any, is done, leaving the bulk of the orthodontic treatment to be carried out in the shortest possible time when the full permanent dentition is present.

- At 12–16 years dental suitability and motivation to cooperate with orthodontic treatment is assessed prior to the commencement of full fixed appliance treatment.
- Rapid palatal expansion and/or fixed appliance orthodontic treatment is undertaken at the optimum time – occasionally elective extraction of teeth for orthodontic reasons is indicated.
- Further orthodontics in conjunction with orthognathic surgery may be required in the event of a significant skeletal dysplasia.
- Definitive orthodontic treatment once active skeletal growth has ceased.
- Presurgical and postsurgical orthodontics in conjunction with orthognathic surgery.

Orthognathic surgery

If a maxillary/mandibular skeletal discrepancy exists at the time of physical maturity an osteotomy may be required along with any further soft-tissue revision which is also undertaken at the same time if needed.

- A Le Fort I osteotomy with modification may be performed to correct the occlusion and facial appearance (Tideman et al 1980).
- More severe skeletal deformities require a staged procedure involving a Le Fort II, and subsequently, a Le Fort I osteotomy and frequently, an additional mandibular procedure.

When a patient is referred late, and has not had the benefit of bone grafting at the optimal time, the osteotomies may be combined with the alveolar bone grafting as a single-stage procedure. If necessary, an aesthetic rhinoplasty, and cheiloplasty should be performed as a final surgical stage. Occasionally, however, functional lip and nose revision is combined with alveolar bone grafting at an earlier stage to reduce the impact of the aesthetic deformity on the growing child and to take advantage of the remaining growth potential in the midface.

The above procedures are only some of the many that are needed by a patient with cleft lip and palate. The acquisition of the clinical skills required to treat affected children, and the need to regularly practise them, are essential if the care that is to be delivered is to be of a sufficiently high quality.

Importance of dental care in overall management

Children with cleft conditions require extensive interdisciplinary care throughout early life and the highest standard of oral health must be maintained because the presence of dental disease can severely compromise both surgical and orthodontic success. Therefore, the specific role of paediatric dentists will be emphasized here because they are effective coordinators of multidisciplinary care. It is essential that the paediatric dentist, or their representative, reviews the child with a cleft lip and palate at least every 6 months.

Initial consultation

Examination of baby

The baby is examined and a record made of the type of cleft or other deformity present and the relation of the lip, alveolar and palatal clefts (i.e. arch form etc.) with a note of any collapse of segments, distortion of premaxilla, etc. Any erupted teeth are charted and a note made of any natal or neonatal teeth in the cleft or other regions.

The parent interview

If the parents are not present when the baby is examined, a separate appointment must be made with them. The parent interview is one of the most important aspect of the initial consultation.

The approach in speaking to parents at this consultation should be relaxed and informative – a mostly 'getting to know you' introduction of the dental team as a preparation for later visits. It must be remembered that because of the emotional impact of the facial abnormality on the mother, father and family, they may not be fully receptive to advice at this early visit or remember much of what is said. At this interview it is important to explain:

- The dental aspects of the clefting process.
- The likely course of dental management. The involvement of different specialties including restorative, radiological, orthodontic and possible later oral surgical care.
- The probability of the absence of the normal tooth in the region of the cleft, and conversely the possibility of one or more supernumerary teeth in the cleft region should be mentioned (Figure 12.8).
- The likelihood of the presence of crown and/or root morphologic abnormalities and enamel hypoplasia of the incisor and canine teeth adjacent to the cleft should be indicated with the positive reassurance that these can be treated relatively simply soon after they appear.
- The absolute importance of sound preventive care and regular dental visits should be emphasized.

It will almost certainly be necessary to reinforce the introductory information and advice given at this visit at many subsequent outpatient visits over the years of treatment. Many cleft palate clinics produce parent handbooks that are particularly useful.

Medical history

A full medical history must be taken at this time. Many clefts are merely one component in one of the 300 'clefting syndromes' (Figure 12.9) – and is it quite common for other congenital abnormalities to be present in addition to the cleft (e.g. congenital heart disease).

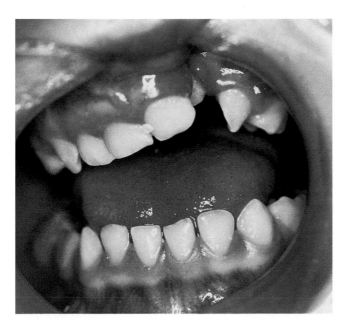

Figure 12.8 A tooth erupting in the cleft. Such teeth often become carious, but should be repaired and retained until bone grafting is performed. Where permanent teeth are congenitally absent, especially the lateral incisor, the supernumerary may be used if of adequate size.

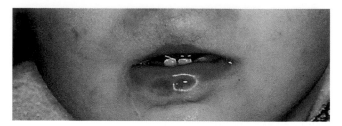

Figure 12.9 There are over 300 syndromes of the head and neck which manifest clefting. Congenital lip pits and hypodontia are seen in van der Woude syndrome and, although uncommon, are an important malformation associated with clefting of the palate.

Dental records
- Photographs should be taken at all major review visits.
- Periodically dental impressions should be taken.
- An initial screening panoramic radiograph is useful at 5–6 years of age (or earlier if pathology is present or suspected) and bitewing radiographs to check for dental caries.
- All children should have study models, panoramic, bitewing and lateral cephalometric radiographs at 8–9 years of age.

Role of the paediatric dentist
The role of the paediatric dentist is one of coordinator. Between the ages of 12 and 18 months the child should be seen by the paediatric dentist at regular intervals no greater than 12 months. In Australia, the child is enrolled in the Cleft Palate Scheme at the first visit. This scheme provides government health benefits to be paid for orthodontic, surgical and some general dental treatment. Parental support groups such as Cleft Pals are present in many countries and contact should be arranged as soon as possible with these organizations.

First follow-up visit
- Dental charting is carried out including a record of the time of eruption of the first tooth.
- Body growth should be checked and height/weight entered on a growth chart. (Details can be obtained from the child's health record book.)

These visits are essential for the general monitoring of growth and development and control of dental disease. Updating of photographic, study model and radiological records will also be done. The paediatric dentist will generally coordinate all dental care aspects with those of other disciplines.

Preventive dental care
Preventive dental care is essential for these patients using all known techniques including:
- Tooth brushing.
- Home application of topical fluoride agents.
- Fissure sealing of both primary and permanent teeth.

- Oral hygiene technique instruction.
- Dietary advice to child and parents by paediatric dentist (or dietitian if necessary).

The prevention of dental caries and periodontal disease will help with cooperation for ultimate definitive orthodontic treatment, by reducing unpleasant visits for treatment in early childhood. Motivation is especially important for later orthodontic treatment in these patients. This should be assessed early, and enhanced during preventive visits during childhood so as to ensure compliance.

General dental practitioner care

The role of the general practitioner is paramount. Children with craniofacial anomalies have significantly greater rates of dental disease, all of which is preventable and will affect the prognosis and course of future treatment. The child should if possible attend a general dental practitioner at 6-monthly intervals for preventive care, dietary advice and oral hygiene technique follow-up, together with routine restorative care if necessary. In addition, the parents should 'agree' to attend the local dentist regularly. One of the most important duties is to establish early contact with the cleft palate team or surgeon and maintain a frequent dialogue.

Dental extractions and minor oral surgery

- Except in an emergency, dental extractions should not be performed for these children by the general dentist without first checking and clearing this with the supervising paediatric dentist or orthodontist.
- Primary molars should be retained by pulpotomy, or the space maintained after extraction as advised by the paediatric dentist.
- Erupted supernumerary teeth should be retained until 6–7 years of age, unless impossible to clean, resulting in progressive dental caries, gingival or mucosal inflammation.

Extraction of such teeth should then, in most cases, be carried out in the supervising hospital under either local or general anaesthetic. If a general anaesthetic is required for restorative treatment of other purpose, superficial or obstructing unerupted supernumerary teeth may be removed at the same time but only after discussion with the coordinating paediatric dentist. If a bone graft is planned for the alveolar cleft, it may be necessary to retain primary teeth that are adjacent to the graft site. This, if done 3–4 weeks prior to the grafting procedure, ensures that the healing of the mucoperiosteal flap is not compromised by leaving a deficiency where the tooth has been extracted at the time of grafting. If the child's behaviour does not permit the extraction of teeth prior to grafting then they may be removed by the maxillofacial or plastic surgeon at the time of bone grafting.

Dental anomalies

Dental anomalies are extremely common in children with orofacial clefting. The most commonly affected tooth is the maxillary lateral incisor on the cleft side. This is due, in part, to disruption of the dental lamina. Anomalies may include:

- Agenesis of teeth.
- Supernumerary teeth.
- Concurrent agenesis and supernumerary teeth within or adjacent the cleft.
- Disorders of morphogenesis (size and shape).

- Supernumerary teeth may occur in either the medial or distal segment and much less frequently in both segments (Figure 12.8).

Cosmetic restoration of malformed anterior teeth and alveolar cleft

The appearance of the teeth should be improved early for these children who may have a poor self-image.

- Composite resin restorations may be placed for hypoplastic or morphologically abnormal permanent incisor teeth adjacent to the cleft(s) soon after eruption, however, enamel-bonded crowns or veneers should be reserved until after passive eruption and establishment of the gingival margin at the cementoenamel junction.
- As a temporary measure, and in suitable cases, a Maryland acid-etch bridge may be placed as a temporary measure. This form of prosthesis is a superior alternative to a removable partial denture. An osseointegrated implant remains the ultimate treatment solution when space cannot be closed orthodontically. Speech may also be improved by the use of fixed prosthodontics.

References and further reading

Abyholm FE, Bergland O, Semb G 1981 Secondary bone grafting of alveolar clefts. Scandinavian Journal of Plastic and Reconstructive Surgery 15:127–140

Bergland O, Semb G, Abyholm FE 1986 Elimination of the residual alveolar cleft by secondary bone grafting and subsequent orthodontic treatment. Cleft Palate Journal 23:175–205

Bixler D 1981 Genetics and clefting. Cleft Palate Journal 18:10–18

Bohn A 1963 Dental anomalies in hare lip and cleft palate. Acta Odontologica Scandinavica 21:(Suppl 38)

Brine EA, Rickard MS, Liechty EA et al 1994 Effectiveness of two feeding methods in improving energy intake and growth of infants with cleft palate: a randomised study. Journal of the American Dietetic Association 94:732–738

Bütow KW 1984 Treatment of cleft lip and palate. Part II: the jaw-orthognathial suction and drinking plate. Journal of the Dental Association of South Africa 39:331–334

El Deeb M, Messer LB, Lehnert MW et al 1982 Canine eruption into grafted bone in maxillary alveolar cleft defects. Cleft Palate Journal 19:9–16

El Deeb M, Hinrichs JE, Waite DE et al 1986 Repair of alveolar clefts with autogenous bone grafting: periodontal evaluation. Cleft Palate Journal 23:126–136

Enemark H, Pederson S 1983 Surgical-orthodontic treatment of severe lateral open bite and cross bite in unilateral cleft lip and palate patients. International Journal of Oral Surgery 12:277

Hall HD, Posnick JC 1983 Early results of secondary bone grafts in 106 alveolar clefts. Journal of Oral and Maxillofacial Surgery 41:289–294

Hall RK 1986 Care of adolescents with cleft lip and palate: the role of the general practitioner. International Journal of Dentistry 36:120–130

Heggie AC, West RA 1988 Co-ordinated treatment of secondary cleft deformities. Australian Dental Journal 33:116–128

Hellquist R, Svardstrom K, Porter B 1983 A longitudinal study of delayed eruption due to the cleft alveolus. Cleft Palate Journal 20:277–288

King NM 1986 Advice to the parents of a neonate with cleft lip and palate. HK Dental Journal 3:186–192

Kinnebrew MC, McTigue DJ 1984 Submucous cleft palate: review and two clinical reports. Pediatric Dentistry 6:252–258

McWilliams BJ, Morris HL, Shelton RL 1990 Patterns of malformation associated with clefting. In: McWilliams BJ, Morris HL, Shelton RL, eds. Cleft palate speech, 2nd edn. Mosby, St Louis: 31–46

Samman N, Cheung LK, Tideman H 1994 A comparison of alveolar bone grafting with and without simultaneous maxillary osteotomies in cleft palate patients. International Journal of Oral and Maxillofacial Surgery 23:65–70

Shah CP, Wong D 1980 Management of children with cleft lip and palate. Canadian Medical Association Journal 122–129

Shaw WC, Bannister RP 1999 Assisted feeding is more reliable for infants with clefts: a randomised trial. Cleft Palate-Craniofacial Journal 36:262–268

Stengelhofen J 1989 The nature and causes of communication problems in cleft palate. In: Stengelhofen J, ed. Cleft palate: the nature and remediation of communication disorders. Churchill Livingstone, Edinburgh: 1–30

Tideman H, Stoelinga PJ, Gallia L 1980 Le Fort I advancement with palatal osteotomies in patients with cleft palates. Journal of Oral Surgery 38:196–199

Vanderas AP 1987 Incidence of cleft lip, cleft palate and cleft lip and palate among races: a review. Cleft Palate Journal 24:216–225

Young JL, O'Riordan M, Goldstein JA et al. 2001 What information do parents of newborns with cleft lip, palate, or both want to know? Cleft Palate-Craniofacial Journal 38:55–58

Speech, language and swallowing

Contributors
Julie Reid, Sarah Starr

Introduction

The ability to communicate effectively is vital to a person's functioning in society. Speech and language acquisition is a developmental process occurring most dramatically in the first years of life but one that proceeds throughout a person's lifetime. Difficulties may be encountered at any point during the language acquisition process. Children may experience problems acquiring the sounds of the language, learning how to combine words meaningfully or comprehending others' questions and instructions. In all cases, a speech and language pathologist is the primary healthcare professional responsible for the identification and treatment of individuals with communication problems. Paediatric dentists should be aware of the symptoms and problems associated with communication impairment, particularly when it relates to orofacial or dentofacial anomalies. They should know how to refer children and their families to a speech pathologist.

Communication begins at birth and continues throughout a child's life through adolescence and into adult life. A child's communication development is influenced by many variables including neurological status and motor development, oromotor status (anatomical and physiological), cognition, hearing, birth order, environment, communication modelling and experiences as well as their personality.

This chapter will briefly describe some of the main communication disorders that can present with particular focus for paediatric dentists.

Communication disorders

There are six main areas to be considered when assessing a child's communication:
- Oral motor and feeding problems.
- Articulation.
- Language.
- Voice.
- Fluency.
- Pragmatics.

Oral motor and feeding problems

Problems in this area constitute the earliest at which children are referred to a speech pathologist. Significant problems can result when an infant does not develop control of the oral mechanism sufficient for successful feeding. Early reflex development typically facilitates feeding behaviour, but neuromotor factors, prematurity, cleft lip and palate, long-term non-oral feeding and other reasons may interfere with a child's development of the movement patterns essential for sucking, swallowing and feeding. Since these patterns form the scaffolding of movement for early speech sound development, children with a history of feeding difficulties may have subsequent difficulties in producing sounds for speech.

Reasons for referral

- Sucking, swallowing or chewing difficulties.
- Gagging, coughing or choking with feeds.
- Moist vocal quality during or after feeds.
- Poor cough or gag reflex.
- Persistent drooling (not coincident with teething).
- Recurrent chest infections.
- Presence of a craniofacial malformation.
- Parental report of feeding difficulty or refusal.
- Poor oral intake and associated poor weight gain in infants and young children.

Articulation

Articulation refers to the production of speech sounds by modification of the breath stream using the various valves along the vocal tract: lips, tongue, teeth and palate. Problems in these areas can vary from a fairly mild distortion of sounds such as a lisp, where the child's speech is still easy to understand through to a more severe speech production problem where all speech attempts are unintelligible or where the child makes very few speech attempts. Errors can be classified in the following ways:

- Speech sound omissions:
  - 'cu' for 'cup'
  - 'te-y' for 'teddy'.
- Substitutions of sounds:
  - 'wed' for 'red'
  - 'tun' for 'sun'.
- Distortions:
  - lateral lisps – 's' that sounds slushy.

Children learn to produce sounds in a developmental sequence, with adult-like sound systems expected by 8 years of age (Table 11.1). For example, it is quite acceptable for a 2-year-old to mispronounce an 's' sound, but it would be considered a problem if a similar error were made by a 7-year-old.

Language

In contrast to the fairly straightforward examples listed above to illustrate speech sound learning, language development is much more complex. Skills emerge in two parallel levels.

Receptive language

This is the ability to understand language.

Expressive language

This refers to the ability to produce verbal and non-verbal communication in the form of words and sentences and may include speech and written language.

Table 13.1 Development of sounds with age

Age (years)	Sounds correctly produced	Comments
2	m,n,h	Speech is sometimes difficult to understand, especially for unfamiliar people
2½	p, b, ng, w, d, g	
3	y, k, f, sh	By 3 years of age, 80–90% of a child's speech should be easily understood
3½	t, ch, dge	
4	l, s, zh (measure)	Blends of sounds (i.e. st, cl, dr) are acquired later than the individual sounds but are usually mastered by 5 years
5	r	
5½	z	The ages quoted here are only a guideline as to when the average child acquires the sound, but by 8 years of age, all sounds should be mastered
7½	th	
8		

A child with a language disorder may present with difficulties in both comprehension and expression of language or in only one area of language learning. Language learning proceeds in a predictable order but there is more variability in the emergence of these skills than the acquisition of speech sounds. Vocabulary grows as does a child's ability to progressively understand more complex language. Words are combined into phrases and eventually sentences and comprehension becomes more adult-like over time. Eventually, language that is heard and said becomes the language of literacy, reading and writing. School success is highly correlated with language learning, especially in the early years.

Children may experience language learning problems at any stage of the acquisition process. There may be:

- Difficulties interpreting the meaning of words and gestures.
- Delays in the production of first words and phrases.
- A lack of understanding of questions and instructions.
- An inability to produce sentences that are grammatically correct.
- An inability to participate in conversations.

A delay at any single stage may not necessarily constitute a long-standing problem, although it should be investigated further. Problems with language acquisition are the most subtle indicators of difficulties with childhood development and therefore, should never be ignored.

Voice

Voice is produced when the vocal cords in the larynx are vibrated. Changes in air flow and the shape of the vocal folds can affect loudness, pitch and voice quality. Once voice is produced, its tone (resonance) and quality is modified by the throat, oral and nasal cavities. A child with a voice problem may present with the following:

Abnormal voice quality
Rough, breathy or hoarse voice in the absence of upper respiratory tract infection.

Abnormal resonance
Hypernasality (excessive nasal tone usually due to problems closing the velopharyngeal port during speech) or hyponasality (lack of nasal resonance usually due to some type of nasopharyngeal obstruction).

Inappropriate loudness levels
Voice too soft to be heard or so loud that it is distracting from the message of the speaker.

Problems with pitch
Pitch too high or low for age or sex.
  Voice problems may be caused by:
- Poor vocal use, e.g. excessive yelling or screaming (in some cases producing vocal nodules).
- Neurological problems (e.g. cerebral palsy).
- Vocal pathology such as polyps or cysts.
- Muscular pathology.
- Vocal cord paralysis.
- Vocal irritants such as exposure to smoking, chemicals or aerosol sprays.
- Physical conditions including cleft palate, laryngectomy and hearing loss.

Fluency
Fluency refers to the smooth flow of speech. Where there are interruptions in the flow of speech, stuttering occurs. Many children experience brief periods of stuttering as they learn to speak in longer sentences and this early form of dysfluency is not considered a disordered pattern as it will usually pass. Early developmental dysfluency is best resolved by reacting to the message the child is attempting to convey rather than the dysfluency. When stuttering persists beyond the normal time period of approximately 3–6 months, and/or there is strong family history of stuttering or when it is becoming stressful for the child, referral to a speech pathologist is indicated.
  A child or an adult with a stutter experiences involuntary repetition of words, prolongations of sounds in words and blocks where no sound is produced at all. Some speakers with a stutter will use words like 'um' to help them initiate speaking. Sometimes secondary features such as eye blinking and facial grimacing occur with the stutter.
  Stutterers do not have more emotional or psychological problems when compared with the general population, nor is there evidence of decreased mental aptitude. Approximately 3% of the population stutter with a predominance of males (3 : 1). The disorder usually has its onset in the early years of life and treatment is most successful in the preschool years. Hence, the importance of prompt and early referral.

Pragmatics
Pragmatics refers to *how* we communicate with others through our verbal and non-verbal language as well as our tone of voice, stress, pausing, pitch and loudness. Pragmatics relates to our social use of language including how we initiate, engage

and maintain others in a communication dialogue through our eye contact, body language, physical space, choice and use of words, conversational turn taking and responses to others.

Pragmatic skills allow us to develop friendships and effectively communicate our messages in a social, educational and workplace setting. They are crucial to effective communication and develop from birth throughout our adult life. Pragmatic skills develop as part of normal cognitive development and are influenced by environmental and cultural modelling. Disorders in pragmatic skills can be isolated or part of a language, developmental, psychological or specific condition (e.g. autism).

Structural anomalies and their relationship to speech production and eating and drinking

The speech language pathologist is actively involved in the evaluation of orofacial, pharyngeal and laryngeal structures and functioning important for speech production and deglutition. Evaluation techniques may be perceptual or instrumental (e.g. video-fluoroscopic X-ray studies of swallowing) and are often a combination of both with input from other members of a multidisciplinary team. Results of diagnostic structural and/or functional testing direct which management strategies are available to the patient.

Speech sounds may be acoustically or visually distorted due to abnormal structure and/or function of the articulators (most commonly the lips, tongue, teeth and palate). There are three main ways in which speech sound production is influenced and these can coexist thus differential diagnosis is important in decision making for management.

1. Speech sounds may be omitted, substituted or added during early childhood as mature speech patterns are mastered. For example, 3-year-old children often substitute alveolar sounds for velar sounds (cap → tap, go → do). Some children continue these substitutions for longer than expected and need speech therapy to learn mature speech patterns.
2. Speech sounds may be distorted due to underlying neurological impairment or oro-motor planning/coordination problems. Speech may be termed dysarthric (neurological) or dyspraxic (motor planning) depending on aetiology and characteristics noted.
3. Structural problems may affect speech (and swallowing) in a number of ways. These are outlined below.

Dental anomalies
Malocclusion has the potential to greatly affect speech production although the ability of patients to compensate for abnormal dental relationships should never be underestimated. However, there is no definite proof that altering the position of a tooth may improve speech (Johnson & Sandy 1999).

Hypodontia/missing teeth causing interdental spacing
Chewing difficulties may result and a lateral or forward displacement of tongue during speech may occur, resulting in distortion of sounds. The presence or absence of teeth

and the position of these teeth in the dental arch is thought to be more significant for speech production than the condition, size or texture of the teeth (Shprintzen & Bardach 1995). In general, lingual-alveolar sounds (e.g. /s/, /z/) followed by lingual-palatal sounds ('j', 'sh', 'ch') are most affected by spaces in the dental arch. The tongue tends to move forwards into the interdental space causing a central or lateral 'lisp'. The speech sounds most resistant to changes in the dental arch are the velar consonants /k/ and /g/ (Bloomer 1971).

Class III malocclusion

A severe Class III malocclusion may be associated with distortion or interdentalization ('lisping') of sibilant and alveolar speech sounds (/s/, /z/, /t/, /d/, /n/, /l/) due to difficulty elevating the tongue tip to the alveolar ridge. The sound most likely to be affected is /s/. This is probably because production relies on precise placement of the tongue tip and blade in addition to sufficient space being available anterior to the tip in the anterior portion of the palate (Bloomer 1971). Forward tongue placement can also be associated with a tongue thrust swallow and more cumbersome oral preparation of food with poor lateral tongue transfers and imprecise tongue tip elevation during swallowing.

Class II malocclusion

A severe Class II malocclusion may interfere with lip closure during eating and drinking. Bilabial speech sounds (/p/, /b/, /m/) may be distorted or produced in a labiodental manner (with the upper incisors articulating with the lower lip). The speech sounds may be 'visually' distorted that is they may look different but be acoustically acceptable (sound near normal).

Anterior open bite

An anterior open bite allows the tongue to move forward into the interdental space causing interdentalization ('lisping') or distortion of speech sounds, particularly those which involve the tongue tip contacting the alveolar ridge (/t/, /d/, /n/, /l/) and palate (/s/, /z/).

Swallowing may also be different for children with an anterior open bite compared to those with a normal occlusion. For example, genioglossus muscle activity is significantly higher in patients with anterior open bite than those without (Alexander & Sudha 1997). Difficulty biting with middle incisors is common when an anterior open bite is present with overfilling of the mouth, tearing of food or compensatory biting with more lateral teeth noted.

Maxillary collapse

This condition sometimes occurs after cleft palate surgery and leads to distortion of sounds requiring tongue and palatal contact ('s', 'z', 'sh', 'ch', 'j').

Speech and feeding problems are not always associated with these dental conditions. Each patient must be considered individually in light of their abilities to compensate for dental or occlusal anomaly. In cases where problems are identified, speech therapy is coordinated with dental and orthodontic management. Some children may not be able to improve their speech or feeding until their dental treatment is complete.

Lip anomalies
Cleft lip
Sometimes tissue deficiency and excessive tightness or scarring of tissue affect speech. The speech sounds most likely to be affected are the bilabials (/p/, /b/, /m/). Problems with the facial nerve affecting speech have been reported in syndromes such as hemifacial microsomia and Moebius syndrome (Shprintzen & Bardach 1995).

Depending on the nature of the lip abnormality and range of lip movement, lip closure and protrusion during drinking (e.g. cup/straw drinking) or speech may be affected. Poor lip closure may relate to imprecise labial sounds (p, b, m) and poor lip protrusion associated with distortion of sounds such as 'w', 'oo', 'er'.

Palatal anomalies
The soft palate and pharyngeal walls work simultaneously to close the nasopharynx during speech production and swallowing (i.e. velopharyngeal closure). This action prevents excessive airflow into the nasal cavity during speech, maintains negative intra-oral pressure during sucking and swallowing and prevents nasal regurgitation of food or fluid during the swallow. If there is a palatal abnormality, velopharyngeal closure cannot take place efficiently, and there is often associated poor sucking, slow feeding and possible escape of food and liquid into the nose. Speech is nasal and breathy, sounds are unclear and volume may be reduced.

Palatal anomalies may include:
- Cleft palate (with or without cleft lip).
- Submucous cleft palate, characterized by a bifid uvula, notching of the posterior margin of the hard palate, zona pellucida and abnormal insertion of the levator musculature into the free bony edge of the hard palate.
- Congenital palatal anomalies including short palate, deep nasopharynx, uncoordinated or inefficient velopharyngeal movement.
- Acquired palatal abnormalities resulting from neurological damage, surgery or neoplasms.
- Neurological abnormalities influencing palatal movement (e.g. cerebral palsy, cranial nerve IX and X abnormalities, muscular dystrophy).

Children with palatal anomalies are best referred to a specialist cleft palate clinic where they can receive coordinated multidisciplinary assessment and management (see Chapter 12).

Lingual anomalies
Abnormalities of the tongue may affect the precision, range and speed of tongue movement, resulting in speech or feeding difficulties. The most common problem is ankyloglossia or tongue tie.

Ankyloglossia (Figure 13.1)
Tongue tie may occur with varying degrees of severity, which does not always correlate with severity of functional impairment. Some children have no problems with eating/drinking or speech and others do. Some of the possible are:
- Feeding difficulties such as difficulty sucking in infancy, poor tongue movement and chewing due to restricted tongue movement laterally and persistent messy eating (due to the child being unable to clear food from the buccal cavities and the lips).

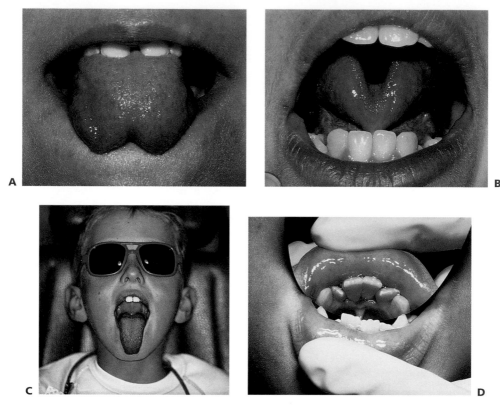

Figure 13.1 Ankyloglossia. **A, B** Notice the tethering of the frenum to the anterior tip of the tongue restricting elevation and protrusion. It is important to assess the position of the frenum into the body of the tongue as well as any attachment into the gingival margin that may cause periodontal complications. **C** Extent of protrusion after lingual frenectomy. **D** Another indication for frenectomy is where the attachment inserts into the free gingival margin causing potential periodontal problems.

- Substitution and distortion of tongue tip (alveolar) sounds /l/, /t/, /d/, /n/, /s/, /z/ caused by restricted elevation of the tongue tip.
- Slower than normal speech rate or reduced speech intelligibility in conversational speech.
- Reduced speech precision during shouting. (Shouting requires the mouth to open more widely and thereby may result in the tongue tie having a more negative effect on speech precision.)
- Difficulty breastfeeding in infancy and persistent messy eating in later childhood (due to the child being unable to clear food from the buccal cavities and the lips).

If a child's speech or feeding appears to be affected by tongue tie an assessment by a speech pathologist and a paediatric dentist is useful to determine whether or lingual frenectomy is required.

Macroglossia

An abnormally large tongue may be associated with syndromes such as Beckwith–Wiedemann syndrome. Children with macroglossia may have difficulty correctly articulation dento-lingual sounds (e.g. 'th'), lingual–alveolar sounds /t/, /d/, /n/, /l/ and palatal–lingual sounds (e.g. 'ch', 'j', 'sh') In severe cases the blade of the tongue may contact the upper lip affecting vowels and glides (e.g. /r/ and /w/).

Microglossia

An abnormally small tongue may be associated with syndromes such as hypoglossia-hypodactyly. In these cases the tongue tip may not contact the teeth, palate or alveolus sufficiently for precise consonant production. Compensatory articulation of sounds may need to be developed.

Maxillofacial surgery and its relation to speech production

When orthognathic surgery is being considered, a consultation with a speech pathologist should be made to determine the possible consequences of the procedure on speech production.

Maxillary advancement procedures

When the maxilla is advanced anteriorly, the hard palate and soft palate are also displaced forwards, increasing the distance that the soft palate must move to achieve velopharyngeal closure. Most patients seem able to compensate for this alteration in nasopharyngeal relationships and their speech and swallowing are not affected. Some patients, however, are 'at risk' for deterioration in speech and swallowing characteristics (e.g. those with a repaired cleft palate). Forward displacement of the palatal structures may result in velopharyngeal insufficiency (VPI) and hypernasal speech production. Forward placement of the maxilla also means that the tongue contact on the palate may be altered for some sounds. Therefore tongue placement and sound production may be improved in cases with severe Class III malocclusion.

Given the potential impact of surgical interventions on velopharyngeal function the careful timing and selection of surgical techniques is recommended (Jacques et al 1997). Postsurgical speech review and possible speech therapy may also be warranted.

Referral to a speech pathologist

When the presence of a communication or feeding problem is suspected, referral should be made as soon as possible.

Dentists should refer any child who experiences the difficulties outlined below.

Feeding and swallowing

- Has difficulty sucking, swallowing and chewing.
- Is coughing, gagging or choking during feeds.

- Is drooling excessively.
- Has reported breast, bottle, drinking or eating difficulties.

Articulation
- Is not babbling a wide variety of sounds by 8–10 months.
- Is not easily understood by caregivers by 2 years.
- Is not easily understood by familiar adults by 3 years.
- Is having difficulty in producing sounds accurately by 5 years.

Language
- Is not understanding simple instructions and questions by 18 months.
- Is not using single words by 18 months.
- Is not combining two words by 2 years (i.e. 'more drink').
- Has difficulty following instructions or answering questions.
- Gives inappropriate answers or frequently ignores language spoken to them.
- Is constructing sentences that are incorrect or immature by 3–4 years (i.e. 'me go to him house').
- Cannot maintain a topic of conversation by 4 years.

Voice
- Has a hoarse or breathy voice or often loses their voice.
- Has a nasal voice.
- Often sounds as though they have a cold.
- Has a voice that seems too high or low for their sex or age.
- Continually speaks abnormally loudly or softly.
- Has a sudden onset of any of these problems.

Fluency
- Persistent stuttering at any age.

Pragmatics
- Does not initiate or engage others in communication at any age.
- Has poor eye contact.
- Constantly interrupts others.
- Displays inappropriate social use of language (e.g. inappropriate use of words for a situation).
- Talks excessively does to take conversational turns or goes off on a tangent when speaking.

Referral procedures
It will be necessary to locate the most appropriate service to meet your patient's needs. Most often, access to a speech pathologist through a local community health centre or hospital will be all that is required. Some patients may require a more specialized service such as a developmental disability service, cleft palate clinic, feeding specialist or feeding clinic. Some patients may prefer the services of a private practitioner.

Referral is most efficient when the dentist provides a written referral outlining the areas of concern. Following an assessment, a treatment plan will be devised according to the individual needs of the patient. Treatment can be provided in individual or group sessions and it may extend over a period of time, depending on the nature and severity of the condition. Most speech, language and feeding problems are best treated with parental participation. Preschool or school-based programmes are important for older children.

References and further reading

Alexander S, Sudha P 1997 Genioglossus muscle electrical activity and associated arch dimensional changes in simple tongue thrust swallow pattern. Journal of Clinical Pediatric Dentistry 21:213–222

Bloomer JH 1971 Speech defects associated with dental malocclusions and related abnormalities. In: Travis LE, ed. Handbook of speech pathology and audiology. Prentice-Hall, Englewood Cliffs, NJ

Jacques B, Herzog G, Muller A et al 1997 Indications for combined orthodontic and surgical (orthognathic) treatments of dentofacial deformities in cleft lip and cleft palate patients and their impact on velopharyngeal function. Folia Phoniatrica et Logopaedica 49:181–193

Johnson NC, Sandy JR 1999 Tooth position and speech – is there a relationship? Angle Orthodontist 69:306–310

Shprintzen RJ, Bardach J 1995 Cleft palate speech management: a multidisciplinary approach. Mosby, St Louis

Appendices

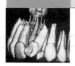

Contributors
Angus Cameron, Richard Widmer, Neil Street, Peter J Cooper, Mark Schifter,
Christopher Olsen, Kerrod B Hallett

Appendix A: Normal values of blood chemistry

Laboratory examination may be divided into two general categories: screening and diagnostic. Screening studies are intended to identify individuals with disease in the early and asymptomatic stages. By definition, screening studies must be relatively simple and inexpensive, and are useful only when used to identify a disease which is relatively frequent (diabetes mellitus, anaemia, syphilis, blood disorders). Diagnostic examinations provide more specific information. The distinction between screening and diagnostic laboratory examination is not always rigid or absolute.

It must be remembered that laboratory examinations provide information that contributes to the diagnostic process. Seldom is this information of value by itself. The results must be interpreted in conjunction with other information that is available about the patient. It should also be noted that a laboratory value outside the normal range does not necessarily indicate disease. That value may represent normal for that specific patient. Usually normal values are determined by testing supposedly healthy people, and these results are used to calculate the mean and normal range. Variables are not considered, and as a consequence normal ranges are not always valid for all patients. Conversely, if a clinical diagnosis appears valid and is not substantiated by laboratory results, the tests should be repeated to rule out the possibility of laboratory error.

Haematology
Full blood count
A full blood count (FBC) usually includes a white blood cell count (WBC), red cell blood count (RBC), haemoglobin (Hb), haematocrit (Hct) and red blood cell indices (mean corpuscular haemoglobin, mean corpuscular volume, mean corpuscular haemoglobin concentration and platelet count).

Platelet function tests are rarely ordered, usually only in consultation with a haematologist. If one asks for FBC and 'differential', one will also receive a breakdown of the RBC and WBC as listed on the form. If an FBC detects anaemia, then one should request serum ferritin, red cell folate and serum vitamin B_{12}. However, in interpretation of these results one should seek counsel, as they are difficult.

Coagulation and bleeding tests
Problems relating to bleeding are relatively infrequent in dental practice. Most inherited defects will usually have been identified early in life, and so it is usually acquired bleeding problems about which the dentist must be aware. Screening studies will identify whether there is a bleeding problem, and in which of the three systems it is, namely, platelets, coagulation, or vascular abnormalities.

Table A.1   Normal blood values

	Children		Adults	
White blood cells	$4.0–15.0 \times 10^9$/L		$4.0–11.0 \times 10^9$/L	
Neutrophils	$1.5–7.5 \times 10^9$/L	50%	$2.0–8.0 \times 10^9$/L	60%
Lymphocytes	$1.0–8.6 \times 10^9$/L	42%	$0.5–4.0 \times 10^9$/L	33%
Monocytes	$0.5–1.5 \times 10^9$/L	5%	$0.2–1.0 \times 10^9$/L	4%
Eosinophils	$0.3–0.8 \times 10^9$/L		$0.04–0.5 \times 10^9$/L	
Basophils	$<0.1–0.2 \times 10^9$/L		$<0.01–0.2 \times 10^9$/L	
Red blood cells	$4.0–5.5 \times 10^{12}$/L	(3–12 years)	$4.5–6.5 \times 10^{12}$/L	Male
			$3.8–5.8 \times 10^{12}$/L	Female
Haemoglobin	115–145 g/L	(3–12 years)	130–180 g/L	Male
			115–165 g/L	Female
Mean corpuscular volume	70–90 fL		80–96 fL	
Mean corpuscular haemoglobin	23–31 pg		27–32 pg	
Platelets	$150–450 \times 10^9$/L			
Erythrocyte sedimentation rate	0–10 mm/h		0–5 mm/h	Male
			0–20 mm/h	Female
Reticulocytes	2.0–6.0% or	Infants	0.2–2.0%	
	mean 150×10^9/L			
	$10–100 \times 10^9$/L	Children		
Red cell folate	340–2500 nmol/L			
Serum folate	7–40 nmol/L			
Vitamin B$_{12}$	150–700 pmol/L			

Table A.2   Tests for bleeding problems

Activated partial thromboplastin time (APTT)		24–38 s
Prothrombin time		11–17 s
Factor VIII assay		50–200%
	Mild haemophilia	20–25%
	Moderate	2–5%
	Severe	<1%
Skin bleeding time		<9 min

Clinical chemistry

It is not appropriate to simply request a multi-blood analysis in the hope of finding a diagnosis or abnormality. The following abbreviations are often used when ordering tests, but will obviously differ from one institution or laboratory to another.

EUC   electrolytes, urea, creatinine
LFTs   liver profile, including serum proteins
CA   calcium
PHOS   inorganic phosphate, alkaline phosphatase

Blood chemistry

Table A.3 Normal blood chemistry	
Sodium	136–146 mmol/L
Potassium	3.4–5.5 mmol/L
Chloride	94–107 mmol/L
Total CO_2	24–31 mmol/L
Urea	2.5–6.5 mmol/L
Creatinine	60–125 mmol/L
Glucose: fasting	3.9–6.1 mmol/L
2 h postprandial	<7.8 mmol/L
Maintenance range for IDDM	4–10 mmol/L
Calcium	2.13–2.63 mmol/L
Phosphate	0.18–1.45 mmol/L
Osmolality	275–295 mmol/L
Lactate	0.63–2.44 mmol/L
Alkaline phosphatase	60–391 U/L

Liver function tests

Table A.4 Liver function tests	
Total bilirubin	2–21 mmol/L
Total protein	63–79 g/L
Albumin	35–53 g/L
Alkaline phosphatase (ALP)	30–115 U/L
γ-Glutamyl-transpeptidase (γGT)	
Male	8–43 U/L
Female	5–30 U/L
Alanine aminotransferase (ALT)	7–47 U/L

Iron studies

These tests are used when there is a suspicion of an underlying anaemia. The request for iron studies provides information regarding serum iron, total iron binding capacity, and percentage iron saturation.

Table A.5	
Ferritin	
Male	30–300 mg/L
Female: premenstrual	15–150 mg/L
Female: postmenstrual	25–200 mg/L
Iron	7.0–29.0 mmol/L
Transferrin	2.1–3.9 g/L
Saturation	0.09–0.52

Urine chemistry

Table A.6	
Sodium	40–220 mmol/L
Potassium	25–120 mmol/L
Creatinine	8.0–18.0 mmol/L
Total protein	<0.15 g/dL

Arterial blood gas

Table A.7	
pH	7.35–7.45
pCO_2	35–45 mmHg
pO_2	75–100 mmHg
HCO_3	22–26 mmol/L
Base excess	–3 to +3 mmol/L
SaO_2	0.95–0.98

Appendix B: Fluid and electrolyte balance

Fluid and electrolyte replacement can be conveniently divided into:
- Maintenance replacement – The fluid and electrolyte losses occur during a normal day. These values are modified by other factors such as patient and environmental temperatures, age weight and metabolic rate.
- Deficit replacement – To replace any existing or ongoing abnormal losses such as dehydration from vomiting or diarrhoea and blood loss.

Maintenance replacement

The need for water and electrolytes is a function of the metabolic rate as they are substrates for metabolism. Thus, the younger the child, the higher the metabolic rate on a weight basis and the higher the turnover of water and electrolytes.

Water requirements

Table A.8		
Infants	Day 1	60 mL/kg/day
	Day 2	80 mL/kg/day
	Day 3	100 mL/kg/day
	Day 4 to 1 year	120 mL/kg/day
Children	<10 kg	4 mL/kg/hour
	10–20 kg	2 mL/kg/hour + 40 mL/hour
	>20 kg	1 mL/kg/hour + 60 mL/hour

Modifying factors
Increased maintenance requirement
- Fever – add 12% per degree above 37.5°C.
- Hyperventilation.
- Extreme activity.
- High environmental temperature.

Decreased maintenance requirement
- Cardiac failure.
- Inactivity (patient sedated in ICU) – decrease by 30%.
- Hypothermia – decrease 12% per degree <37.5°C.
- Head injury – decrease by 30%.
- Renal failure – decrease by 70% + urine output.

Electrolyte requirements
Normal electrolyte requirements are shown in Table A.9.

Table A.9 Electrolyte requirements

	0–10 kg	11–20 kg	>20 kg
Fluids (mL/kg/day)	100	50	20
Energy (cal/kg/day)	100	50	20
Na (mmol/kg/day)	3.0	1.5	0.6
K (mmol/kg/day)	2.0	1.0	0.4

N/4 Saline (0.225% sodium chloride + 3.75% dextrose) at normal maintenance rates will supply adequate sodium and chloride. Potassium should only be added to intravenous fluids if replacement is to continue for more than 24 hours and adequate urine output is present. Infants under 3 months of age will also require supplements of dextrose if they are to fast for longer than 4–6 hours.

Fluid deficit

Fluid deficit is usually expressed as a percentage of body weight. This allows for easy calculation of replacement fluids. Fluid imbalance may be as a result of any of the following.

Water loss
- Decreased intake.
- Increased respiratory loss (especially seen in children with high respiratory rates).
- Renal concentration impairment.

Water and salt loss
- Vomiting.
- Diarrhoea.
- Increased sweating.

Blood volume loss
- Haemorrhage.
- Septic shock.
- Anaphylaxis.
- Burns.

Assessment of deficit

Deficit assessment is difficult even for experienced paediatricians. Some idea of the deficit can be gained from the history of the abnormal loss. For example:
- Has the vomiting persisted for more than 24 hours?
- Has the child passed urine in the past 12 hours?
- Is the child thirsty?
  Dehydration is generally assessed by estimating weight loss.

Mild dehydration (2–3% acute weight loss)
- Thirst.
- Mild oliguria.
- No physical signs.

Moderate dehydration (5% acute weight loss)
- Slight decrease in skin tone.
- Sunken fontanelles in infants.
- Slight decrease in ocular tension.
- Tachycardia.

Severe dehydration (7–8% acute weight loss)
- Marked tachycardia.
- Loss of skin tone.
- Loss of ocular tension.
- Sunken eyes.
- Restlessness and apathy.

Profound dehydration (>10% acute weight loss)
- Circulatory collapse.
- Delirium and coma.
- Hyperpyrexia.
- Cyanosis.

Replacement of deficit

Usually the deficit is replaced with the fluid that most closely approximates the fluid that has been lost. Replacement therapy is aimed at restoring the fluid compartments in the following order. If there is significant loss of blood volume, then this must be replaced as rapidly as is safely possible to preserve brain, heart and kidney perfusion.

Blood volume loss
- Blood: packed red cells or whole blood.
- Colloid: 4% Albumex or Haemaccel.
- Hartmann's solution or normal saline.
- Inotropes if needed.

Salt and water loss
- Hartmann's solution or normal saline.
- 0.45% sodium chloride + 2.5% dextrose (N/2 Saline).

Water loss
- 0.255% sodium chloride + 3.75% dextrose (N/4 Saline).
- Maintenance fluids should be added to the deficit losses and given over the normal period.

Calculation of deficit

Deficit (mL) = % dehydration × weight (kg) × 10

Examples

Mild dehydration

Where there is no circulatory compromise, the loss will be water and electrolytes from all body compartments. This can be replaced with dextrose saline solution over many hours.

Severe dehydration

There is loss of intracellular, interstitial and most importantly blood volume. The priority is to rapidly restore blood volume and with that, cardiac output with colloid or blood (10–20 mL/kg over 20–30 min) or saline solutions (20–40 mL/kg) to allow adequate vital organ perfusion. After this is achieved, electrolyte and water deficits should be replaced as calculated with dextrose saline solutions over a longer period of time (several hours to 24 hours).

Severe blood loss

In cases of trauma or bleeding, there will initially be loss of blood volume. This is treated in the same way as above, i.e. restoring circulating blood volume with colloids or blood and reassessment of losses. If the blood loss is unknown, then initial therapy is to start with 20 mL/kg over 10–20 minutes and then reassess. If the blood pressure has returned to normal and fallen again or has not responded to this initial bolus, then a repeat of the initial bolus of fluid is indicated, followed by reassessment. The signs of adequate fluid replacement without the aid of central venous pressure or urine output measurement are the return to normal values of blood pressure and heart rate without the need for further boluses of fluid.

Notes on rehydration

The above guidelines apply to previously healthy children. Those children with cardiac disease or significant systemic disease require intensive intravascular monitoring in a paediatric intensive care unit.

- Constant reassessment of fluid therapy is essential throughout replacement.
- Measurement of electrolytes is essential in the replacement of greater than moderate deficits and applies especially to potassium.
- Measurement of acid–base status with arterial blood gases is often necessary as fluid deficit causes organ hypoperfusion and subsequent metabolic acidosis. This will usually correct itself with correction of blood volume and cardiac output over many hours.
- Fluid balance and acid–base disturbances are often very complex and life-threatening, if there is any doubt as to management, then specialist paediatric or anaesthetic advise should be sought.

Transfusion

Volume (mL) = weight (kg) × g% Hb rise required × 3

Table A.10 Composition of intravenous crystalloid fluids

	Na⁺ (mmol/L)	Cl⁻ (mmol/L)	Lactate (mmol/L)	Ca²⁺ (mmol/L)	Dextrose (g/L)
Normal saline	150	150			
0.45% NaCl + 2.5% Dextrose	75	75			25
0.225% NaCl + 3.75% Dextrose	37.5	37.5			37.5
0.18% NaCl + 4% Dextrose	30	30			40
Hartmann's solution	130	110	5	3	

Table A.11 Composition of intravenous colloid fluids

	Na⁺ (mmol/L)	Cl⁻ (mmol/L)	K⁺ (mmol/L)	Ca²⁺ (mmol/L)	Colloid (g/L)
Haemaccel	145	145	5.1	6.25	Polygeline 35
Gelofusine	144	120			Gelatin 40
4% Albumex	140	128			Albumin 40

Appendix C: Management of anaphylaxis

Anaphylaxis
A symptom complex accompanying the acute reaction to a foreign substance to which the patient has been previously sensitized.

Anaphylactoid
Same symptoms but the reaction is non-immunological or unknown.

Incidence
- Anaesthesia – 1:5000 to 1:30000 (mortality 4% of reactions).
- X-ray contrast – 2%.
- Antibiotics– 1:5000.
- Latex allergy – 0.13%.
- Local anaesthetics – rare (usually to preservative).
- Foods, insects.

Latex sensitization in the general population is about 1%. Certain groups have a much higher incidence such as the healthcare workforce in which sensitization is estimated to be between 5% and 12% and children with spina bifida who are repeatedly exposed to latex from birth.

Timing
98% occur within 5 minutes of drug administration, but may occur up to hours later.

Clinical presentation
Prodrome
- Metallic taste.
- Apprehension.
- Coughing.
- Choking sensation.
- Paraesthesia.
- Arthralgia.

Cutaneous
- Blushing.
- Urticaria.
- Angio-oedema.
- Pallor and cyanosis.

Cardiovascular
- Tachycardia.
- Hypotension.
- Shock.

Respiratory
- Bronchospasm.
- Laryngeal obstruction.
- Pulmonary oedema.

Gastrointestinal tract
- Nausea, vomiting, diarrhoea.
- Abdominal cramps.

Others
- Disseminated intravascular coagulation.
- Fitting.

Treatment
Adrenaline and colloid infusion are the mainstay of the treatment of anaphylaxis. Follow-up is essential. The patient must be transferred to an intensive care unit as symptoms may return up to hours later. A letter must be sent with the patient describing the event and all the drugs used until skin testing can identify the offending drug. Skin testing of all drugs used is performed 3 months after the reaction. A MedicAlert bracelet should be worn by the child, identifying relevant drug reactions.

Notes on management (see Figure A.1)
Adrenaline is the main drug used in the treatment of anaphylaxis and anaphylactoid reactions. Adrenaline *must* be used if anaphylaxis is suspected.

Table A.12	
Children (<12 years)	Dilute 1 ampoule into 9 mL of saline
	1:1000 becomes 1:10000 (1 mg/10 mL)
	Inject 0.25 mL per year of age intramuscularly; this approximates 5 µg/kg
Adults	Inject 1:1000 intramuscularly
Small adults (<50 kg)	0.25 mL
Average adults (50–100 kg)	0.50 mL
Large adults (>100 kg)	0.75 mL
	Intravenous access lines must be large gauge, preferably 16 gauge or larger.
	Colloid 10–20 mL/kg stat

Note
- The doses of adrenaline and colloid must be repeated if the patient's vital signs have not improved.

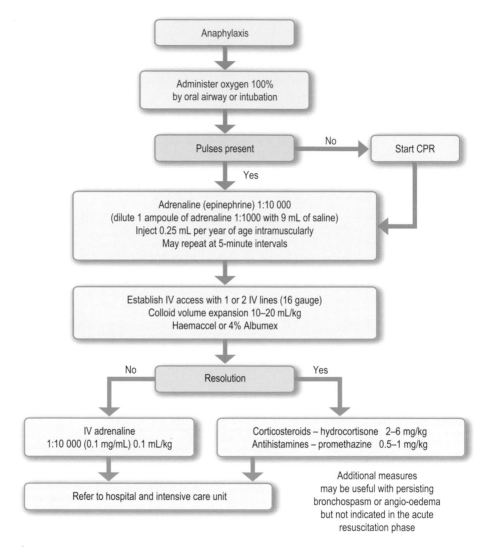

Figure A.1 Management of anaphylaxis.

Appendix D: Management of acute asthma

Asthma is one of the most common childhood diseases in Australia and accounts for significant mortality and morbidity. The emphasis of treatment today is on prophylaxis rather than merely treating attacks. Most children with known asthma will have treatment plans prescribed by their doctor for use in acute episodes. However, there are children who have undiagnosed asthma who are at risk of acute attacks.

Essential equipment for asthma kit
- Ventolin puffer (Figure A.2A).
- Bricanyl Turbuhaler.
- Ventolin nebules (2.5 mg).
- Ventolin nebules (5 mg).
- Nebulizer unit and tubing for wall oxygen.

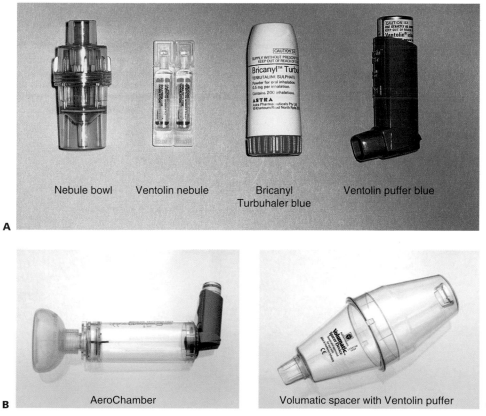

Nebule bowl   Ventolin nebule   Bricanyl Turbuhaler blue   Ventolin puffer blue

A

AeroChamber   Volumatic spacer with Ventolin puffer

B   C

Figure A.2 A–C Drugs and devices used in the management of asthma.

- Child mask for nebulizer.
- Small volume spacer with face mask.
- Volumatic spacer or small volume spacer with mouthpiece.

Bronchodilators (Figure A.2A)
Ventolin
- Inhaler (blue): 100 µg/puff.
- Dose: 4–12 puffs (weight dependent) via spacer.
- Nebules: 2.5 mg or 5 mg given via nebulizer.

Bricanyl
- Turbuhaler: 500 µg/inhalation.
- In acute situations – preferable to use puffer and a spacer.

Apparatus for administration of bronchodilators
Small volume spacer: children 4 years and under (Figure A.2B)
- Position AeroChamber with mask over child's face.
- Four puffs from Ventolin puffer, patient inhales four to six times for each puff.

Volumatic spacer: children over 4 years (Figure A.2C)
- Position spacer between lips.
- Four puffs from Ventolin puffer, patient inhales four to six times for each puff.
- Encourage child to breath deeply for 6–10 seconds.

Nebulizer
- For very young children or in older children when condition is not improved by puffer with spacer after 10 minutes.
- <5 years: 2.5 mg nebule.
- >5 years: 5 mg nebule.
- Place contents of nebule in bottom of nebule bowl, fix to face mask and apply oxygen or air to mask at 6–8 L/min flow rate. Add normal saline to Ventolin Nebule solution to make up to 4 mL total.
- A fine mist will form, which the child breathes deeply for about 10 minutes.

Management
See Figure A.3.

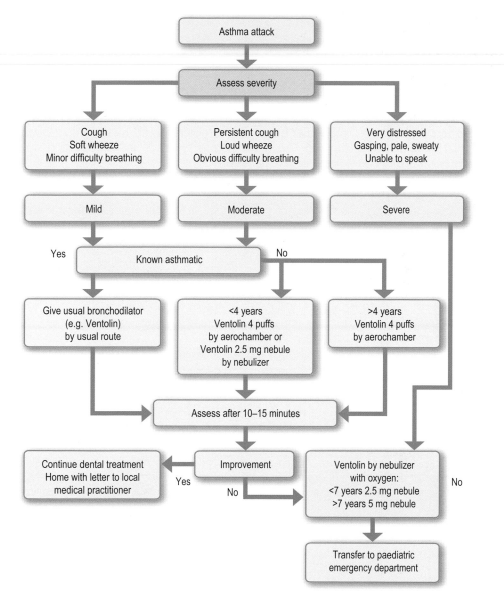

Figure A.3 Management of acute asthma.

Appendix E: Antibiotic prophylaxis protocols for the prevention of infective endocarditis

Infective endocarditis is a rare and potentially life-threatening disease with a reported annual incidence of 0.3 per 100 000 children in Western countries, which has remained unchanged in the past 40 years. Despite the advent of antibiotics, infective endocarditis still has a high rate of mortality, up to 25%, and is associated with significant morbidity.

Approved antibiotic prophylaxis is required for potentially at-risk patients receiving dental treatment as there is strong circumstantial evidence that endocarditis may follow dental treatment in susceptible patients.

Pathogenesis
- Characterized by inflammation of the inner surface of the heart (endocardium).
- Generally due to bacterial infection.
- Most commonly affecting the heart valves.
- May also involve non-valvular areas.
- Implanted cardiac mechanical devices also affected, such as prosthetic heart valves.

Three conditions need to be met for infective endocarditis to occur:
- Pre-existing damage to the heart valve surface.
- Bacteraemia, that is the introduction and circulation of bacteria in the bloodstream.
- Presence of bacteria of sufficient virulence to evade the body's innate defences, and able to attach, colonize, invade and so cause infection of the damaged heart valve surface.

Epidemiology
The at-risk population consists of principally those with:
- Rheumatic fever. Previously, the commonest cause of heart valve damage was childhood rheumatic fever. Improved sanitation and living conditions and the availability of antibiotics has significantly reduced the incidence of rheumatic fever. In those areas with social and economic deprivation, rheumatic heart valve disease is still prevalent.
- Congenital heart disease.
- Prosthetic aorto-pulmonary shunts.
- Prosthetic heart valves.
- Patients with a previous history of endocarditis
- Immunocompromised patients with long-term central venous lines.

Antibiotic prophylaxis
It has been long recognized that invasive dental procedures, typically extractions, cause an acute, substantive bacteraemia. However, there are increasing concerns regarding the cumulative bacteraemia associated with the activities of daily living, such chewing or tooth brushing, particularly in the presence of chronic dental disease. In spite of this, infective endocarditis is uncommon.

In an attempt to reduce the significant mortality and morbidity rates seen with infective endocarditis, numerous protocols recommending the prophylactic use of antibiotics have been published. Two of the most authoritative bodies, namely, the American Heart Association (AHA) and the Working Party of the British Society for Antimicrobial Chemotherapy (BSAC) have recently published significantly revised protocols for antibiotic prophylaxis for susceptible patients.

Cardiac conditions associated with the highest risk of adverse outcome from endocarditis for which prophylaxis with dental procedures is recommended:

- Previous history of infective endocarditis.
- Prosthetic cardiac valve replacement.
- Cardiac transplant recipients who develop valvulopathy.
- Specified congenital heart disease involving the presence or placement of shunts or conduits:.
  - unrepaired cyanotic shunts, including palliative shunts or conduits
  - completely repaired congenital heart defects with prosthetic material or device for at least 6 months after the procedure
  - repaired congenital heart disease with residual defects or adjacent to a site of prosthetic patch or material.

At-risk dental procedures

Antibiotic prophylaxis is now indicated for *any and all* dental procedures that involve manipulation of the gingival, mucosal or periapical tissues that is likely to cause bleeding (i.e. extractions, scaling, root canal instrumentation beyond the apex). The following procedures and events *do not* need prophylaxis:

- Routine anaesthetic injections through non-infected tissue.
- Taking dental radiographs.
- Placement of removable prosthodontic or orthodontic appliances.
- Adjustment of orthodontic appliances.
- Placement of orthodontic brackets.
- Shedding of deciduous teeth.
- Bleeding from trauma to the lips or oral mucosa.

Guidelines for clinicians
Past and current medical history

It is essential that the patient's medical status and history be assessed with respect to their cardiac problem. Consultation with the patient's doctor or cardiologist is essential. Dentists should be prepared to discuss with the treating doctor any issues surrounding the dental care of their patient.

Considerations in selecting appropriate antibiotics

- Anaphylaxis must be considered a risk in all patients taking any antibiotic, but particularly with any of the penicillins.
- Does the patient have a convincing history of allergy to any of the recommended antibiotics?
- Is the patient on long-term antibiotics? Or have they recently been taking an antibiotic? Alternative agents should be used.
- Does the patient have impaired renal function that will necessitate dose modification?

- Is the patient able to accept oral medications? Is there a history of vomiting with oral antibiotics? If so, consider parenteral medication.

Treatment planning
- 'Group' together a number of invasive dental procedures to be done in the minimal number of appointments to reduce the need for repeated courses of antibiotics.
- The same antibiotic should not be prescribed within 14 days.
- Is a general anaesthetic indicated? Consideration should be given to completing all possible treatment in one appointment.

Recommendations for use of protocols for antibiotic prophylaxis

The authors do not make a recommendation about the efficacy of one particular protocol over another. There are problems associated with prophylaxis regimens in that no two sets of guidelines are the same. Less than 10% of patients with endocarditis have had a recent invasive dental procedure and there is no direct evidence in humans that antibiotic prophylaxis is effective. Currently there is disagreement over the efficacy of different protocols, which patients and what dental procedures should be covered. It is accepted that the two most widely used protocols (those

Table A.13 Current protocols for susceptible patients

Situation	Agent	Regimen Single dose 30–60 minutes before procedure	
		Adults	**Children‡**
Oral	Amoxicillin	2 g	50 mg/kg to adult dose
Unable to take oral medications	Ampicillin *or*	2 g IV or IM	50 mg/kg IV or IM
	Cefazolin or ceftriaxone	1 g IV or IM	50 mg/kg IV or IM
Oral but allergic to penicillins or ampicillin	Cefalexin*† *or*	2 g	50 mg/kg
	Clindamycin *or*	600 mg	20 mg/kg
	Azithromycin *or* clarithromycin	500 mg	15 mg/kg
Allergic to penicillins or ampicillin and unable to take oral medications	Cefazolin or ceftriaxone *or*	1 g IV or IM	50 mg/kg IV or IM
	Clindamycin	600 mg IM or IV	50 mg/kg IV or IM

After Wilson et al 2007.
*Or other first or second generation cephalosporin in equivalent adult or paediatric dose.
†Cephalosporins should not be used in an individual with a history of anaphylaxis, angio-oedema or urticaria with penicillins or ampicillin.
‡Child dose must not exceed adult dose.
IM, intramuscular; IV, intravenous.

of the AHA and BSAC) have each been formulated with due regard to the current literature and clinical practice. As this edition is going to print, the National Institute for Health and Clinical Excellence has published new guidelines for the United Kingdom. The major recommendation of this group is that antibiotic prophylaxis is not recommended for people undergoing dental procedures. The use of specific protocols will also differ from one institution to another and in different countries, and therefore it is the responsibility of clinicians to determine which protocol is the most suitable to their individual patient.

Paediatric dosing
- The dose for any child should be calculated up to, but not exceeding the maximum adult dose.
- Dosage should always be prescribed according to weight (dose per kg).

Other considerations
- It is expected that some cases of endocarditis will occur despite the use of optimal prophylaxis protocols.
- In circumstances where appropriate prophylaxis has not been given, antibiotics prescribed up to 6 hours after a procedure may give effective cover.
- Good history taking is essential.
- If in doubt, consult relevant medical authorities.

References and further reading

Gould FK, Elliott TS, Foweraker J, Fulford M, Perry JD, Roberts GJ, and others. Guidelines for the prevention of endocarditis: report of the Working Party of the British Society for Antimicrobial Chemotherapy. J Antimicrob Chemother 2006; 57(6):1035–1042.

National Institute for Clinical Excellence. Prophylaxis against infective endocarditis. NICE Guildline 64. March 2008.

Sroussi HY, Prabhu AR, Epstein JB 2007 Which antibiotic prophylaxis guidelines for infective endocarditis should Canadian dentists follow? Journal of the Canadian Dental Association 73:401–405

Therapeutic Guidelines: Oral and Dental, Version 1, 2007. Therapeutic Guidelines Limited. Melbourne. Available at: www.tg.com.au

Wilson W, Taubert KA, Gewitz M et al 2007 Prevention of infective endocarditis. Prevention of infective endocarditis: Guidelines from the American Heart Association. A guideline from the American Heart Association Rheumatic Fever, Endocarditis and Kawasaki Disease Committee, Council on Cardiovascular Disease in the Young, and the Council on Clinical Cardiology, Council on Cardiovascular Surgery and Anesthesia, and the Quality of Care and Outcomes Research Interdisciplinary Working Group. Journal of the American Dental Association 138:739–760

Appendix F: Vaccination schedules*

Table A.14 Vaccination schedule*

Age	Vaccine	Disease/organism
Birth	hep B	Hepatitis B
2 months	dTPa-hepB Hib (PRP-OMP) IPV 7vPCV Rotavirus	Diphtheria, tetanus, pertussis + Hepatitis B *Haemophilus influenzae* type b Poliomyelitis Pneumococcal pneumonia Rotavirus (diarrhoea)
4 months	dTPa-hepB Hib (PRP-OMP) IPV 7vPCV Rotavirus	
6 months	dTPa-hepB Hib (PRP-OMP) IPV 7vPCV Rotavirus	
12 months	hep B MMR Hib (PRP-OMP) MenCCV	 Measles, mumps, rubella Meningococcal C
18 months	VZV	Chickenpox (varicella)
4 years	dTPa MMR OPV	
10–13 years	hep B VZV	
15–17 years	dTPa	

*Sources: Australian Government, Department of Health and Ageing, National Immunisation Program Schedule – Immunise Australia Program 1 July 2007; National Health and Medical Research Council. Australian Immunisation Handbook 8th edn., 2003, available at: www9.health.gov.au/immhandbook/ (accessed November 2007).

Table A.15 Prescription of tetanus toxoid boosters

History of vaccination	Time since last dose	Type of wound	Tetanus toxoid	Tetanus immunoglobulin
≥3 doses	<5 years	All wounds	No	No
≥3 doses	5–10 years	Clean minor	No	No
≥3 doses	5–10 years	All others	Yes	No
≥3 doses	>10 years	All wounds	Yes	No
<3 doses		Clean minor	Yes	No
<3 doses		All others	Yes	Yes*

*TIG dose 250 IU if <24 hours, otherwise 500 IU.

Appendix G: Isolation and exclusion from school for childhood infectious diseases

Table A.16		
Condition	**Isolation period**	**Incubation time**
Acute conjunctivitis	Until all discharge has ceased	
Chickenpox	For at least 7 days after the first appearance of spots No open sores should be present	10–21 days
Diphtheria	Immediate isolation until certified by a medical practitioner	3–6 days
Infectious mononucleosis	Until fully recovered or certified by a medical practitioner	2–6 weeks
Infectious hepatitis	Until all symptoms have disappeared or until a medical practitioner certifies recovery At least 7 days from the first signs of jaundice	15–50 days
Measles	At least 5 days from the appearance of the rash	10–12 days
Rubella	Until fully recovered For at least 5 days after the appearance of the rash	14–21 days
Pertussis	Immediate isolation Exclude from school for at least 3 weeks from the onset of the whoop, until full recovery or a medical certificate is obtained	5–21 days
Impetigo	Attendance at school is permitted if the sores are being treated and properly covered with a clean dressing Exclusion from school is required if the sores are not covered and are on exposed areas such as the scalp, hands or legs until healed	2–5 days
Pediculosis (head lice)	Until treatment with anti-lice lotion or shampoo has been undertaken Hair should be free of eggs	
Ringworm	Until appropriate treatment has begun	
Scabies	Until appropriate treatment has begun	

*NSW Department of Health, Australia, NSW Public Health Act 1991.

Appendix H: Somatic growth and maturity

As soon as the child enters the surgery, assessment should begin. At the outset, the dentist should always look at a child's size, development, appearance and behaviour in relation to their chronological age. Dental examination will initially include an assessment of dental age (based on time of exfoliation, eruption status and root development) in relation to the chronological age. Any marked discrepancies should then be investigated further.

Basic indicators of somatic growth and development
Height and weight
Height measurement
- Measure the child with shoes off, standing straight, with the Frankfort plane horizontal to the floor.
- Measurement is taken on deep inspiration of the patient.
- Sequential measurements are ideally taken at the same time of day.

Weight measurement
- Taken in light indoor clothing, with shoes off, ideally at the same time of day as height measurements.

Height abnormalities
- Short stature <3rd percentile, tall stature >97th percentile over a 6-month period, or
- Rate of growth <3–5 cm/year, consider referral to specialist growth unit at a paediatric hospital.
- Measurements must be considered in relation to height of parents and skeletal age.
- Height prediction possible using methods of Tanner and Whitehouse (1983) or Bayley and Pinneau (1952).
- Prediction of adolescent growth spurt is achieved by serial measurements, and may influence the subsequent timing of myofunctional orthodontic treatment.

Weight abnormalities
- Children with an endomorphic appearance tend to mature early, while those who are ectomorphic (especially boys) tend to mature late.
- Underweight – consider anorexia/bulimia.
- Overweight – may indicate nutritional problems.
- When children are markedly outside norms for age, early referral to paediatrician or dietitian is essential.
- Gross obesity may significantly alter drug metabolism and will affect the calculation of drug dosages.

Skeletal assessment
- It has been consistently shown that bone age as determined from hand-wrist radiographs using the Greulich and Pyle or Tanner and Whitehouse systems has a high correlation with stature and general body development.
- Other rarely used methods of bone-age calculation include the FELS method, use of knee joint or cervical vertebrae.

- Convention for anthropometric measurements uses the left hand.
- These methods assume bones of all patients consistently go through the same sequence of development, albeit at different rates. The Greulich and Pyle system is the most skeletally advanced for any age group as it was derived in the USA from healthy children from a high socioeconomic group.

Greulich and Pyle method
Each bone is matched with a similar appearing bone in a series of standard radiographs of increasing age. Thus each bone has a bone age assigned to it and the modal (or most frequent) of these bone ages is taken as the bone age of the hand and wrist. Frequently the step of assigning bone ages to each separate bone is omitted and instead the patient's hand-wrist radiograph is matched to the nearest standard radiograph, thereby determining the patient's skeletal age. Radiographic standards are provided at 6- and 12-monthly intervals for both males and females.

Tanner and Whitehouse method
This method scores specified bones according to their stage of development, using a written description and a radiographic standard of each stage of development. The total score for all bones is used to derive a skeletal age from tables provided. Generally the TW-2 (13 bone score) is used in preference to the Tanner and Whitehouse 20-bone method as it is about as accurate and quicker to use. A computerized image analysis system for estimating TW-2 bone age has been shown to be more reliable than the manual rating system. The Tanner and Whitehouse TW-2 method is easier and more accurate than the Greulich and Pyle method for the occasional user.

Significance
- Used to calculate potential for further increase in height.
- Used to predict adolescent growth spurt for timing of orthodontic treatment.
- Monitor growth abnormalities.

Dental development
Eruption times
- The emergence of teeth in the primary and permanent dentitions is unreliable because of environmental influences (i.e. early extraction of primary teeth will delay eruption of the succedaneous tooth, while late extraction of a primary tooth will hasten the eruption of the permanent successor).
- Eruption is not a continuous event.
- Racial variations – published data on eruption times are generally of northern European populations. Earlier eruption times may be the norm in Asian peoples, and later eruption times the norm in eastern and southern European groups.

Root development
- Use the scoring systems of Nolla, Moorees, Fanning, Demirijan and others. These quantify tooth development from initial calcification to final root closure as seen on radiographs.

Sexual development: peak height velocity

- Hägg and Taranger (1982) observed that menarche occurred a mean 1.1 years after peak height velocity (PHV).
- Menarche is a highly reliable but not absolute indicator that PHV has been reached or passed.
- Menarche occurs at a bone age of 13.1 years.
- Boys attained a 'pubertal voice' (the pitch of the voice had changed noticeably but had not yet acquired adult characteristics) 0.2 years before PHV, and the 'male voice' (pitch of the voice had acquired adult characteristics) 0.9 years after PHV.
- Tanner (1978) found that in males breaking of the voice happens relatively late in puberty and is due to the increased length of the vocal cords which follows the growth of the larynx. Voice breaking is often a gradual process and is not reliable as a criterion of puberty. Facial hair appears in boys usually somewhat later than the PHV.

Correlation between dental development and other maturity indicators

Evidence so far indicates that the skeletal system, as well as height and the onset of puberty, develop largely independently of the dental system. Teeth are partly of epithelial origin, whereas bone is derived from mesoderm. Serious endocrinopathies, while severely retarding somatic growth and maturation, exert only a minor effect on the dentition. Demirijan (1978) found a very low correlation between dental age (root development) and skeletal age.

General observations on somatic growth

- Growth is nutrition dependent and a well-fed infant gains length before it gains weight.
- The pubertal growth spurt is governed by growth hormone and anabolic steroids (testosterone and oestrogens).
- Girls enter the growth spurt about 2 years earlier than boys; however, they complete the growth spurt only about a year earlier than boys.
- The growth spurt is of greater magnitude and of shorter duration in boys than girls as testosterone has a greater anabolic effect than oestrogen.
- Growth ceases from the feet upwards, so limb growth stops before spine growth.
- The pubertal growth spurt adds 25–30 cm to final height over the childhood growth curve. Boys on average end 12–13 cm taller than girls as their growth spurt occurs after an additional 2 years of childhood growth.

References

Bayley N, Pinneau S 1952 Tables for predicting adult height from skeletal age. Journal of Pediatrics 14:432–441.

Demirjian A 1978 Dentition. In: Falkner F, Tanner JM, eds. Human growth. 2: Postnatal growth. Plenum Press, New York: 413–444.

Fishman LS 1988 Radiographic evaluation of skeletal maturation: a clinically oriented method based on hand wrist films. Angle Orthodontist 52:88–112

Hagg U, Taranger J 1980 Skeletal stages of the hand and wrist as indicators of the pubertal growth spurt. Acta Odontologica Scandinavica 38:187–200

Hassel BA, Farman AG 1995 Skeletal maturation evaluation using cervical vertebrae. American Journal of Orthodontics and Dentofacial Orthopedics 107:58–66

Tanner JM 1978 Fetus into man. Harvard, Cambridge, MA

Tanner JM, Gibbons RD 1994 A computerized image analysis system for estimating Tanner–Whitehouse 2 bone age. Hormone Research 42:282–887

Tanner JM, Whitehouse RH, Cameron WA et al 1983 Assessment of skeletal maturity and prediction of adult height (TW2 method), 2nd edn. Academic Press, London

Appendix I: Growth charts

Birth to 36 months: Boys
Length-for-age and Weight-for-age percentiles

NAME _____

RECORD # _____

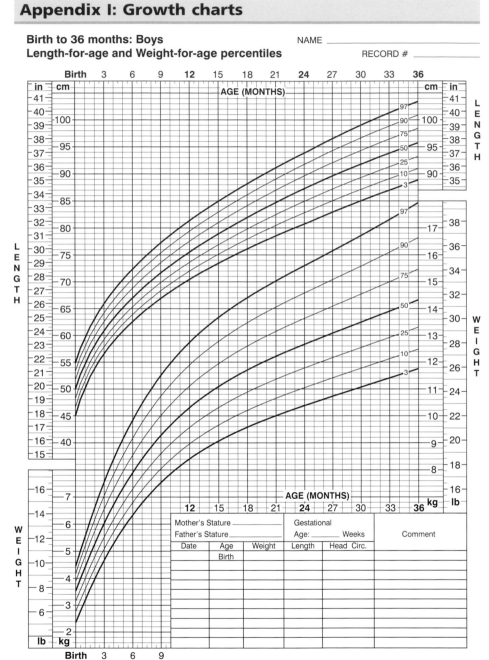

Published May 30, 2000 (modified 4/20/01).
SOURCE: Developed by the National Center for Health Statistics in collaboration with
the National Center for Chronic Disease Prevention and Health Promotion (2000).
http://www.cdc.gov/growthcharts

CDC
SAFER·HEALTHIER·PEOPLE™

Figure A.4

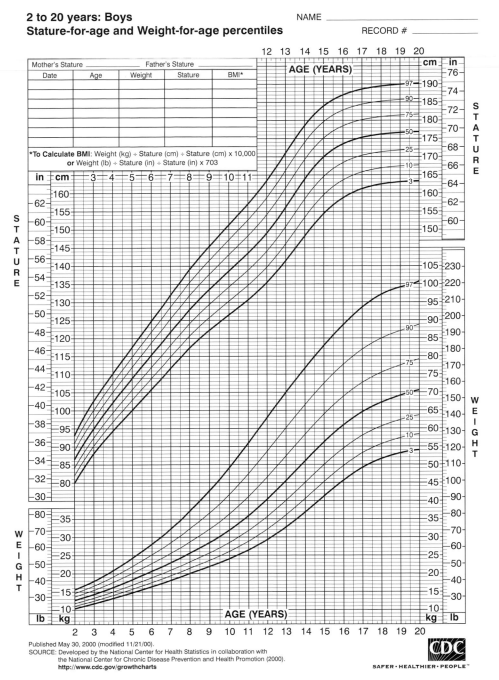

2 to 20 years: Boys
Stature-for-age and Weight-for-age percentiles

NAME _____

RECORD # _____

Published May 30, 2000 (modified 11/21/00).
SOURCE: Developed by the National Center for Health Statistics in collaboration with
the National Center for Chronic Disease Prevention and Health Promotion (2000).
http://www.cdc.gov/growthcharts

Figure A.5

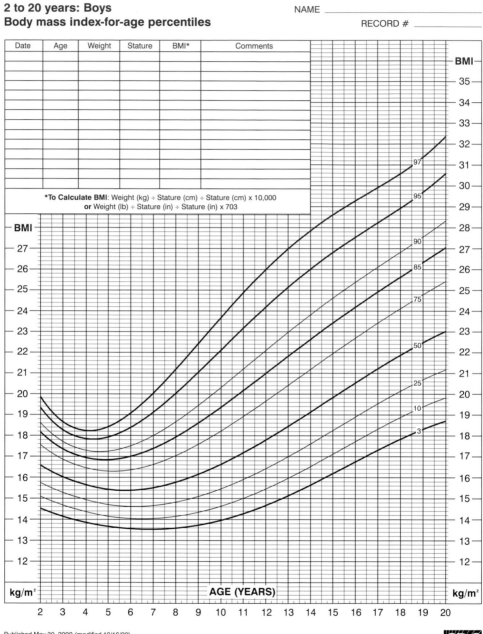

2 to 20 years: Boys
Body mass index-for-age percentiles

NAME _____

RECORD # _____

*To Calculate BMI: Weight (kg) ÷ Stature (cm) ÷ Stature (cm) x 10,000
or Weight (lb) ÷ Stature (in) ÷ Stature (in) x 703

Published May 30, 2000 (modified 10/16/00).
SOURCE: Developed by the National Center for Health Statistics in collaboration with
the National Center for Chronic Disease Prevention and Health Promotion (2000).
http://www.cdc.gov/growthcharts

Figure A.6

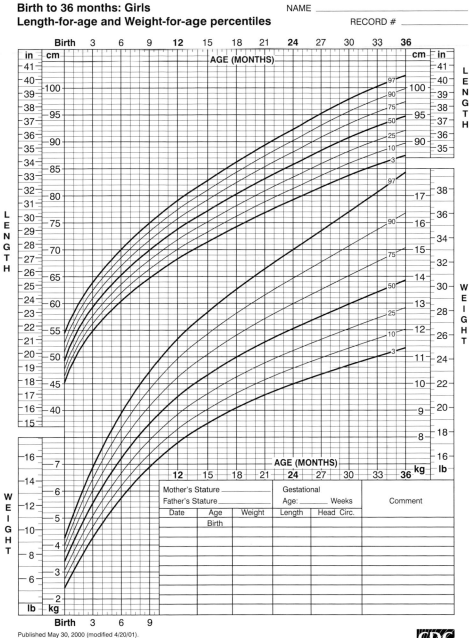

Birth to 36 months: Girls
Length-for-age and Weight-for-age percentiles

NAME _____

RECORD # _____

Published May 30, 2000 (modified 4/20/01).
SOURCE: Developed by the National Center for Health Statistics in collaboration with
the National Center for Chronic Disease Prevention and Health Promotion (2000).
http://www.cdc.gov/growthcharts

SAFER · HEALTHIER · PEOPLE™

Figure A.7

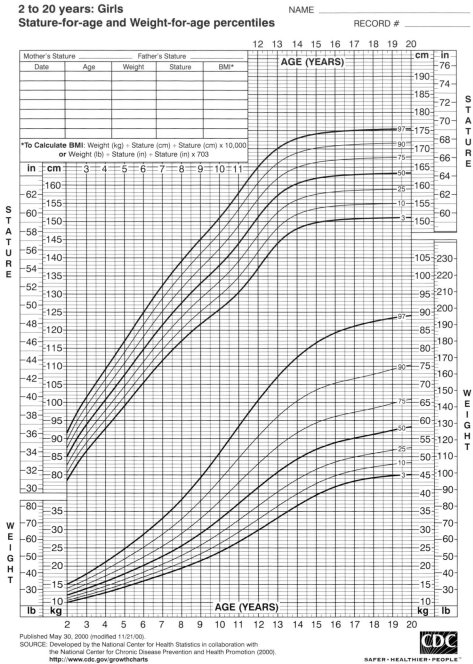

2 to 20 years: Girls
Stature-for-age and Weight-for-age percentiles

Published May 30, 2000 (modified 11/21/00).
SOURCE: Developed by the National Center for Health Statistics in collaboration with
the National Center for Chronic Disease Prevention and Health Promotion (2000).
http://www.cdc.gov/growthcharts

Figure A.8

2 to 20 years: Girls
Body mass index-for-age percentiles

NAME _____

RECORD # _____

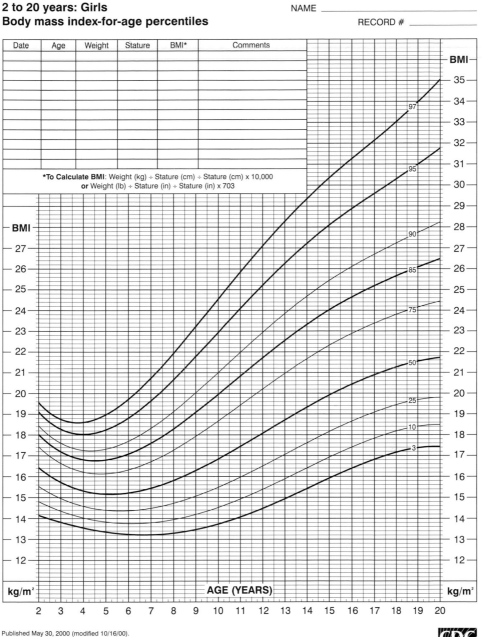

*To Calculate BMI: Weight (kg) ÷ Stature (cm) ÷ Stature (cm) x 10,000
or Weight (lb) ÷ Stature (in) ÷ Stature (in) x 703

Published May 30, 2000 (modified 10/16/00).
SOURCE: Developed by the National Center for Health Statistics in collaboration with
the National Center for Chronic Disease Prevention and Health Promotion (2000).
http://www.cdc.gov/growthcharts

SAFER·HEALTHIER·PEOPLE™

Figure A.9

Appendix J: Differential diagnosis of radiographic pathology in children

Periapical radiolucencies
- Periapical granuloma, abscess, surgical defect, scar.
- Radicular cyst.
- Dentigerous cyst.
- Traumatic bone cyst.

Radiolucencies associated with the crowns of teeth
- Dentigerous cyst.
- Inflammatory follicular cyst.
- Eruption cyst.
- Ameloblastic fibroma.
- Adenomatoid odontogenic tumour.
- Ossifying fibroma.
- Odontogenic keratocyst.

Separate isolated radiolucencies
- Primordial cyst.
- Traumatic bone cyst.
- Aneurysmal bone cyst.
- Odontogenic keratocyst.
- Fissural cysts.
- Median palatine cyst.
- Incisive canal cyst.
- Nasolabial cyst.
- Central giant cell granuloma.
- Hyperparathyroidism.
- Ossifying fibroma.

Multiple or multi-locular radiolucencies
- Central giant cell tumour.
- Cherubism.
- Giant cell lesion of hyperparathyroidism.
- Langerhans' cell histiocytosis.
- Central haemangioma of bone.
- Odontogenic myxoma.
- Ewing sarcoma.
- Desmoplastic fibroma.
- Metastatic tumours (especially rhabdomyosarcoma).

Generalized bony rarefactions
- Hyperparathyroidism.
- Thalassaemia.
- Langerhans' cell histiocytosis.
- Fibrous dysplasia.

Mixed lesions with radiopacities and radiolucencies
- Odontoma.
- Ameloblastic fibro-odontoma.
- Calcifying odontogenic cyst.
- Odontogenic fibroma.
- Adenomatoid odontogenic tumour.
- Fibrous dysplasia.
- Garré's osteomyelitis.
- Osteogenic sarcoma.

Radiopacities in the jaws
- Focal sclerosing osteomyelitis.
- Retained roots.
- Gardner's syndrome.
- Cleidocranial dysplasia.

Appendix K: Piaget's four stages of intellectual development

Stage one: the sensorimotor period (0–2 years)
Children in this period learn primarily through the senses of taste, touch, sight, sound, and manipulation. Mouthing of objects is a common method of learning. Intelligence is related to sensation, not reflective thought.

Stage two: the preoperational period (2–7 years)
While children in this state are capable of some intuitive thought, intelligence is based primarily on perception. The classic Piagetian experiment in this stage is the pouring of water into two test tubes. Children are shown that the exact same amount of water is poured into a tall thin tube and a short wide tube. Those children between the ages of 2 and 7 will typically argue that the taller one has more water, because their reasoning is tied to perception. Preoperational children believe what they see and hear.

Stage three: the concrete operational period (7–11 years)
Children in this stage develop the ability to reverse their thinking and to employ basic logic. They begin to question whether their perceptions are true. For example, whereas a 4-year-old will believe that Santa Claus exists because they saw him in a shopping centre, the 9-year-old will question the existence of Santa Claus because actions such as flying in a sleigh defy logic.

Stage four: the formal operational period (11–15 years)
With the beginning of adolescence comes the possibility of reaching the highest level of intellectual development: the ability to think abstractly. This stage is not reached by all individuals. Intellectually, those in the formal operational period are capable of thinking in propositions. Subjects like algebra and geometry require this type of abstract thought.

Implications for dentists
- Effective communication with a child or adolescent requires some understanding of their intellectual development.
- For example, consider how the following joking comment might differentially affect a 4-year-old and an 11-year-old:
  'Sit really still so I don't accidentally drill through your head!'
- An 11-year-old might see the humour in what the dentist has said. At 11 years, the child has reached the 'concrete operational' stage and can therefore employ logic to realize that the dentist is exaggerating.
- The 'preoperational' 4-year-old, on the other hand, may become frightened by the sarcastic comment. Children at this stage often take at face value the words that adults tell them.

Appendix L: Glasgow Coma Scale

The Glasgow Coma Scale (GCS) is a rating score for head injury and the score gives an indication of degree of injury and level of consciousness. The table below has been modified for children by the Adelaide Women's and Children's Hospital as the response scores are usually lower in children. Children between 6 months and 2 years may localize pain but not obey commands, and before 6 months the best score is withdrawal from pain or abnormal extension and flexion. There is no modification of the adult eye opening scale. Verbal responses should be consistent with age.

Modified Glasgow Coma Scale

Table A.17 Modified Glasgow Coma Scale			
	Response	**Response for infants**	**Score**
Eye opening	Spontaneously	Spontaneously	4
	To speech	To speech	3
	To pain	To pain	2
	None	None	1
Verbal	Orientated	Coos and babbles	5
	Words	Irritable cries	4
	Vocal sounds	Cries to pain	3
	Cries	Moans to pain	2
	None	None	1
Motor	Obeys commands	Normal spontaneous movements	6
	Localizes	Withdraws to touch	5
	Withdraws from pain	Withdraws from pain	4
	Abnormal flexion to pain	Abnormal flexion	3
	Extension to pain	Abnormal extension	2
	None	None	1
Best possible score			15

Outcomes

In children with GCS scores of 3 or 4, there are significant mortality rates (between 20% and 70%), whereas in those with scores over 5 there is low mortality and morbidity (<30%). If a child does not die within the first 24 hours, the risk of death falls to between 10% and 20%. Sixty-four per cent of children who do not open their eyes spontaneously within 24 hours will die or survive in a vegetative state. It is important to note that over 90% of children who are comatose initially with a GCS score greater than 3 will recover to an independent state, although 50% will have neurological impairment. If coma persists greater than 3 months there is almost always neurological and cognitive damage.

Appendix M: Common drugs usage in paediatric dentistry

Table A.18 Common drug usage in paediatric dentistry

Drug	Route	Dose	Frequency	Max dose	Indications	Contraindications/notes
Antibiotics						
Amoxicillin	PO	15–25 mg/kg/dose	tds	4 g/day	Antibiotic of first choice, except in allergic patients	Syrup or chewable tablets for young children
	IV	25 mg/kg/dose	tds	8 g/day	Antibiotic of first choice, except in allergic patients	
	PO IV	50 mg/kg up to adult dose 2 g	60 min prior stat	2 g adult dose	ENDOCARDITIS PROPHYLAXIS	
Amoxicillin plus clavulanic acid	PO	22.5 mg/kg/dose	bd	1.5 g/day	Severe/persistent dental infections	For β-lactam resistant organisms only
Ampicillin	IV	25 mg/kg/dose	qid	12 g/day		
	IV	50 mg/kg up to adult dose 2 g	stat	2 g adult dose	ENDOCARDITIS PROPHYLAXIS	
Benzylpenicillin	IV	30 mg/kg/dose	qid	1.2 g/dose	First IV drug of choice for odontogenic infections	
Phenoxymethylpenicillin potassium	PO	10–12.5 mg/kg/dose	qid	500 mg/dose		Must be given on an empty stomach
Cefalexin	PO	12.5–25 mg/kg/dose	qid	1 g/dose		
	PO	50 mg/kg up to adult dose 2 g	60 min prior	2 g adult dose	ENDOCARDITIS PROPHYLAXIS	
Cefalotin	IV	25 mg/kg/dose	qid	2 g/dose		Not for use in pregnancy
Cefazolin	IV	50 mg/kg up to adult dose 1 g	stat	1 g adult dose	ENDOCARDITIS PROPHYLAXIS	

Drug	Route	Dose	Frequency	Max dose	Indication	Notes
Metronidazole	IV	12.5 mg/kg/dose	bd	500 mg/dose	Supplement to penicillins in cases of severe or protracted infection	Not for use in pregnancy
	PO	10 mg/kg/dose	tds	400 mg/dose		
Clindamycin	PO IV	10 mg/kg/dose	tds	450 mg/dose	Antibiotic of first choice in penicillin-allergic patients	Low risk of pseudo-membranous colitis with protracted use
	PO IV	20 mg/kg up to adult dose 600 mg	60 min prior stat	600 mg adult dose	ENDOCARDITIS PROPHYLAXIS	Oral 1 hour or IV stat before procedure
Azithromycin Clarithromycin	PO	15 mg/kg up to adult dose 500 mg	60 min prior	500 mg adult dose	Alternative for ENDOCARDITIS PROPHYLAXIS	Macrolide antibiotics – supersedes erythromycin
Antifungals						
Nystatin	PO	<2 years 50000–100000 U >2 years 100000–500000 U	qid		Topical antifungal	Drops – apply to affected area Tablets – chew slowly
Miconazole	PO	½ tbsp	bd–qid		Topical antifungal	Oral gel – apply to affected area
Fluconazole	PO IV	3–6 mg/kg/day	daily	400 mg/day	Systemic antifungal Candidiasis prophylaxis and treatment in immunosuppressed patients	Warfarinised and renal patients. Change to oral as soon as possible. Multiple drug interactions
Amphotericin B	PO	10 mg/dose (NOT kg)	6-hourly		Topical antifungal	Lozenge – patient to chew slowly
	PO	100 mg/mL	6-hourly		Topical antifungal	Suspension – apply to affected area
	PO	3%	6-hourly		Topical antifungal	Ointment – apply to affected area

Table A.18 Continued

Drug	Route	Dose	Frequency	Max dose	Indications	Contraindications/notes
Antivirals						
Aciclovir	PO IV	20 mg/kg/dose 10 mg/kg/dose	5-hourly tds		Early primary herpetic gingivostomatitis	Immunosuppressed patients, should be prescribed within 72 hours of infection
Analgesics						
Xylocaine (viscous)	PO	2% 5 mL	3-hourly			Rinse mouth/gargle for 30 seconds No food or drink for 1 hour after
Aspirin						Should not be used in children under 12 years of age due to the risk of Reye's syndrome
Paracetamol	PO PR	15 mg/kg/dose	q4–6-hourly	60 mg/kg/day up to 4 g/day		Hepatotoxic if overdose Be aware of different presentations of paracetamol
Ibuprofen	PO	5–10 mg/kg/dose	q6–8-hourly	40 mg/kg/day (2 g/day)		
Naproxen	PO	10–20 mg/kg/day	q8–12-hourly	1 g/day		
Diclofenac	PO PR	1 mg/kg/dose	q8–12-hourly	3 mg/kg/day (150 mg/day)		Only in children >10 kg
Codeine phosphate	PO	0.5–1 mg/kg/dose	q4–6-hourly	60 mg/kg/dose		Similar side effects of narcotics including nausea and constipation
Oxycodone	PO	0.1–0.25 mg/kg/dose	q4–6-hourly			
Morphine	PO IV IM	0.2–0.5 mg/kg/dose 100–200 µg/kg/dose	q4–6-hourly q2–4-hourly	15 mg/dose		Should only be used in admitted patients

Drug	Route	Dose	Frequency	Maximum	Indication	Notes
Tramadol	PO	1–2 mg/kg/dose	q6-hourly	6 mg/kg/day (400 mg/day)		
Naloxone	IM IV	5–10 μg/kg	Single dose	10 mg total	Narcotic overdose	May be repeated at 2–3 minute intervals if necessary
Midazolam	PO PN IV	0.3 mg/kg 0.2 mg/kg 0.1–0.2 mg/kg	Single dose	10 mg 5 mg	Sedation	
Flumazenil	IV	5 μg/kg repeated every minute up to 40 μg/kg	Every minute	Total 2 mg/dose	Benzodiazepine reversal	Complex to administer – refer to product information sheet. Requires IV access in emergency resuscitation
Chloral hydrate	PO	10–20 mg/kg/dose 30–50 mg/kg	6-hourly Single dose	500 mg/dose 1 g	Sedation Hypnotic or premed	Avoid with renal or hepatic impairment
Temazepam	PO	0.3 mg/kg/dose	Single dose	20 mg/dose	Single dose for sedation	
Antiemetics						
Metoclopramide	PO IM IV	0.1–0.15 mg/kg	Single dose	0.5 mg/kg/day (30 mg/day)	Antinauseant/antiemetic	Single dose after narcotic if vomiting or nausea Dystonic extrapyramidal reactions may occur
Ondansetron	IV	0.1–0.15 mg/kg	Single dose	4 mg/dose	Antinauseant/antiemetic Postoperative nausea and vomiting	Centrally acting Often used in chemotherapy recipients
Corticosteroids						
Kenalog in Orabase	PO	Triamcinolone 0.1%	4–6-hourly	–	Mild-moderate oral ulceration	Ointment – apply to ulcers but do not rub in

Table A.18 Continued

Drug	Route	Dose	Frequency	Max dose	Indications	Contraindications/notes
Betamethasone in Orabase	PO	0.1% compound 1:1 w/w with Orabase	4–6-hourly		Moderate to severe ulceration	Ointment – severe ulceration Apply to ulcer but do not rub in
Dexamethasone	PO IV	0.1 mg/ml 0.1–0.2 mg/kg/dose	4–6-hourly Single dose		Moderate to severe ulceration Reduction in postsurgical inflammation	Mouthwash for very severe mucosal ulceration 5 mL rinse for 5 minutes and spit out well
Prednisolone	PO	'Pulse' dose of up to 2 mg/kg/day	6–12-hourly		Severe intractable immune-mediated oral ulceration	Week-long course, rapid taper
Antifibrinolytics						
ε aminocaproic acid (EACA)	IV	30 mg/kg	stat			Patients haemorrhagic diathesis loading dose of 100 mg/kg
Tranexamic acid	PO	15–20 mg/kg	qid			
Tranexamic acid	PO	10% compounded mouthwash	qid			Mouthwash – 5 mL rinse, then spit out well
DDAVP	IV	0.3 mg/kg	Slowly infuse over 60 min	20 μg/dose	Give before surgery	Infused over 1 hour before surgery

Clinicians are warned to prescribe and administer any drug carefully. The dosages in the table above are provided as a guide to the usage of medications in paediatric dental practice and clinicians should also consult their relevant pharmacopeia. Take care when determining maximal dose and frequency of administration.

Appendix N: Eruption dates of teeth

Table A.19	Development of primary teeth				
Tooth	**Initiation (weeks in utero)**	**Calcification begins (weeks in utero)**	**Crown formation at birth (38–42 weeks)**	**Crown complete (months)**	**Eruption (months)**
Central incisor	7	13–16	5/6 maxilla 3/5 mandible	1–3	6–9
Lateral incisor	7	14–16	2/3 maxilla 3/5 mandible	2–3	7–10
Canine	7.5	15–18	1/3	9	16–20
First molar	8	14.5–17	Cusps united Occlusal surface complete 1/2 to 3/4 crown height	6	12–16
Second molar	10	16–23.5	Cusps united 1/4 crown height	10–12	23–30

From: Logan & Kronfeld (1933); Shour & Massler (1940).

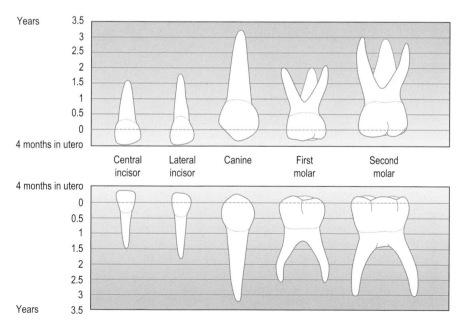

Figure A.10 Chronological development of primary dentition. (After Pindborg 1970 Pathology of the dental hard tissues. WB Saunders, Philadelphia, with permission.)

Table A.20 Development of permanent teeth

Tooth	Initiation	Calcification begins	Crown complete (years)	Eruption (years)
Mandible				
Central incisor	5–5.25 miu	3–4 months	4–5	6–7
Lateral incisor	5–5.25 miu	3–4 months	4–5	7–8
Canine	5.5–6 miu	4–5 months	6–7	9–11
First premolar	Birth	1.75–2 years	5–6	10–12
Second premolar	7.5–8 months	2.25–2.5 years	6–7	11–12
First molar	3.5–4 miu	Birth	2.5–3	6–7
Second molar	8.5–9 months	2.5–3 years	7–8	11–13
Third molar	3.5–4 years	8–10	12–16	17–12
Maxilla				
Central incisor	5–5.25 miu	3–4 months	4–5	7–8
Lateral incisor	5–5.25 miu	11 months	4–5	8–9
Canine	5.5–6 miu	4–5 months	6–7	11–12
First premolar	Birth	1.25–1.75 years	5–6	10–11
Second	7.25–8 months	2–2.5 years	6–7	10–12
First molar	3.5–4 miu	Birth	2.5–3	6–7
Second molar	8.5–9 months	2.5–3 years	7–8	12–13
Third molar	3.5–4 years	7–9 years	12–16	17–25

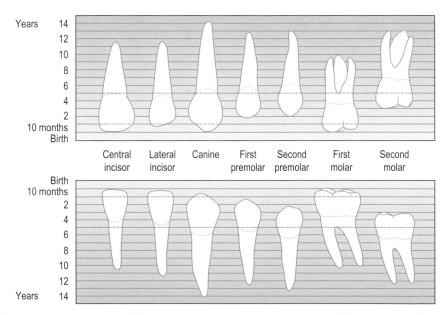

Figure A.11 Chronological development of permanent dentition. (After Pindborg 1970 Pathology of the dental hard tissues. WB Saunders, Philadelphia, with permission.)

Notes on eruption of teeth

All these values are based on work that was published over 50 years ago. To this date there has been very little up-to-date work on the eruption of teeth. It should be noted that there is extreme variability within normal populations and it is of more value to compare the eruption pattern of the whole dentition rather than one particular tooth. Eruption sequence is of particular importance and may be indicative of pathology, for example a supernumerary tooth blocking the eruption of a central incisor.

References

Logan WH, Kronfield R 1933 Development of the human jaw and surrounding structures from birth to the age of 15 years. Journal of the American Dental Association 20:379–427

Shour I, Massler M 1940 Studies in tooth development. The growth pattern of human teeth. Journal of the American Dental Association 27:1918–1931

Appendix O: Construction of family pedigrees

Pedigrees are a useful presentation of families in clinical notes. It displays information about past generations and the transmission of genetic traits through families. The symbols used in constructing pedigrees are shown in Figure A.12.

The affected individual at examination is termed the proband and an arrow is placed indicating this patient. Generations are numbered with roman numerals and arabic numerals are used to indicate individuals within each generation. An example of a family pedigree displaying a sex-linked transmission is shown in Figure A.13.

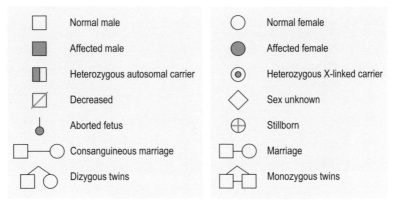

Figure A.12 Symbols used in the construction of pedigrees. (From Pindborg 1970 Pathology of the dental hard tissues. WB Saunders, Philadelphia, with permission.)

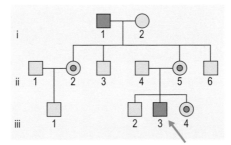

Figure A.13 A pedigree of a family with ectodermal dysplasia, demonstrating sex-linked inheritance. In the first generation, the grandfather (I1) of the proband (III3) (arrow) had no hair, was hyperthermic and only had three permanent teeth. Of his offspring, all the females were heterozygotes (II2 and II5). The younger had sparse hair and eczema and was missing seven teeth including the lower canines. It is important to note that there is no male to male transmission. The daughter then passed the mutation to one of her sons (III3), who fully expresses the gene, and one of her daughters, who is a carrier. (From Pindborg 1970.)

Appendix P: Calculating fluoride values for dental products

The basic unit used for measuring and comparing fluoride products is 'parts per million' (ppm). This is a water engineering term that has been adopted by the dental profession. One ppm is equal to 1 mg in 10^6 mg (or 1 kg). One ppm is 1 mg dissolved in 1 L of water; 1 L of water weighs 1 kg.

Some useful analogies for thinking about 1 ppm are as follows:

- 1 inch in 16 miles.
- 1 minute in 2 years.
- 1 cent in Aus$10000.
- 1 drop in 10 gallons.
- 1 mL in 1000 mL.

The molecular weight ratio (MWR) is used to calculate the fluoride content of fluoride products. Most fluoride products are labelled with the concentration of the compound (e.g. 2% NaF), rather than the fluoride content. An exception to this labelling occurs with the 1.23% APF gels that are unusual in being labelled with the fluoride concentration (i.e. 1.23% F or 12300 ppm F).

Sample calculations

Sodium fluoride

A NaF compound contains:

- Na (atomic weight: 23) and F (atomic weight: 19)
- NaF then contains $19 + 23 = 42$ (combined atomic weight).

In this compound:

- F then represents $19/42 = 0.45$ (MWR for F)
- Na represents $23/42 = 1.8$ (MWR for Na).

Consider a 2%NaF product:

In order to calculate the % F in this product, the numerical % concentration is multiplied by the MWR for F: $2 \times 0.45 = 0.91\%F$.

To convert 0.91% F to ppm, multiply by 10^4 (since 1%F = 10,000ppmF):

- $0.91 \times 10^4 = 9100$ ppmF.

Sodium monofluorophosphate (MFP)

Na_2FPO_3:

- 2Na (atomic weight: 46)
- F (atomic weight: 19)
- PO_3 (atomic weight: 79).

In this compound:

- F represents $19/144 = 0.132\%$ F
- 0.76% MFP toothpaste contains: $0.76 \times 0.132 = 0.1\%$ F or 1000 ppm F.

Appendix Q: Bisphosphonate-related osteonecrosis of the jaws

Osteonecrosis is a recently described complication of bisphosphonate therapy in adults. While here have been no reported cases yet of bisphosphonate-related osteonecrosis (BRON) in children, there has been a significant increase in the use of these drugs in the management of children with connective tissue disorders and decreased bone density including:

- Congenital osteoporosis – osteogenesis imperfecta.
- Secondary osteoporosis – immobility, steroid induced.
- Focal orthopaedic conditions – avascular necrosis (AVN), Perthes' disease; fracture non-union; Ilizarov limb lengthening; bone cysts.

There is an increased association of BRON with any invasive dental procedure such as extractions. While the risks for children is unknown, clinicians should be aware of this potentially destructive condition.

The duration of bisphosphonate treatment is variable:

- Osteogenesis imperfecta : 2–5+ years.
- Osteoporosis: 1–2 years.
- AVN /Perthes': 1–1.5 years.
- Delayed bone healing/bone cyst: 2–3 treatments (0.3 years).

Risk factors for BRON

- Drug related – such as potency and route of administration, dose, duration of treatment (>3 years oral; >6 months intravenous).
- Local factors – dentoalveolar surgery (extractions, implants, periodontal surgery) 7 × increase in risk, active infection (periodontitis, odontogenic infection).
- Demographics – increasing age.
- Concurrent medication – glucocorticoids, chemotherapy.
- Comorbidity – diabetes, smoking, alcohol, poor oral hygiene, cancer type (very high for multiple myeloma), osteopenia/osteoporosis.

Current management of established BRON

Stage 1 conservative: chlorhexidine 0.12% tds.
Stage 2 conservative + symptomatic: chlorhexidine 0.12% tds; antibiotics.
Stage 3 conservative + surgery: as above + sequestrectomy/resection.

Prevention of BRON in children requiring invasive dental procedures

Pre-bisphosphonate therapy: dental evaluation within 3 months of starting treatment with radiographic screening.

Management for children requiring dental interventions:

- If possible stop bisphosphonate 3 months prior to and for 3–6 months after procedure.

- Prophylactic antibiotics 10 days prior to and after procedure.
- Consider primary closure of wounds.
- Chlorhexidine mouthwash 10 days prior to and after procedure.
- Regular monitoring until complete healing.

Dental follow-up for children receiving bisphosphonates: 6-monthly dental reviews with 1–2-yearly radiographic survey as required.

Appendix R: Charting form

Western Sydney **HEALTH**
Area Health Service

DR-003

Hospital			M.R.N.
Title Surname			
Given names			
DOB	Sex	AMO	Ward/Unit

TREATMENT PLAN

Condition on Initial Examination

	18	17	16	15	14	13	12	11	21	22	23	24	25	26	27	28	
1																	2
				55	54	53	52	51	61	62	63	64	65				
	RIGHT													LEFT			
				85	84	83	82	81	71	72	73	74	75				
4																	3
	48	47	46	45	44	43	42	41	31	32	33	34	35	36	37	38	

Initial Perio Exam

17—14	13—23	24—27
47—44	43—33	34—37

Treatment Required — Perio

Restorations Required:

	18	17	16	15	14	13	12	11	21	22	23	24	25	26	27	28	
1																	2
				55	54	53	52	51	61	62	63	64	65				
	RIGHT													LEFT			
				85	84	83	82	81	71	72	73	74	75				
4																	3
	48	47	46	45	44	43	42	41	31	32	33	34	35	36	37	38	

Fissure Tx ______ Endo ______

GIC ______ Inlay/Onlay ______

Composite ______ Crown/Bridge/Veneer ______

Amalgam ______ Other ______

Removable Pros ______

Treatment Sequence: ______

Date   Clinician/Student (PRINT)   Staff Signature

4/92

Figure A.14

Appendix S: Neurological observation chart

Western Sydney HEALTH
Area Health Service

WSMR-1303

Hospital/Community Health Centre			M.R.N.
Title	Family name		
Given names			
DOB	Sex	Consultant	Ward/Unit

Neurological observation chart

DATE			
TIME			
COMA SCALE	**EYES OPEN** Closed by swelling = C	Spontaneously	4
		To speech	3
		To pain	2
		None	1
	VERBAL RESPONSE E T Tube or Trach = T	Orientated	5
		Confused	4
		Inapprop words	3
		Incompreh sounds	2
		None	1
	MOTOR RESPONSE Usually record best arm response	Obeys command	6
		Localizes pain	5
		Withdraws	4
		Flexion to pain	3
		Extension to pain	2
		None	1
TOTAL SCORE			
LIMB MOVEMENT	ARMS: Record right & left separately if there is a difference between each side	Normal power	
		Mild weakness	
		Severe weakness	
		Spastic flexion	
		Extension	
		No response	
	LEGS: Record right & left separately if there is a difference between each side	Normal power	
		Mild weakness	
		Severe weakness	
		Extension	
		No response	
EYE SIGNS	**EYES** + Reacts − No C Closed	right	Size
			Reaction
		left	Size
			Reaction
	PUPIL SIZE: 2, 3, 4, 5, 6, 7, 8, 9	OTHER COMMENTS	

ANY CHANGES MUST BE REPORTED IMMEDIATELY

2/99

Figure A.15

Index

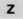